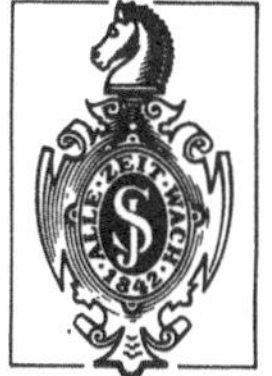

Clinical Practice in Urology
Series Editor: Geoffrey D. Chisholm

Titles in the series already published

Urinary Diversion
Edited by Michael Handley Ashken

Chemotherapy and Urological Malignancy
Edited by A. S. D. Spiers

Urodynamics
Paul Abrams, Roger Feneley and Michael Torrens

Male Infertility
Edited by T. B. Hargreave

The Pharmacology of the Urinary Tract
Edited by M. Caine

Forthcoming titles in the series

Urological Prostheses, Appliances and Catheters
Edited by J. P. Pryor

Percutaneous and Interventional Uroradiology
Edited by Erich K. Lang

Adenocarcinoma of the Prostate
Edited by Andrew W. Bruce and John Trachtenberg

Bladder Cancer

Edited by
E. J. Zingg and D. M. A. Wallace

With 50 Figures

Springer-Verlag
Berlin Heidelberg NewYork Tokyo

E. J. Zingg, MD
Professor and Chairman, Department of Urology,
University of Berne, Inselspital,
3010 Berne, Switzerland

D. M. A. Wallace, FRCS
Consultant Urologist, Department of Urology,
Queen Elizabeth Medical Centre,
Birmingham, England

Series Editor

Geoffrey D. Chisholm, ChM, FRCS, FRCSEd
Professor of Surgery, University of Edinburgh;
Consultant Urological Surgeon,
Western General Hospital,
Edinburgh, Scotland

ISBN-13:978-1-4471-1364-5 e-ISBN-13:978-1-4471-1362-1
DOI: 10.1007/978-1-4471-1362-1

Library of Congress Cataloging in Publication Data
Main entry under title:
Bladder Cancer
(Clinical Practice in Urology)
Includes bibliographies and index. 1. Bladder – Cancer. I. Zingg, Ernst J.
II. Wallace, D.M.A. (David Michael Alexander), 1946–
DNLM: 1. Bladder Neoplasms. WJ 504 B6313
RC280.B5B632 1985 616.99'462 85–2572
ISBN-13:978-1-4471-1364-5 (U.S.)

Softcover reprint of the hardcover 1st edition 1985

Typeset by Wilmaset, Birkenhead, Merseyside
Printed by Page Bros. (Norwich) Limited, Mile Cross Lane, Norwich

2128/3916–543210

Series Editor's Foreword

Cancer of the bladder has a bad reputation: the combination of urinary problems and malignancy gives just cause for continuing concern. Not only is this common cancer a burden to the patient but, because of the need for regular follow-up, it creates a large workload on the urological services.

It might be imagined that the bladder would give early warning signals of disease, and indeed it may do so; yet it can also be hesitant to reveal its severity. Thus there are many problems that create challenges in the diagnosis and management. Prevention is still the first goal of an oncologist, with early detection of early disease being the next best option. Early bladder cancer is amenable to several therapeutic approaches, but we have still to determine the best approach. The management of more advanced invasive bladder cancer all too often leads to disappointment, and we remain uncertain as to the optimum approach—surgery, radiotherapy, chemotherapy or some combination of these. Although none of these problems may be fully answered either now or in the near future, many people are working towards their solution, and the rate of progress needs to be documented from time to time. This volume aims to set the standard for the present state of our knowledge on bladder cancer.

The editors, Professor Ernst Zingg and Mr. Michael Wallace, have gathered together the best opinions on a wide range of topics relating to bladder cancer. All the contributors have written from a considerable depth of experience and their combined comments represent the balance of current thinking and established practice. There is obvious significance in the unusual method chosen for presenting the management of invasive cancer. This chapter, with its four subsections, reveals the divergence of opinion and illustrates how a single individual cannot express a judgement on this much debated subject. Readers will have to draw their own conclusions, and, for many, these will be related to their local facilities and expertise.

The topic of urinary diversion was the subject of a previous volume in this series; however the sections on urinary diversion in malignant disease and stoma care remain as relevant as before.

By assembling such a strong team of experts the editors have easily achieved the aim of this series, namely to provide a useful contribution to the clinical practice of Urology.

Edinburgh, March 1985 Geoffrey D. Chisholm

Preface

Bladder cancer is the second commonest urological malignancy and is one of the major problems in urology. There is already an enormous volume of literature on bladder cancer, covering a wide variety of related subjects, and these papers appear in a wide variety of journals and monographs. It is an almost impossible task for the clinician to keep abreast of the literature because of the constant flow of new ideas, information and results. This is especially true in the biology of bladder tumours, in improvements of diagnostic methods and in the treatment of superficial tumours. In contrast, the results of the treatment of invasive bladder cancer show very little improvement and we appear to be reaching the limits of our current therapy with surgery and/or radiotherapy. This, however, remains a highly controversial area with clinicians differing widely in their opinions over present management, but united in their belief that the search for more effective systemic therapy is now the most important task in the treatment of this disease. When this has been found then we expect that most of the present arguments over treatment will become obsolete. Conducting clinical trials and evaluating data on invasive bladder cancer is notoriously difficult, and the results of most studies have been disappointingly inconclusive. We must try to understand the causes of these failures and learn from the mistakes of the past so that any new therapy can be rapidly and critically evaluated.

With the increasing complexity of diagnostic and therapeutic methods there is a growing need for patients, particularly those with invasive disease or poor prognostic factors, to be referred to specialised urological units that are equipped to undertake all aspects of investigation and treatment of such patients. This calls for close cooperation and understanding between the urologist, the general practitioner and all the specialists involved in the management of such patients.

This volume provides a review of the present management of bladder cancer which, in addition to covering the practical aspects of treatment, also emphasises the importance of understanding the biology, pathology and classification of these tumours when making therapeutic decisions. It is intended that this volume will be of use, not just to urologists, but to radiotherapists, oncologists, general surgeons and all medical practitioners who may be involved in what must now become the multidisciplinary management of patients with bladder cancer.

We are pleased that we have been able to gather such a team of highly qualified contributors to this book from many different centres. It has been a stimulating and rewarding venture, although many difficulties have had to be overcome in producing and editing such a multinational work. We make no apology for there being some repetition and divergence of opinion expressed herein. Our theme has been to present the evidence, especially in those areas of controversy, so that the readers may decide how best to treat the patient in their hands and in their departments; every patient must be treated as an individual.

Acknowledgements

We would like to thank our contributors for all the work that they did in the preparation of their manuscripts and for their cooperation and forbearance with the editors while they were preparing this volume. Our thanks also go to Dr. P. Davies from Nottingham City Hospital, Dr. A. Dixon from Cambridge University Medical School and Dr. R. Resnik from St. Bartholomew's Hospital, London, for providing some of the radiological illustrations, and to Mark de Pienne for the line drawings in Chapter 8. Much secretarial work has been required and all those who laboured over the typescripts deserve our praise, in particular Marina Heron and Karin Wallace. We are extremely grateful to Judith Watt for her careful copy editing and to Michael Jackson of Springer-Verlag and Geoffrey Chisholm from Edinburgh for their constant encouragement, help and guidance. Finally, we would like to thank our wives and families for making yet more sacrifices whilst we worked on this volume.

January 1985

D. M. A. Wallace
E. J. Zingg

Contents

Contributors

R. Ackermann, MD
Professor and Chairman, Department of Urology, University of Düsseldorf, D-4000 Düsseldorf, Federal Republic of Germany

M. C. Bishop, MD, FRCS
Consultant Urological Surgeon, Department of Urology, City Hospital, Hucknall Road, Nottingham, England

J. P. Blandy, DM, MCh, FRCS, FACS
Professor of Urology, The London Hospital Medical College, Turner Street, London, England

J. B. deKernion, MD
Associate Professor, Division of Urology, Department of Surgery, UCLA School of Medicine, 10833 LeConte Avenue, Los Angeles, California, USA

U. Engelmann, MD
Department of Urology, Johannes Gutenberg-University Hospital, Mainz, Federal Republic of Germany

T. B. Hargreave, MS, FRCS
Senior Lecturer in Urology, University of Edinburgh, Honorary Consultant Urological Surgeon, University Department of Surgery/Urology, Western General Hospital, Crewe Road, Edinburgh, Scotland

R. Hohenfellner, MD
Professor and Chairman, Department of Urology, Johannes Gutenberg-University Hospital, Mainz, Federal Republic of Germany

G. H. Jacobi, MD
Professor of Urology, Department of Urology, Johannes Gutenberg-University Hospital, Mainz, Federal Republic of Germany

K. H. Kurth, MD
Department of Urology, Erasmus University
3015 GD Rotterdam, The Netherlands

W. Lutzeyer, MD
Professor and Chairman, Department of Urology,
Rheinisch-Westfälische Technische Hochschule, 5100 Aachen,
Federal Republic of Germany

E. Messing, MD
Assistant Professor, Division of Urology/Department of Surgery,
University of Wisconsin School of Medicine, 600 Highland Avenue,
Madison, Wisconsin 53792 USA

P. C. Peters, MD
Professor and Chairman, Division of Urology, Southwestern Medical
School, The University of Texas, Dallas, Texas 85253 USA

P. N. Plowman, MA, MD, FRCP, FRCR
Consultant in Radiotherapy and Oncology, St. Bartholomew's
Hospital and the Hospital for Sick Children, London, England

H. Rübben, MD
Department of Urology, Rheinisch-Westfälische Technische
Hochschule, 5100 Aachen, Federal Republic of Germany

D. M. A. Wallace, FRCS
Consultant Urologist, Department of Urology, Queen Elizabeth
Medical Centre, Birmingham, England

J. N. Webb, MA, MD
Chairman, Department of Pathology,
Western General Hospital, Crewe Road, Edinburgh, Scotland

E. J. Zingg, MD
Professor and Chairman, Department of Urology, University of
Berne, Inselspital, 3010 Berne, Switzerland

Chapter 1

The Epidemiology and Aetiology of Bladder Cancer

H. Rübben, W. Lutzeyer and D. M. A. Wallace

Introduction

An association between an environmental agent and the development of a malignant tumour was first made by Percival Pott in 1775 when he described the scrotal cancer of chimney sweeps. There have been many reports since then of increased risks of developing certain cancers as a result of exposure to various environmental factors. Rehn, in 1895, was the first to report a cluster of cases of bladder cancer occurring in a chemical dye factory. This was later followed by many similar reports from different countries. Rehn was a practising clinician, and many of the later reports that have led to the identification of urothelial carcinogens have been made by clinicians who have observed unusual clusters of cases and investigated why they have occurred.

Epidemiological studies have now become so large and complex that they can only be undertaken by specialist epidemiologists; yet the clinician must retain his interest in the aetiology of bladder cancer as he represents the front line of treatment for the patients. The clinician should continue to inquire into the aetiology of every patient's bladder cancer for the following reasons:

1. *To detect and report cases of bladder cancer caused by occupational exposure to the known bladder carcinogens*. Not all these carcinogens have been eliminated from the environment worldwide, though legislation now exists in nearly all countries for banning the use and manufacture of the most potent urothelial carcinogens. However, the latent period is long and we are likely to see cases of occupational bladder cancer presenting for at least another decade.
2. *To advise and manage the patient*. We have a duty to advise the patient and his or her family when possible occupational exposure has occurred so that they can be fully investigated and compensation sought.
3. *To detect new urothelial carcinogens*. Many potentially carcinogenic substances are being introduced into the environment each year. Some of these could be urothelial carcinogens which may present as unexpected clusters of cases of bladder cancer.

4. *To identify the aetiological factors which may influence the course of the patient's disease*. Most cases of bladder cancer are under urological surveillance for several years and during this time new tumours may develop, become invasive and metastasise. There is much evidence that urothelial carcinogenesis is a multistage process that takes place in man over many years, and, while the initiating event may not be relevant to the patient's management, an understanding of the later events that cause the promotion and propagation of tumour growth may direct and influence the patient's therapy.

Epidemiology

It is a fundamental principle of epidemiology that a disease does not occur randomly, and it is the aim of epidemiological studies to identify these non-random occurrences. These studies can be either descriptive or analytical.

Descriptive studies

Descriptive studies document for each anatomical site the morphology, stage and grade of tumour and provide information about the incidence, prevalence and mortality with respect to such parameters as age, sex, race, geographical distribution and changes over periods of time. The main sources of information for these studies are:

1. *Population statistics*. These are available for most countries and may give much information about the whole population and its subdivisions.
2. *Mortality statistics*. These have usually been derived from death certificates, which are frequently inaccurate, especially with respect to a disease that may not be the direct cause of death.
3. *Specific registries*. In these registries the data are collected from patients indentified by a particular disease. In many countries, or regions within countries, all cancer cases are being entered into such registries and classified according to organ site and tissue type.

Analytical studies

Analytical studies can give much more information than the purely descriptive studies because they can be designed to answer specific questions. An analytical study may be carried out either as a cohort study or as a case control study. In a cohort study the cohort is identified by the exposure to the possible carcinogen over a set period of time, whereas in a case control study the group is identified by the disease itself. The definition of the study populations and the recruitment of both cases and fully matched controls are laborious and costly and therefore their application is limited.

The interpretation of such studies and comparisons between studies must be undertaken with caution. Differences in the classification of diseases and changes in classification must be taken into account, as has occurred, for example, with the use of the term 'papilloma of the bladder', and the introduction of the Ta and T1 categories of bladder tumour in the TNM system. The standards of diagnosis, medical treatment and reporting may vary from region to region and will change over periods of time. There may also be age and sex differences caused by population shifts over the time of the study.

Incidence

Age and Sex

The incidence of bladder cancer in a population can be given as either the age-specific rate or as the age-standardised incidence for the whole population and is expressed as the number of new cases per 100000 of population, per year. The age-specific incidence rates for the USA are similar to those of Western Europe and are presented in Table 1.1. Bladder cancer is extremely rare in the first two

Table 1.1. Age-specific and age-standardised incidence rates for the white population of the USA (Cutler and Young 1975)

Age	Male	Female
0–19	0.2	0.2
20–29	1.0	0.3
30–39	2.5	1.0
40–49	10.3	2.7
50–59	32.4	10.5
60–69	91.2	25.9
70–79	172.3	42.2
80–	201.5	62.5

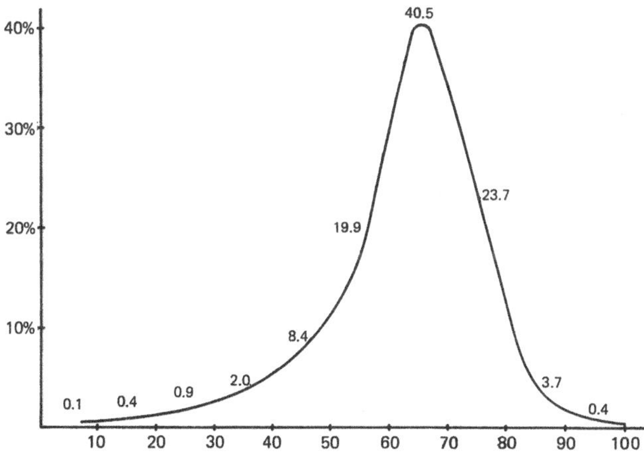

Fig. 1.1. Relative incidence of bladder carcinoma by age at the time of first diagnosis; n=2624 (RUTTAC 1981)

decades of life, and the incidence begins to rise sharply after the fifth decade of life (Fig. 1.1). The male to female ratio in most western countries is approximately 3:1. The incidence is lower in blacks in the USA as compared with whites, but some of these differences can be explained by the use and the standard of the medical services.

Time Trends

Data from the US National Cancer Survey show that the incidence of bladder cancer among white males has increased from 14.1 in 1939 to 21.3 in 1971, with a similar increase of 3.8 to 9.8 for black males; however, there was no increase among black or white females (Devesa and Silverman 1978). The Connecticut data (Connecticut Tumour Registry 1963–1973) also showed an increase for males but not females, but Morrison (1978) did find the incidence in females to be increasing, and this he attributed to increased cigarette smoking. There has been no change in the age at diagnosis in either men or women from the data collected before or after 1970 in the registry for urinary tract tumours at Aachen (RUTTAC 1981).

Demography of Bladder Cancer

The incidence of bladder cancer varies considerably between different continents and countries and between different regions of a single country. The age-adjusted mortalities for both sexes for a number of countries are shown in Table 1.2. In Hawaii the incidence for Caucasians (18.7) is higher than for Japanese (11.1). Israelis born in the USA or Europe have a higher incidence than Israelis born in

Table 1.2. Age-adjusted mortality for various countries by sex (Segi and Kurihara 1972)

Country	Male	Female	Ratio
South Africa	7.9	1.7	4.6:1
England and Wales	7.6	2.0	3.8:1
Denmark	7.3	2.4	3:1
Scotland	7.1	2.5	2.8:1
Belgium	6.5	1.6	4:1
Netherlands	5.9	1.7	3.5:1
Israel	5.6	1.5	3.7:1
Italy	5.6	1.2	4.7:1
Canada	5.5	1.8	3:1
USA (white)	5.1	1.7	3:1
France	5.1	1.3	3.9:1
Northern Ireland	4.9	1.6	3:0
New Zealand	4.9	1.2	4:1
Switzerland	4.9	1.4	3.5:1
Australia	4.8	1.6	3:1
Finland	4.7	1.3	3.6:1
USA (non-white)	4.6	2.7	1.7:1
Sweden	3.9	1.4	2.8:1
Ireland	3.5	1.5	2.3:1
Japan	2.4	1.1	2.2:1

Israel, while migrants to the USA from Italy, Poland and Sweden have a lower incidence than those born in the USA. The explanation of all these observations is uncertain, but it is likely to be complex, in view of the numerous possible environmental factors that may be operating. The incidence ratio of urban to rural populations is 2:1 and this is probably due to the greater risks of exposure to industrial carcinogens (Morrison and Cole 1976).

Aetiology—the Exogenous Factors

Aromatic Amines (Arylamines)

The first report by Rehn (1895) of four cases of bladder cancer occurring at a chemical dye works was followed by similar reports from other countries in Europe and from the USA. Rehn himself was able eventually to collect 23 cases of bladder cancer from the same chemical factory (Rehn 1904). All these reports were highly controversial and usually disputed by the chemical industry. The first experimental evidence that an aromatic amine could cause bladder tumours came when Hueper et al. (1938) published the results of feeding 2-naphthylamine to dogs and showed that this caused the development of solid and papillary transitional cell tumours of the bladder. These results prompted the chemical industry to initiate a full epidemiological survey in the industry; this was carried out by Case (Case et al. 1954). In his survey of the British chemical manufacturing industry he showed that those workers who were exposed to 1-naphthylamine, 2-naphthylamine or benzidine had an increased risk of developing bladder cancer and that this risk was proportional to the intensity and duration of the exposure. He also showed that workers who were engaged in the manufacture of the dyes auramine and magenta had an increased risk, but he did not find that there was an increased risk for either the manufacture or use of aniline (Case and Pearson 1954). It was the original theory of Rehn that the aniline was the agent responsible for the development of the bladder cancers, and aniline dyes have since become almost synonymous with occupational bladder cancer. As part of this study Case also showed that there was an increased risk of developing bladder cancer among workers in the rubber industry. This was found to coincide with the use of an antioxidant containing 2-naphthylamine, and again the risks were related to the intensity and duration of the exposure.

As a result of this evidence the chemical industry stopped the manufacture of these compounds in the UK, but other industries continued to use them until the early 1960s. Japan was the last country to be manufacturing 2-naphthylamine, and this was stopped in 1972 (Ohkawa et al. 1982).

Melick (1955) reported another carcinogen 4-aminobiphenyl (xenylamine) which had caused cases of bladder cancer at two factories in the USA. After 17 years of follow-up the incidence of bladder cancer among exposed workers was between 16.1% and 18.5% (Melick et al. 1971).

Carcinogenic Aromatic Amines

The chemicals that have been shown to be urothelial carcinogens in man (Table 1.3) are all aromatic amines and have a similar chemical structure. They are

Table 1.3. Known human bladder carcinogens

2-Naphthylamine	Phenacetin
Benzidine	Chlornaphazine
4-Aminobiphenyl	Cyclophosphamide
Dichlorobenzidine	
Orthodianisidine	
Orthotolidine	

absorbed through the gastrointestinal tract, respiratory mucosa and even through the skin. These chemicals were used in many industries in a variety of different preparations and with many different names; therefore, to determine if there has been exposure to one of these chemicals may be a complex and difficult process requiring expert help.

Occupations Exposed to Aromatic Amines

The occupations where workers have been exposed to aromatic amines are listed in Table 1.4. In nearly all these occupations the risks have been recognised and the chemicals withdrawn or strictly controlled. However, the latent period is long and is, on average, nearly 20 years and may extend up to 40 years. We can therefore expect to continue to see cases of occupationally induced bladder cancer presenting for many years after the exposure to the carcinogen has ceased.

Table 1.4. Occupations which have exposed workers to the known bladder carcinogens

Chemical dye manufacture and other chemicals
Manufacture of rubber articles (tyres, cables)
Gas works producing coal gas
Rodent operator
Laboratory work
Sewage work
Manufacture of firelighters
Textile printing
Kimono painting

There is also a number of occupations where an increased risk of developing bladder cancer has been observed but exposure to the known urothelial carcinogens has not been established. These include leather working, aluminium refining, hairdressing, tailoring, textiles and printing in general.

Although the parent compounds may have all been withdrawn or strictly controlled, their products or closely related compounds may still be used and represent a continuing hazard. Of special importance are the azo dyes which are formed from benzidine. These may be broken down by the action of bacteria in the gut to release benzidine. This is the reason for the high incidence of bladder cancer in the Japanese kimono painters who licked their paint brushes and thereby ingested the azo dyes.

Mechanisms of Urothelial Carcinogenesis by Aromatic Amines

The pathways by which aromatic amines are metabolised to urothelial carcinogens have now mostly been established and have been reviewed by Lower (1982). The first metabolic step occurs in the liver, where these compounds are either activated as urothelial carcinogens or they are inactivated. The activation of aromatic amines requires hydroxylation at the *N*- position (Radomski and Brill 1970; Cramer et al. 1960) and the *N*-hydroxymetabolite is then conjugated with glucuronic acid, in which form it is excreted in the urine. In man and other mammals the aromatic amines are inactivated by the enzyme system *N*-acetyl transferase, and this enzyme system can be either a fast or a slow system. The ability to inactivate aromatic amines by this enzyme system and the rate at which it works vary from species to species; they also vary between individuals of the same species. This may account for the different susceptibilities of species of animals to the development of bladder tumours after exposure to aromatic amines, and may also account for the differing susceptibilities to the development of bladder cancer among workers exposed to aromatic amines (Cartwright et al. 1982). However, there is no clear correlation in man between slow acetylators and the development of bladder cancer.

The conjugated *N*-hydroxy metabolites must be deconjugated in the urine before they can interact with the urothelial cells. Enzymes in the urine such as β-glucuronidase, which comes from the kidney and from the urothelium, can deconjugate and release the active carcinogen. Attempts to block the action of β-glucuronidase in experimentally induced tumours (Boyland et al. 1960) and in bladder cancer patients (Boyland et al. 1964) did not prove successful.

In acid urine, *N*-hydroxylamines lose water to yield electrophilic arylnitrenium ions which react covalently with cellular nucleic acids (Kadlubar et al. 1978). This causes damage to the DNA—the essential feature of carcinogenic initiation. This damage may be repaired by the cell, but if this is not successfully repaired the alteration in the DNA may be passed on through cell divisions and thereby becomes accumulative and persists for the life span of the host. This damage alone may be enough to result in the development of a tumour, but it is more likely that the cells will have to undergo a further series of events which will cause them to go through a progression of changes that will eventually result in a malignant growth (see p. 16).

Cigarette Smoking

Many retrospective and prospective studies have shown that there is an increased risk for cigarette smokers of developing bladder cancer. The relative risk for a smoker of developing bladder cancer as compared with a non-smoker has been calculated by various authors to be between two and six times. The percentage of cases of bladder cancer that can be attributed to cigarette smoking is between 30% and 40% (Cole 1973; Wynder and Goldsmith 1977). Cohort studies carried out by Armstrong and Doll (1974) have shown that the increase in bladder cancer mortality in male cohorts born since 1870 can be attributed to cigarette smoking. This increase was only found in men over the age of 40 years, which may mean that it requires over 20 years of cigarette smoking to increase the mortality. Hoover and Cole (1971) found the same association for both sexes, for different nationalities and for both urban and rural groups. The risk of developing bladder cancer has a dose-response relationship to cigarette smoking and probably requires more than 20 years' exposure. Stopping cigarette smoking reduces the risk, but this takes between 7 and 15 years (Wynder and Goldsmith 1977). There is probably no increased risk for pipe and cigar smokers.

Analysis of cigarette smoke has shown that it contains many aromatic amines, including 2-naphthylamine and several nitrosamines (Hoffman et al. 1969; Hecht et al. 1976; Patrianakos and Hoffman 1979). Bladder tumours were produced in one experiment in which tobacco tar was painted on the buccal mucosa of mice (Holsti and Ermala 1955), but this has not been repeated.

Very little is known about the effects of continued smoking on the clinical course of bladder cancer. The reason for this is that it would be virtually impossible to get two comparable groups of bladder cancer patients with one continuing to smoke and the other giving up smoking. However, in a retrospective report from Anthony and Thomas (1970) more deaths from bladder cancer were found in the group that had continued to smoke as compared with the group of patients that had stopped smoking when they were diagnosed as having bladder cancer. In view of the strong evidence for a causal relationship between cigarette smoking and bladder cancer, all patients who are smokers should be strongly advised to stop smoking when bladder cancer is diagnosed.

Urinary Infection

An increased incidence of bladder cancer has been reported in patients with long-standing urinary infections, particularly when this is associated with either a bladder calculus or long-term catheter bladder drainage (Wynder and Goldsmith 1977). The tumours that develop are usually squamous cell carcinomas. Paraplegic patients with permanent indwelling catheters are a group that are particularly at risk. Olsen and de Vere White (1979) reported squamous cell carcinomas in 5 out of 100 paraplegic patients, and Kaufman et al. (1977) reported that 6 out of 62 paraplegic patients developed diffuse squamous cell carcinomas of the bladder. Five of these patients had had indwelling catheters for more than 10 years.

The nitrosamines are a group of compounds that have been shown from experimental studies to contain some of the most potent and specific urothelial carcinogens. Hawksworth and Hill (1971) showed that nitrosamines could be produced by the action of bacteria, such as *Escherichia coli* and *Proteus* species, from amines and nitrates in vitro. Later this was shown to occur in vivo both in experimental animals (Hawksworth and Hill 1974) and in man (Radomski et al. 1978; Hicks et al. 1977). Nitrosamines are an extremely large family of compounds, only some of which are carcinogenic to the urothelium, and these are at present very difficult to analyse in the urine. Therefore screening for nitrosamines in the urine is impracticable. The co-carcinogenic or promoting action of intravesical stones or pellets has been well demonstrated in experimental animals (Clayson 1974; Harzmann et al. 1980). In the catheterised patient the initiation may therefore be the result of the production of carcinogens by the action of bacteria in the urine and the promotion by the chronic irritation of the catheter.

Bilharzia

Bilharzia is endemic in many regions of Africa and Arabia, and in some of these areas, particularly in Egypt, there is an association with bladder cancer. In other areas of Africa such as Uganda and Tanzania squamous cell carcinomas of the bladder are common, but bilharzia is not endemic in these regions (Dodge 1962); in West Africa the incidence is similar in areas where bilharzia is endemic and where it is absent (Payet 1962).

In the acute phase of the infestation with *Schistosoma haematobium* granulomatous polyps may develop and even form papillomatous tumours, but these follow a benign course and resolve with effective therapy for the bilharzia. When the infestation is chronic, epithelial hyperplasia, dysplasia and squamous metaplasia occur and eventually squamous carcinomas may develop (Morrison and Cole 1982). Bilharzia characteristically damages the whole bladder wall, and the urine in these patients is invariably infected. Hicks et al. (1977) have proposed that the initiation of bilharzial bladder cancer is by the formation of nitrosamines in the infected urine and is promoted by the chronic irritation of urothelium caused by the passage of the ova. They found very high levels of nitrosamines in the urines of a series of Egyptian patients with bladder cancer. Patients with bilharzia of the bladder should therefore be followed up with regular urine cultures (and cytology if this is practicable), and should have their bacterial urinary infections treated.

Exstrophy of the Bladder

There have been several reports of primary adenocarcinomas of the bladder occurring in patients with exstrophy of the bladder (Abeshouse 1943; Engel and Wilkinson 1970). One case of a primary adenocarcinoma of the bladder has been reported in a patient with epispadias, a minor variant of this anterior closure defect of the urinary tract (Altamura et al. 1982). The exstrophic bladder usually shows changes of cystitis cystica and cystitis glandularis, and in the exstrophic bladder these should be regarded as premalignant lesions.

Non-nutritive Sweeteners

The non-nutritive sweeteners saccharine and cyclamate have been in use for many years as food additives and artificial sweeteners and their use has increased markedly since the early 1960s. Whether these non-nutritive sweeteners are bladder carcinogens has now become a debate of major public health importance. Saccharine and cyclamate were first shown to produce bladder tumours when implanted in cholesterol pellets into the mouse urinary bladder. Then in prolonged feeding studies they were shown to cause a low incidence of bladder tumours in male rats (Price et al. 1970; Arnold et al. 1980). Several two-stage experiments have been performed where rats have been exposed to an initiating but sub-carcinogenic dose of a known bladder carcinogen such as the intravesical instillation of *N*-methyl-*N*-nitrosourea or after being fed on *N*-[4-(5-nitro-2-furyl)-2-thiazolyl] formamide (FANFT; see p. 13). The animals that were then fed on saccharine or cyclamate developed a higher incidence of bladder tumours, and it is therefore postulated that these non-nutritive sweeteners act as tumour promoters rather than initiators (Hicks et al. 1978; Cohen et al. 1979).

There is, to date, no good evidence that the use of these non-nutritive sweeteners is carcinogenic to humans, and there has been no increase so far in the mortality from bladder cancer that can be attributed to the introduction of saccharine (Armstrong and Doll 1974). However, it may be too early to reach such a conclusion as the use of saccharine only became widespread after 1960; it may be that a latent period of approximately 20 years is required before any promoting effect on bladder cancer can manifest itself. Diabetics, who use more saccharine than other people, were found to have a lower, rather than a higher, incidence of bladder cancer (Armstrong and Doll 1974). There have been nine case control studies investigating the risk of developing bladder cancer amongst users of artificial sweeteners (IARC 1980), and nearly all these studies have shown no excess risk, except for the study by Howe et al. (1977), who reported a relative risk of 1.6, which was dose dependant.

If there is any causal relationship between bladder cancer and non-nutritive sweetener consumption it is very weak and there will still be the question as to whether the risk of increasing calorie intake by withdrawing them will outweigh the advantages of a small reduction in the incidence of bladder cancer.

Coffee Consumption

The case control study reported by Cole (1971) suggested that there was an increased risk of developing bladder cancer in those who drank more than one cup of coffee per day. Several other studies have also suggested that there is a weak association between coffee drinking and bladder cancer, particularly for men (Weinberg et al. 1983). No dose-response relationship was found in a study by Morgan and Jain (1974), nor by Morrison et al. (1982) in a large case control study from the USA, Japan and England, which was adjusted for cigarette smoking. Cigarette smoking is strongly correlated with coffee drinking and this may have influenced the results in some of these studies. If there is an association between coffee drinking and bladder cancer, then it is likely to be very weak.

Iatrogenic Causes

Drugs

Three drugs have been clearly associated with the development of bladder cancer and one of these is still regularly prescribed.

Chlornaphazine. This drug is chemically very similar to β-naphthylamine and was used in the treatment of polycythaemia in Denmark up until 1963. Out of 61 cases treated, 10 developed bladder cancer and a further 5 had atypical cells in their urine at the time of follow-up (Thiede and Christensen 1969).

Phenacetin. This drug used to be freely available, which resulted in the habitual consumption of large quantities in certain communities, particularly in certain areas of Sweden, Switzerland and Australia. As well as developing analgesic nephropathy these patients have a high incidence of urothelial carcinomas, most of which develop in the upper tracts. Approximately 5%–10% of patients with analgesic nephropathy will go on to develop urothelial carcinomas (Gonwa et al. 1980). The induction time is again of the order of 15–20 years and probably requires a consumption in excess of 1 g daily. The mean age at which these tumours develop is lower, at 58 years, than for other chemically induced bladder cancers and the sex ratio is equal (Rathert et al. 1975). The active carcinogen is likely to be the *N*-hydroxy metabolite of phenacetin, which is chemically similar to the other aromatic amines.

Cyclophosphamide. There have now been many reports of bladder cancers developing in patients who had previously been treated with cyclophosphamide (Pearson and Soloway 1978; Fairchild et al. 1979). Therapy with cyclophosphamide probably needs to be prolonged rather than intermittent, and the induction period may be much shorter than for other chemically induced bladder cancers. Cyclophosphamide is both mutagenic and teratogenic and has produced a low incidence of bladder tumours in experimental animals after prolonged feeding. Patients who have been on prolonged cyclophosphamide therapy should be kept under surveillance with regular urine cytology.

Radiation

Radiation therapy is known to induce cancers at a number of different sites, and it is likely that radiation therapy to the pelvis may result in bladder cancer. An increased incidence of bladder cancer was reported by Duncan et al. (1977) following pelvic irradiation for gynaecological malignancies. However, it is not possible to be certain that the incidence of bladder cancer in patients who have already developed one malignancy, particularly a gynaecological malignancy, is going to be the same as that of a control population.

Endemic Nephropathy

A high incidence of urothelial cancers has been reported from certain areas of Yugoslavia, Rumania, Bulgaria and Greece in association with the Balkan nephropathy (Petkovic et al. 1971); 90% of the tumours occur in the upper tracts and 10% are bilateral. These tumours are characteristically well-differentiated and non-invasive papillary tumours, and the majority of patients die from their renal failure rather than from the carcinomas. The aetiology is not clear but it appears to be closely related to the climatic conditions, which suggests that it might be caused by a saprophytic fungus which grows in the stored crops and produces nephrotoxic and carcinogenic mycotoxins (Sattler et al. 1977).

Bracken Fern

When cows feed on bracken fern (*Pteridium aquilinum*) they are prone to develop multifocal papillary transitional cell carcinomas of the urinary tract (Pamukcu et al. 1976). The urothelial carcinogen in the bracken fern is not yet identified but is present in the cows' milk, and this has been shown to induce tumours in the bladder, small intestine and kidney when the milk is fed to rats (Pamukcu et al. 1978). Bracken fern is rarely consumed by humans except in Japan, where it has been reported as being associated with an increased risk of developing carcinoma of the oesophagus (Hirayama 1979).

Endogenous Factors

There is no evidence to suggest that hereditary factors have a significant role in the development of bladder cancer in man. The demographic studies previously mentioned would all suggest that it is the environmental factors that are the most important. A study of cancers in twins by Harald and Hauge (1963) show no increased risk for the twin.

However, much research has been done to try and identify biochemical and metabolic characteristics which might be associated with the development of bladder cancer. One that has already been discussed is the *N*-acetyl transferase system (see p. 7). Another is the metabolism of the amino acid tryptophan.

Metabolism of Tryptophan

Ekman and Strombeck (1947) were the first to propose that the metabolites of tryptophan could be bladder carcinogens. The metabolic pathways of tryptophan are complex, and several of the metabolites have ring structures which resemble the known aromatic amine urothelial carcinogens. When these metabolites were implanted in cholesterol pellets into the mouse urinary bladder, three of them were found to be carcinogenic. These were 3-hydroxykynurenic acid, 3-hydroxyanthranilic acid and 2-amino-3-hydroxyacetophenone. When tryptophan was fed alone to rats no bladder tumours developed (Rauschenbach et al. 1963), but in experiments where tryptophan was added to the diet of rats that were previously treated with a low dose of carcinogens such as 2-acetylaminofluorene (Dunning et al. 1950) or FANFT (Cohen et al. 1979) then the tryptophan was found to have a promoting effect on the growth of bladder tumours.

In man tryptophan is nearly all metabolised to carbon dioxide and water, with only 2% being excreted in the urine as its metabolites. Tryptophan metabolites can be absorbed through the bladder mucosa. Pyridoxine (vitamin B_6) is required for the metabolism of tryptophan, and in pyridoxine deficiency the quantity of abnormal metabolites excreted in the urine rises to 27% (Yess et al. 1964). An increased excretion of tryptophan metabolites has been reported in a number of disease states, including prostatic cancer, chronic urinary infection, rheumatoid arthritis, lupus erythematosis, scleroderma and porphyria and in pregnancy.

There have also been several studies that have shown an increase in the abnormal tryptophan metabolites in the urine of patients with bladder cancer (Boyland et al. 1956; Brown et al. 1960; Price et al. 1965) but other case control studies have failed to confirm this (Friedlander and Morrison 1981). In order to accentuate the difference between those that have normal and abnormal tryptophan metabolism a loading dose of 2 g of tryptophan may be given and the urine collected over the next 24 h.

The effects of pyridoxine therapy on the course of superficial bladder cancer has been reported by Byar and Blackard (1977), who were unable to show that pyridoxine therapy influenced the recurrence rate in patients with superficial bladder cancer; however, these patients were not stratified according to whether they had abnormal tryptophan metabolism or not. There is therefore no clear evidence that abnormal tryptophan metabolites play a significant role in the development of bladder cancer or that pyridoxine therapy has a place in its management.

Experimental Bladder Carcinogenesis

Many chemicals have been shown to be capable of producing bladder tumours in experimental animals (Clayson and Cooper 1970) but only a few of these have been useful in developing animal model systems to study urothelial carcinogenesis. The lines of investigation have now broadened out from the simple identification of bladder carcinogens into the study of the mechanisms of bladder carcinogenesis and also to the development of animal model systems for evaluating various therapeutic modalities. The success of these animal model systems has been due to the identification of specific urothelial carcinogens which can produce a 100% yield of bladder tumours which are dose dependant. The tumours produced resemble the human tumours histologically, though the interpretation of the early changes is difficult and the histological criteria for classifying the various tumours are not standardised. These models all have sub-carcinogenic doses and require prolonged or repeated exposures to the carcinogens to produce tumours. This has made possible the study of the stages of carcinogenesis and, in particular, the study of the mechanisms of tumour promotion. The three most widely used models will be described, as experiments with these models are often quoted in the literature.

N-[4-(5-nitro-2-furyl)-2-thiazolyl]formamide (FANFT). This compound is a nitrofuran which has produced bladder tumours in a wide variety of animal species and is a specific bladder carcinogen. The FANFT is administered usually as 0.1% or 0.2% of the diet. The production of bladder tumours in 100% of animals depends on having a sufficient concentration in the diet and feeding the animals for long enough. When rats are fed 0.2% FANFT for 12 weeks 100% will develop bladder tumours; if feeding is stopped at 6 weeks then the incidence of tumours approaches zero (Arai et al. 1983). The longer the FANFT is administered the more rapidly do the tumours appear. FANFT requires metabolic activation, but its metabolic pathways have not been fully determined. In many respects the FANFT model is the best model to work with as the dose and exposure can be controlled, the response is predictable, the tumours resemble closely the human tumours and their pathogenesis and they are transplantable (Erturk et al. 1969). However, it does have the major disadvantages of dietary carcinogens which are the environmental hazard and the expense of containing this hazard.

Butyl-(4-hydroxybutyl)-nitrosamine (BBN). This is one of several nitrosamines that are urothelial carcinogens in rodents. Like FANFT it is a very potent and specific bladder carcinogen and has a marked dose response (Ito et al. 1969). BBN is either given in the drinking water or it can be given more safely and precisely by repeated doses via a gastric tube. Administration must be for a similar period to FANFT for tumours to develop. BBN is metabolised to the carboxy-propyl derivative, which is probably the ultimate carcinogen.

N-methyl-N-nitrosourea (MNU). This is an extremely potent carcinogen which is carcinogenic to many tissues to which it is directly exposed. It requires no metabolic activation and is very unstable. To produce bladder tumours it is instilled directly into the bladder. The MNU is very cytotoxic to the bladder and the tumours frequently show squamous metaplasia. A single dose produces very few tumours and multiple instillations are required to give a 100% incidence of tumours. Because of its instability MNU is difficult to work with but is much safer than other compounds as it can so readily be decomposed.

Morphological Development of Experimental Bladder Tumours

The urothelium is highly specialised and adapted to its role of forming a barrier to urine and to accommodating large changes in both the volume of the bladder and the tonicity of the urine. One of the characteristic features of urothelium is the asymmetric unit membrane of the luminal surface of the superficial layer of cells (the umbrella cells; Fig. 1.2). The cell turnover of the urothelium is extremely

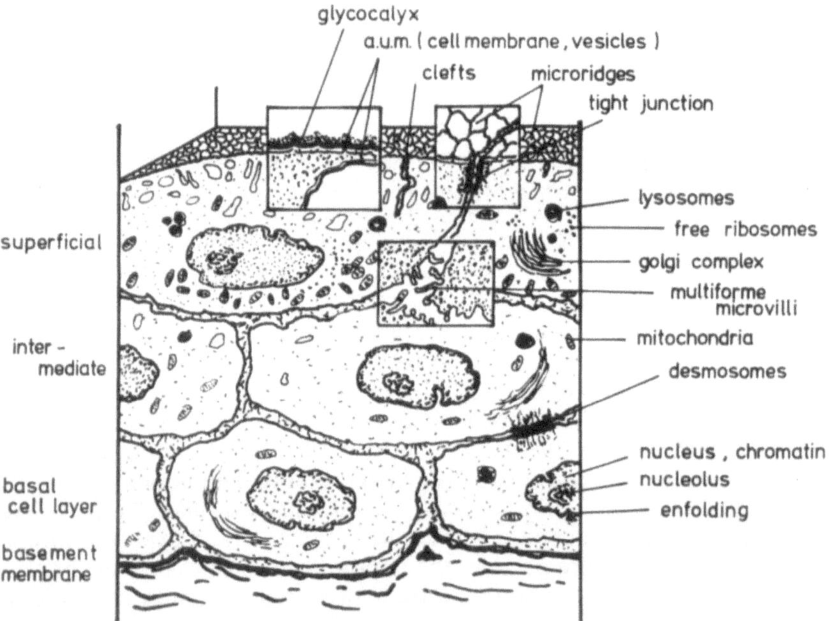

Fig. 1.2. Morphological criteria of the normal bladder urothelium

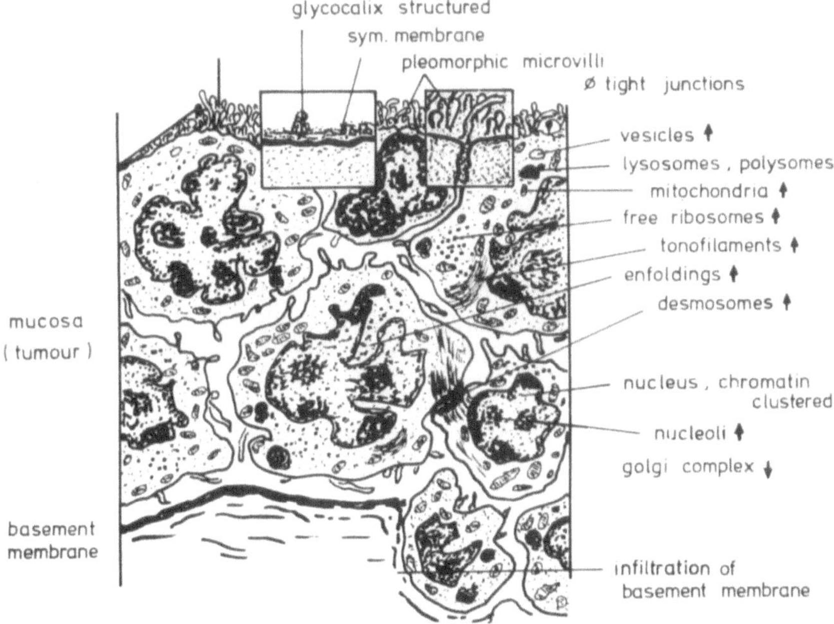

Fig. 1.3. Morphological criteria of the neoplastic bladder urothelium

slow, of the order of 200 days, but it is capable of very rapid proliferation in response to injury.

The initial response following exposure to a carcinogen is a widespread proliferation which results in hyperplasia. This is usually reversible if the carcinogen is withdrawn at a very early stage, but cancer may develop following a single exposure to a carcinogen after a long latent period. If exposure continues, then these hyperplastic lesions become nodular, the subepithelial capillaries proliferate and papillary processes develop. At the time that this process has become irreversible, certain morphological changes occur in the cell surface ultrastructure. The surface layer loses its orderly ridged appearance and becomes covered with pleomorphic microvilli (Fig. 1.3). These microvilli can also be found on benign reversible lesions as well and are not pathognomonic of tumour formation. The papillary tumours continue to proliferate even if the carcinogen is withdrawn, but invasion occurs at a late stage and metastases in all model systems are very rare, probably because the animals die of the local complications of their tumours or else they are sacrificed first. The classification of these early proliferative lesions is difficult and there is no general agreement yet.

Multistage Urothelial Carcinogenesis

The first experiments on staged carcinogenesis were carried out on rodent skin tumours (Berenblum 1941). These experiments first showed that if the exposure to the initiating carcinogen was short, then no tumours would develop, but if the exposure was prolonged or was followed by another agent, not itself a carcinogen, then tumours would develop. The order in which the carcinogen and the promoter are applied is important, but the time interval between the carcinogen exposure and the promoter does not matter, implying that the changes induced by the carcinogen are irreversible. The promotion phase has been further divided into the phase of conversion, where something more than mere proliferation of the target tissue is required after initiation, and a phase of propagation, where only a substance that increases cell proliferation is required (Boutwell 1964; Slaga et al. 1980).

Multistage carcinogenesis experiments have now been performed in the urinary bladder as a result of the development of the above animal models where a subcarcinogenic initiating dose can be given and followed by administration of substances suspected of being promoters. Many experiments have now been performed using the carcinogens FANFT, BBN, MNU and 2-acetylaminofluorene and demonstrating that saccharine, cyclamate, tryptophan and phenacetin can act as tumour promoters (Dunning et al. 1950; Hicks 1980; Cohen 1983). Stones and foreign bodies in the bladder also have a tumour-promoting effect (Chapman et al. 1973).

The role of urine itself in bladder carcinogenesis has now come under scrutiny. At first it was thought that the urine acted only as a carrier for the carcinogens, but the experiments of Rowland et al. (1980) and Oyasu et al. (1981) have shown that urine may have a more direct role and may act as a promoter. If the urine of rats was diverted from the bladder by performing a ureterosigmoid diversion after it had been exposed to an initiating dose of FANFT, then the incidence of tumours fell from 8 out of 19 in the controls to 1 of 18 with the diversion (Rowland et al. 1980). If the bladder was transplanted heterotopically into syngeneic rats after the donor rats had been given an initiating dose of BBN then subsequent treatment of the transplanted bladders with rat urine promoted tumour growth, whereas repeated treatment with saline did not (Oyasu et al. 1981). The nature of the promoting agents in the urine has yet to be identified.

A further question of clinical relevance is whether the proliferative response to non-specific trauma to the urothelium can cause the propagation of tumours. In endoscopic surgery not only is the resection or diathermy causing trauma to the urothelium, but the use of hypotonic cystoscopy fluids are also toxic and cause an increase in cell turnover (Weinstein et al. 1979). Several experiments have now shown that the proliferative responses caused by urothelial injury by freezing, diathermy, catheterisation and cystoscopy fluids can all have a propagating effect on bladder tumour growth in animal models (Murasaki and Cohen 1981, Cohen 1983; Walzer et al. 1983; Wallace et al. 1984). Further work is needed to establish the role of epithelial injury in bladder carcinogenesis and to determine its clinical relevance.

Repeated instillations of the intravesical chemotherapy agents mitomycin C, Adriamycin and *cis*-platinum have all resulted in urothelial proliferations with papillary tumour formation. When Adriamycin was instilled every third day for 30 days, 5 out of 29 rats developed tumours, 3 of which were invading the lamina propria and were also associated with areas of carcinoma in situ (Rubben et al. 1983). These lesions took 6 months to develop from the last instillation. Thus the repeated exposure to certain cytotoxic agents may itself be carcinogenic, provided that the exposure is repeated often enough and the animal followed for a long enough period.

Oncogenes

Very few human tumours are associated with a possible viral aetiology and there is as yet no sound evidence that bladder cancer is caused by a virus. However, in animals there are several tumours that are caused by viruses. It has been the recent advances in the high technology of molecular biology that have opened up the field of research into these viral tumours and the spectacular results that have been produced may now be converging to give us a clearer understanding of the molecular events involved in human carcinogenesis.

Many of the viruses that cause cancer in animals have been shown to contain genes which will cause the morphological transformation of a culture of mouse cells and these will cause tumours to grow if innoculated back into the mouse. The genes that are responsible for the oncogenic properties of the virus—the oncogenes—are not related to the normal viral genes. The oncogenes from many viruses have now been isolated and cloned in bacteria and found to be homologous to genes that are present in normal vertebrate cells (Duesberg 1983). This has immediately raised many important questions as to what are the normal function of these genes, what is their role in human cancer and whether they are indentical to the viral oncogenes.

The DNA from many human tumours has now been studied to see if they also contain oncogenes. The technique used takes the DNA from a cell culture of a human tumour and divides it into gene-sized portions which are then transfected onto cell cultures of mouse cells that are highly susceptible to transfection with DNA. The cells may then become transformed and, if innoculated back into mice, tumours will grow. The genes that cause this transformation have been found in approximately 10% of the human tumours tested and they have all been shown to be homologues of the various viral oncogenes. These human oncogenes may play a role in carcinogenesis because they contain mutations or because they have increased transcription. One of these from a human bladder cancer cell line (T24) has been isolated by molecular cloning techniques and had its base sequence decoded. This was found to contain a single point mutation in the protein coding sequence that substituted a thymidine for a guanine (Reddy et al. 1982; Tabin et al. 1982).

It is probably of little relevance to urologists that it was a bladder cancer cell line, but the real importance of these results may lie in what these experiments are beginning to reveal about the molecular events in malignant transformation. The transformation of cells in culture can only be done with highly abnormal cells, such as the NIH 3T3 cell line, which can perhaps be regarded as having already undergone the initial stages of carcinogenesis. More recent experiments have shown that transformation may be effected in two stages by using two oncogenes, the first of which brings about an 'immortalising' change in an ordinary cell culture and which then allows the other oncogene to cause malignant transformation. This may be an analogous process to the multistage carcinogenesis experiments previously described.

Molecular biology is a field that is rapidly developing and it is hoped that the initial exciting results give ground for optimism that we may be on the threshold of a new era of understanding of the mechanisms of carcinogenesis.

References

Abeshouse BA (1943) Exstrophy of the bladder complicated by adenocarcinoma of the bladder and renal calculi. A report of a case and a review of the literature. J Urol 49: 259–289

Altamura MJ, Gonick P, Brooks JJ (1982) Adenocarcinoma of the bladder associated with epispadias: case report and update. J Urol 127: 322–324

Anthony HM, Thomas GM (1970) Bladder tumours and smoking. Int J Cancer 5: 266–272

Arai M, St John M, Fukushima S, Friedell GH, Cohen SM (1983) Long term dose response study of *N*-[4-(5-nitro-2-furyl)-2-thiazolyl]formamide-induced urinary bladder carcinogenesis. Cancer Lett 18: 261–269

Armstrong B, Doll R (1974) Bladder cancer mortality in England and Wales in relation to cigarette smoking and saccharine consumption. Br J Prev Soc Med 28: 233–240

Arnold DL, Moodie CA, Grice HC, Charbonneau SM, Stavric B, Collins BT, McGuire PF, Zadwidzka ZZ, Munro IC (1980) Long-term toxicity of ortho-toluenesulfonamide and sodium saccharine in the rat. Toxicol Appl Pharmacol 52: 113–152

Berenblum I (1941) The mechanism of carcinogenesis. A study of the significance of cocarcinogenic action and related phenomena. Cancer Res 1: 807–814

Boutwell RK (1964) Some biological aspects of skin carcinogenesis. Progr Exp Tumor Res 4: 207–250

Boyland E, Williams DC (1956) The metabolism of tryptophan. Biochem J 64: 578–582

Boyland E, Kinder CH, Manson D (1960) Effect of 1,4-saccharinolactone on induction of bladder cancer. Annu Rep Br Emp Cancer Campaign 38: 45–49

Boyland E, Wallace DM, Avis PRD, Kinder CH (1964) Attempted prophylaxis of bladder cancer with 1,4-glucosaccharolactone. Br J Urol 36: 563–569

Brown RR, Price JM, Satter EJ, Wear JB (1960) The metabolism of tryptophan in patients with bladder cancer. Acta Un Int Cancer 16: 299–307

Byar D, Blackard C (1977) Comparisons of placebo, pyridoxine and topical thiotepa in preventing recurrence of stage 1 bladder cancer. Urology 10(6): 556–561

Cartwright RA, Glashan RW, Rogers HJ, Ahmad RA, Barham-Hall D, Higgins E, Kahn MA (1982) Role of *N*-acetyltransferase phenotypes in bladder carcinogenesis: a pharmacogenetic epidemiological approach to bladder cancer. Lancet II: 842–846

Case RAM, Pearson JT (1954) Tumours of the urinary bladder in workmen engaged in the manufacture and use of certain dyestuff intermediates in the British chemical industry. Part II; Further consideration of the role of aniline and of the manufacture of auramine and magenta (fuchsine) as possible causative agents. Br J Ind Med 11: 213–216

Case RAM, Hosker ME, McDonald DB, Pearson JT (1954) Tumours of the urinary bladder in workmen engaged in the manufacture and use of certain dyestuff intermediates in the British chemical industry. Br J Ind Med 11: 75–104

Chapman WH, Kirchheim D, McRoberts JW (1973) Effect of the urine and calculus formation on the incidence of bladder tumours in rats implanted with paraffin wax pellets. Cancer Res 33: 1225–1229

Clayson DB (1974) Bladder carcinogenesis in rats and mice: possibility of artifacts. J Natl Cancer Inst 52: 1685–1689

Clayson DB, Cooper EH (1970) Cancer of the urinary tract. Adv Cancer Res 13: 271–381

Cohen SM (1983) Promotion of urinary bladder carcinogenesis. Basic Life Sci 24: 253–272

Cohen SM, Arai A, Jacobs JB, Friedell GH (1979) Promoting effect of saccharin and DL-tryptophan in urinary bladder carcinogenesis. Cancer Res 39: 1207–1217

Cole P (1971) Coffee-drinking and cancer of the lower urinary tract. Lancet I: 1335–1337

Cole P (1973) A population based study of bladder cancer. In: Doll R, Vodopija I (eds) Host environmental interactions in the aetiology of cancer in man. IARC Scientific Publication No. 7. International Agency for Research on Cancer, Lyon, pp 83–87

Connecticut Tumour Registry (1963–1973) Cancer in Connecticut. Connecticut State Dept of Health, Hartford, Conn

Cramer JW, Miller JA, Miller EC (1960) *N*-hydroxylation: A new metabolic reaction observed in the rat with the carcinogen 2-acetylaminofluourine. J Biochem Chem 235: 885–862

Cutler SJ, Young JL (eds) (1975) Third national cancer survey: incidence data. Natl Cancer Inst Monogr 41: 1–454

Devesa SS, Silverman DT (1978) Cancer incidence and mortality trends in United States; 1935–1974. J Natl Cancer Inst 60: 545–571

Dodge OG (1962) Tumours of the bladder in Uganda Africans. Acta Un Int Cancer 18: 548–553

Duesburg PH (1983) Retroviral transforming genes in normal cells? Nature 304: 219–225
Duncan RE, Bennet DW, Evans AT, Aron BS, Schellhas HF (1977) Radiation induced bladder tumours. J Urol 118: 43–45
Dunning WF, Curtis MR, Maun ME (1950) The effect of added dietary tryptophan on the occurrence of 2-acetylaminofluorine induced liver and bladder cancer in rats. Cancer Res 10: 454–459
Ekman B, Strombeck JP (1947) Demonstration of tumorgenic decomposition products of 2,3-azotuolene. Acta Physiol Scand 14: 43–52
Engel RME, Wilkinson HA (1970) Bladder exstrophy. J Urol 104: 699
Erturk E, Cohen SM, Price JM, Bryan GT (1969) Pathogenesis, histology and transplantability of urinary bladder carcinomas induced in albino rats by oral administration of *N*-[4-(5-nitro-2-furyl)-2-thiazolyl]formamide. Cancer Res 29: 2219–2228
Fairchild WV, Spence CR, Solomon HD, Gangai MP (1979) The incidence of bladder cancer after cyclophosphamide therapy. J Urol 122: 163–167
Friedlander E, Morrison AS (1981) Urinary tryptophan metabolites and cancer of the bladder in humans. J Natl Cancer Inst 67: 347–351
Gonwa TA, Corbett WT, Schey HM, Buckalew VM (1980) Analgesic associated nephropathy and transitional cell carcinoma of the urinary tract. Ann Intern Med 93: 249–252
Harald B, Hauge M (1963) Heredity of cancer elucidated by a study of unselected twins. JAMA 186: 749–753
Harzmann R, Gericke D, Altenahr E, Bichler K-H (1980) Induction of a transplantable urinary bladder carcinoma in dogs. Invest Urol 18: 24–28
Hawksworth GM, Hill MJ (1971) Bacteria and the *N*-nitrosation of secondary amines. Br J Cancer 25: 520–526
Hawksworth GM, Hill MJ (1974) The in vivo formation of *N*-nitrosamines in the rat bladder and their subsequent absorption. Br J Cancer 29: 353–358
Hecht SS, Tso TC, Hoffmann D (1976) Selective reduction of tumorgenicity of tobacco smoke. IV Approaches to the reduction of *N*-nitrosamines and aromatic amines. Proceedings of Third World Conference on smoking and health. Dept Health Education and Welfare Publ No. (NIH) 76, pp 535–545
Hicks RM (1980) Multistage carcinogenesis in the urinary bladder. Br Med Bull 36: 39–46
Hicks RM (1983) The canopic worm: role of bilharziasis in the aetiology of human bladder cancer. J R Soc Med 76: 16–21
Hicks RM, Walters CL, El Sebai I, El Asser AB, El Merzabani M, Gough TA (1977) Demonstration of nitrosamines in human urine. Preliminary observations on a possible aetiology for bladder cancer in association with chronic urinary tract infection. Proc R Soc Med 70: 413–417
Hicks RM, Chowaniec J, Wakefield JStJ (1978) Experimental induction of bladder tumours by a two-stage system. In: Slaga TJ, Sivak A, Boutwell RK (eds) Carcinogenesis, vol 2, Mechanisms of tumour promotion and carcinogenesis. Raven, New York, pp 475–489
Hirayama T (1979) Diet and cancer. Nutr Cancer 1: 67–81
Hoffmann D, Masuda Y, Wynder EL (1969) Alpha-naphthylamine and beta-naphthylamine in cigarette smoke. Nature 221: 254–256
Holsti LR, Ermala R (1955) Papillary carcinoma of the bladder in mice, obtained after peroral administration of tobacco tar. Cancer 8: 679–682
Hoover R, Cole P (1971) Population trends in cigarette smoking and bladder cancer. Am J Epidemiol 94 (5): 409–418
Howe GR, Burch JD, Miller AB (1977) Artificial sweeteners and human bladder cancer. Lancet II: 578–581
Hueper WC, Wiley FH, Wolfe HD (1938) Experimental production of bladder tumours in dogs by administration of beta-naphthylamine. J Indust Hyg Toxicol 20(1): 46–84
IARC (1980) Monographs on the evaluation of the carcinogenic risk of chemicals to humans, vol 22. Some non-nutritive sweetening agents. International Agency for Research on Cancer, Lyon
Ito N, Hiasa Y, Tamai A, Okajima E, Kitamura H (1969) Histogenesis of urinary bladder tumours induced by *N*-butyl-N-(4-hydroxybutyl)nitrosamine in rats. Gann 60: 401–410
Kadlubar FF, Miller JA, Miller EC (1978) Guanyl O^6-arylamination and O^6-arylation of DNA by the carcinogen *N*-hydroxy-1-naphthylamine. Cancer Res 38: 3628–3638
Kaufman JM, Fam B, Jacobs SC, Gabilondo F, Yalla S, Kane JP, Rossier AB (1977) Bladder cancer and squamous metaplasia in spinal cord injury patients. J Urol 118: 967–971
Lower GM (1982) Concepts in causality: chemically induced human urinary bladder cancer. Cancer 49: 1056–1066
Melick WF, Escue HM, Naryka JJ, Mezera RA, Wheeler EP (1955) The first reported cases of human bladder tumours due to a new carcinogen—xenylamine. J Urol 74: 760–766

Melick WF, Naryka JJ, Kelly RE (1971) Bladder cancer due to exposure to *para*-aminobiphenyl: a 17 year follow up. J Urol 106: 220–226
Morgan RW, Jain MG (1974) Bladder cancer: smoking, beverages and artificial sweeteners. Can Med Assoc J 111: 1067–1070
Morrison AS, Cole P (1976) Epidemiology of bladder cancer. Urol Clin North Am 3: 13–29
Morrison AS, Cole P (1982) Urinary tract. In: Schottenfeld D, Fraumeni JF, Saunders WB (eds) Cancer epidemiology and prevention. Saunders, Philadelphia, pp 925–937
Morrison AS, Buring JE, Verhoek WG, Aoki K, Leck I, Ohno Y, Obata K (1982) Coffee drinking and cancer of the lower urinary tract. J Natl Cancer Inst 68: 91–94
Morrison R (1978) Cancer of the urinary bladder. Epidemiology and aetiology. Urol Res 6: 183–184
Murasaki G, Cohen SM (1981) Effect of sodium saccharine on urinary bladder epithelial regenerative hyperplasia following freeze ulceration. Cancer Res 43: 182–187
Ohkawa T, Fujinaga T, Doi J, Ebisuno S, Takamatsu M, Nakamura J, Kido R (1982) Clinical study on occupational uroepithelial cancer in Wakayama City. J Urol 128: 520–523
Olson CA, de Vere White RW (1979) Cancer of the bladder. In: Javadpour N (ed) Principles and management of urologic cancer. Williams & Wilkins, Baltimore, pp 337–376
Oyasu R, Hirao Y, Izumi K (1981) Enhancement by urine of urinary bladder carcinogenesis. Cancer Res 41: 478–481
Pamukcu AM, Erturk E, Yalciner S, Bryan GT (1976) Histogenesis of urinary bladder cancer induced in rats by bracken fern. Invest Urol 14: 213–218
Pamukcu AM, Erturk E, Yalciner S, Milli U, Bryan GT (1978) Carcinogenic and mutagenic activities of milks from cows fed bracken fern (*Pteridium aquilinum*). Cancer Res 38: 1556–1560
Patrianakos C, Hoffman D (1979) Chemical studies on tobacco smoke. LXIV On the analysis of aromatic amines in cigarette smoke. J Anal Toxicol 3: 150–254
Payet M (1962) Mortality and morbidity from bladder cancer in West Africa. Acta Un Int Cancer 18: 641–642
Pearson RM, Soloway MS (1978) Does cyclophosphamide induce bladder cancer? Urology 4: 437–447
Petkovic S, Mutavdzic M, Petronic V, Marcovic V (1971) Tumours of the renal pelvis and ureter: clinical and aetiologic studies. J Urol Nephrol (Paris) 77: 429–434
Pott P (1775) Cancer scroti. In: Chirurgical works. Howes Clark & Collins, London
Price JM, Brown RR, Ellis ME (1965) Quantitative studies on the urinary excretion of tryptophan metabolites by human ingesting a constant diet. J Nutr 60: 323–329
Price JM, Biava CG, Oser BL, Vogin EE, Steinfeld J, Ley HL (1970) Bladder tumours in rats fed cyclohexylamine or high doses of a mixture of cyclamate and saccharine. Science 167: 1131–1132
Radomski JL, Brill E (1970) Bladder cancer induction by aromatic amines: Role of *N*-hydroxy metabolites. Science 167: 992–993
Radomski JL, Greenwald D, Hearn WL, Block NL, Woods FM (1978) Nitrosamine formation in bladder infections and its role in the etiology of bladder cancer. J Urol 120: 48–50
Rathert P, Melchior H-J, Lutzeyer W (1975) Phenacetin: a carcinogen for the urinary tract? J Urol 113: 653–657
Rauschenbach MO, Jarova EI, Protasova TG (1963) Blastomogenic properties of certain metabolites of tryptophan. Acta Un Int Cancer 19: 660–672
Reddy EP, Reynolds RK, Santos E, Barbacid M (1982) A point mutation is responsible for the acquisition of transforming properties by the T24 human bladder carcinoma oncogene. Nature 300: 149–152
Rehn L (1895) Blasengeschwülste bei Fuchsin-Arbeits. Arch Klin Chir 50: 588–600
Rehn L (1904) Weitere Erfahrungen über Blasengeschwülste bei Farbarbeitern. Verh Dtsch Ges Chir 33: 231–240
Rowland RG, Henneberry MO, Oyasu R, Grayhack JT (1980) Effects of urine and continued exposure to carcinogen on progression of early neoplastic urinary bladder lesions. Cancer Res 40: 4524–4527
Rübben H, Hautmann R, Dahm HH (1983) Bladder tumour induction by cytotoxic agents. Clinical experience and experimental data. World J Urol 1: 94–99
RUTTAC [Registry for urinary tract tumours RWTH Aachen] (1981) Arbeitssitzung und Jahresberich des 'Register und Verbundstudie fur Harnwegstumoren RWTH Aachen'. In: Verhandlungsbericht der Deutschen Gesellschaft für Urologie. Springer, Berlin Heidelberg New York, vol 33, pp 559–564
Sattler TA, Dimitrov T, Hall PW (1977) Relation between endemic (Balkan) nephropathy and urinary tract tumours. Lancet I: 278–280
Segi M, Kurihara M (1972) Cancer mortality for selected sites in 24 countries. Rep No 6, Nagoya Jpn Cancer Soc

Slaga TJ, Fischer SM, Nelson K, Gleason GL (1980) Studies on the mechanism of skin tumour promotion: evidence for several stages in promotion. Proc Natl Acad Sci USA 77: 3659–3663
Tabin CJ, Bradley SM, Bargmann CI, Weinberg RA, Papageorge AG, Scolnick EM, Dhar R, Lowy DR, Chang EH (1982) Mechanism of activation of a human oncogene. Nature 300: 143–149
Thiede T, Christensen BC (1969) Bladder tumours induced by chlornaphazine. Acta Med Scand 185: 133–137
Wallace DMA, Smith JHF, Billington S, Stemplewski H, Tipton P, Smith M (1984) The promotion of bladder tumours by endoscopic procedures in an animal model. Br J Urol 56: 658–662
Walzer Y, Matheny RB, Blatnik AF, Soloway MS (1983) Urothelial trauma—a mechanism for tumour promotion? World J Urol 1: 100–102
Weinberg DM, Ross RK, Mack TM, Paganini-Hill A, Henderson BE (1983) Bladder cancer etiology. A different perspective. Cancer 51: 675–680
Weinstein RS, Koo C, Pauli BU, Jacobs JB, Friedell GH (1979) Epithelial injury by cystoscopy fluids. Semin Oncol 6(2): 257–259
Wynder EL, Goldsmith R (1977) The epidemiology of bladder cancer: a second look. Cancer 40: 1246–1268
Yess N, Price JM, Brown RR, Swann PB, Linkswiler H (1964) Vitamin B_6 depletion in man: urinary excretion of tryptophan metabolites. J Nutr 84: 229–238

Chapter 2

The Histopathology of Bladder Cancer

J. N. Webb

Introduction

How patients with bladder cancer are managed depends to a great extent on the nature and degree of spread of the neoplasm; the surgical pathologist, therefore, has a crucial role to play in determining the most appropriate treatment in this group of conditions. The classification of tumours in clinical practice is based on the identification of histological type, the degree of differentiation that the tumour exhibits, i.e. its grade, and thirdly the extent of the tumour—that is to say its category or stage. The wide adoption of the World Health Organisation (WHO) Classification for the typing of tumours (Mostofi et al. 1973) and the *Union Internationale Contre le Cancer* Classification (UICC 1978; see also Table 6.1, p. 119) has greatly facilitated the exchange of information, not only between surgeons, clinical oncologists and pathologists, but also between treatment centres throughout the world. This means that it is possible to make valid comparisons of the results of various treatment schedules, which should lead to a steady improvement and refining of the management of this difficult form of cancer. What one is aiming to achieve is to base decisions about treatment on rational and objective criteria. In the case of bladder cancer—a disease of infinitely variable manifestations—it is especially important that one adheres to these complementary, internationally recognised systems of classification.

However, for the pathologist, it is not sufficient to be content simply with classifying disease processes, no matter how precise these may be. On the contrary, it is necessary to attempt to understand how the lesions under consideration develop, their pathogenesis in the broad sense. To this end this chapter will consider bladder cancer not only from the point of view of pathological classification but will also review the problem of the development or evolution of the neoplastic lesion in so far as it is understood at the present time.

The Normal Urothelium

By far the commonest type of bladder cancer is the urothelial carcinoma, derived from the transitional cell epithelium or urothelium. (The terms 'transitional cell epithelium' and 'urothelium' are used synonymously in this chapter). The urothelium is a specialised epithelium forming the lining of the calices, renal pelvis, ureters, bladder and upper urethra. It is a type of epithelium adapted to an organ which constantly expands and contracts. It consists of an epithelium three or four to six cell layers thick (Fig. 2.1); the surface layer is composed of specialised umbrella cells with polyploid nuclei. The cytoplasmic processes of these umbrella cells extend to cover several cells of the layer immediately beneath. Ultrastructural studies reveal a number of special features in these surface cells, namely the surface has a unique angular contour formed by rigid plaque regions in the surface membrane. The membrane in the plaque region is 12 nm thick, as opposed to the membrane elsewhere, which measures 8 nm thick. Scanning electron microscopy emphasises this remarkable surface arrangement of rigid plaques and flexible interplaque areas. The cytoplasm of these cells contains elongated vesicular structures which may represent a reserve of cell membrane material (Hicks and Chowaniec 1978).

There are a number of *epithelial variants* commonly found in normal bladders. Wiener et al. (1979) have investigated their incidence in apparently normal bladders. These normal variants consist of von Brunn's nests, cystitis glandularis and a 'vaginal' type of non-keratinising squamous epithelium. Von Brunn's nests are most commonly found in the trigone of the bladder and consist of solid buds of urothelium which protrude into the lamina propria (Fig. 2.2). These buds may

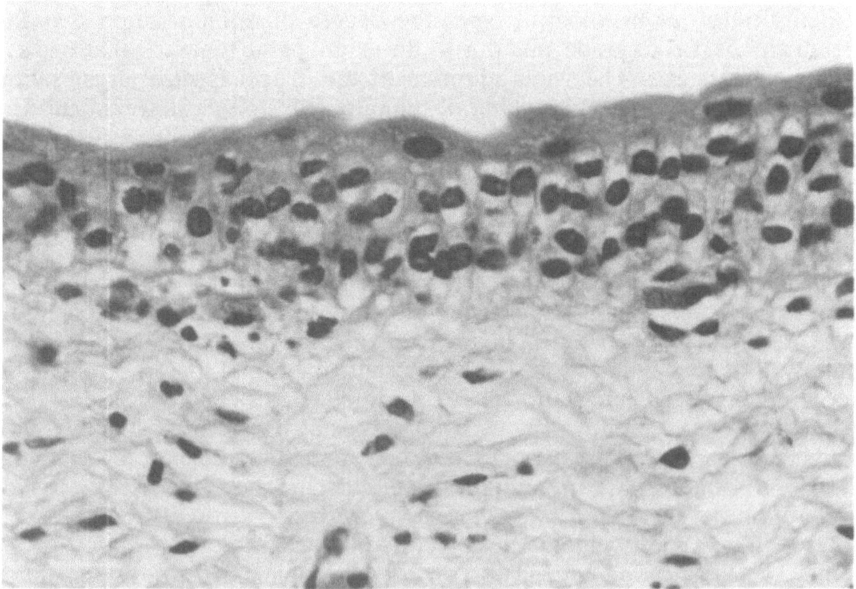

Fig. 2.1. Normal urothelium. × 500

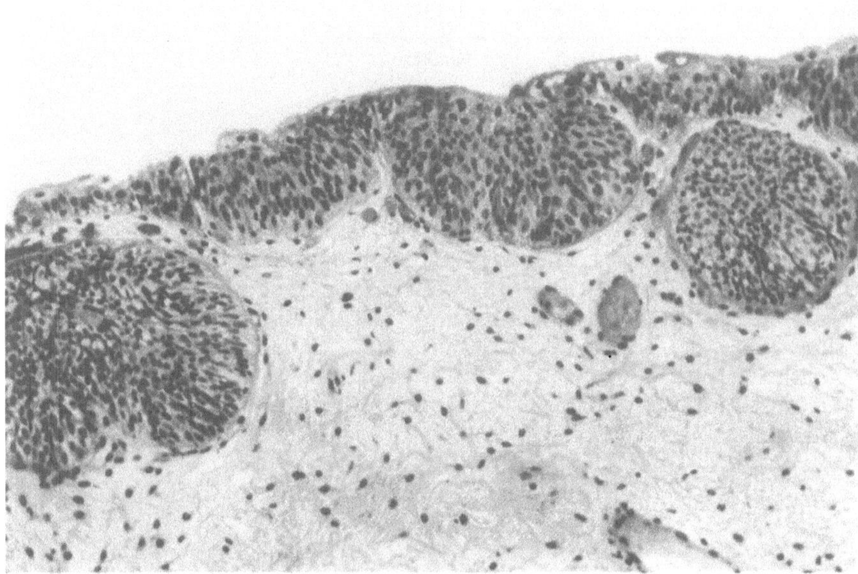

Fig. 2.2. Bladder mucosa with von Brunn's nests. × 160

develop lumina which may come to be lined by columnar epithelium (Fig. 2.3). The lumen may contain mucinous material. These may develop into the full-

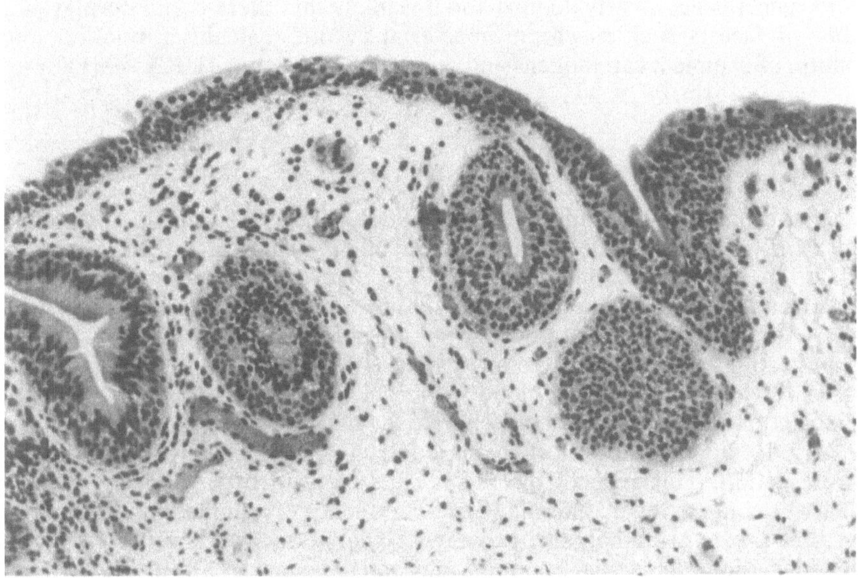

Fig. 2.3. Bladder mucosa, von Brunn's nests with central lumen lined by columnar mucin-secreting epithelium. × 160

Table 2.1. Frequency of epithelial variants in 100 normal bladders, 61 males, 39 females (after Wiener et al. 1979)

Epithelial variants	Male	Female
von Brunn's nests	53	36
Cystitis glandularis	32	28
Vaginal type (squamous)	3	19
None	6	1

blown cystitis glandularis. The third type of epithelial variant, also most commonly found in the trigone, is the vaginal type of squamous epithelium — usually but not exclusively found in females. The studies of Wiener et al. (1979) have shown that the great majority of normal bladders contain one or other of these epithelial types (Table 2.1). There is no reason to suppose that they represent in any way a preneoplastic state. Nor can they, strictly speaking, be regarded as metaplastic processes.

Urothelial Carcinoma

These are by far the commonest type of bladder tumour, although in certain parts of the world, notably Egypt, there is a high incidence of squamous carcinoma of the bladder (El-Bolkainy and Chu 1981). This peculiar geographic incidence has been ascribed to schistosomiasis of the bladder, which is endemic in Egypt (and in other parts of Africa). However, the precise relationship of schistosomiasis to bladder cancer is not clearly defined and it is likely that there is an interplay of a number of factors such as chronic bacterial cystitis, calculus formation, the formation of chemical carcinogens and vitamin A deficiency (UICC 1981).

Growth Pattern

Urothelial carcinomas account for approximately 90%–95% of bladder tumours (Koss 1979). The majority of these are papillary when first seen, variously estimated at between 64% and 80% to 90% of urothelial carcinomas (UICC 1981). Broadly speaking one may subdivide urothelial tumours into superficial papillary tumours—usually of low grade—and solid infiltrating tumours. These solid infiltrating tumours are aggressive carcinomas liable to invade deeply and to metastasise via lymphatics and blood stream. This is in marked contrast to the superficial tumours of low grade which may show no evidence of invasion over a long period of time—the lesions being controlled by repeated fulguration or electroresection. This type of disease is characterised by a tendency for the papillary tumours to recur. This may be re-emergence of a similar papillary lesion at the same site, or else emergence of a new papillary tumour at another site within the bladder. Multiple papillary tumours may emerge concurrently or consecutively, so that the bladder mucosa may come to be covered by widespread papillary tumours which can no longer be controlled by simple methods. These tumours may take on more aggressive characteristics, i.e. develop into a higher grade and invade the bladder wall.

Morbidity and prognosis in this group of tumours is to a great extent dependent on (1) the grade of the tumour, and (2) the extent of invasion—its category. These are largely interdependent properties, in that the high-grade carcinomas are more aggressive in their behaviour and the great majority are likely to be invasive—perhaps deeply invasive—early in the clinical history (Friedell et al. 1976), whereas, as stated above, the low-grade papillary tumour is unlikely to show any invasion. These forms of bladder tumour are common to both the occupational and the sporadic disease (Foulds 1975).

Grading

Urothelial carcinomas are further classified according to the degree of cellular anaplasia, i.e. the grade of the tumour. This system depends predominantly on cytological features, namely loss of polarity, variation in shape and size of cells, crowding of cells, nuclear changes such as hyperchromatism, large nuclei, prominent nucleoli and numerous mitotic figures. Grade 1 tumours are those which show the least degree of atypia, whilst Grade 3 tumours show these altered cytological features in their most pronounced degree. Grade 2 tumours are intermediate in their cytological abnormalities. Table 2.2 summarises the main features for the three grades which are depicted in Figs. 2.4–2.6.

The grade of the tumour not only correlates with the degree of invasiveness but also, as might be expected, the natural history and prognosis. Few Grade 1 tumours are invasive—probably less than 10%—and if invasive at all appear to push or expand into the adjacent lamina propria rather than exhibiting true infiltrative growth. Approximately 50% of Grade 2 tumours are likely to be invasive when first diagnosed, whilst the great majority of Grade 3 tumours are frankly invasive when first seen (Friedell et al. 1976). There is a correlation between grade or invasiveness and prognosis, as shown by Gilbert et al. (1978), who related 5-year survival to the grade of bladder tumour when first diagnosed. The overall 5-year mortality was 26%, but as many as 60% of the patients with

Table 2.2. Morphology of urothelial carcinomas (transitional cell carcinoma)

Features	Grade 1	Grade 2	Grade 3
Increased cell layers	Variable	Variable	Prominent
Superficial cells	Variable	Absent	Absent
'Clear' cytoplasm	Often absent	Often absent	Absent
Cell size	Increased	Increased	Greatly increased
Pleomorphism	Slight	Moderate	Marked
Nuclear polarisation	Slightly abnormal	Abnormal	Absent
Hyperchromatism	Slight	Moderate	Marked
Mitoses	Uncommon	Common	Prominent

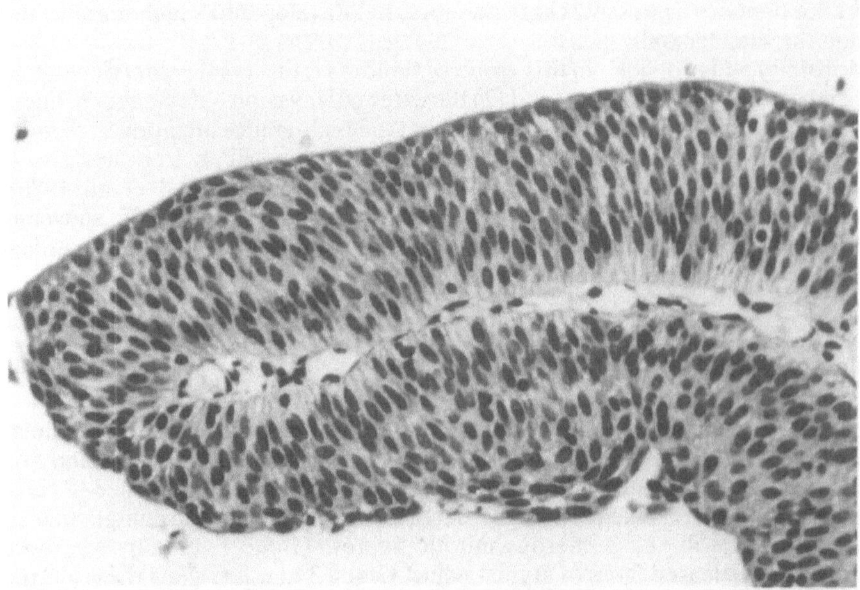

Fig. 2.4. Papillary urothelial (TC) carcinoma, Grade 1. × 320

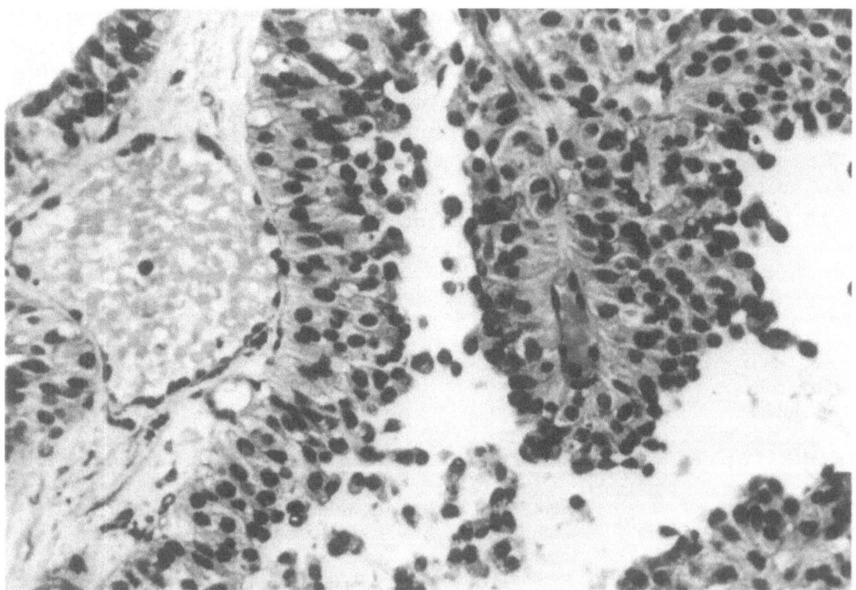

Fig. 2.5. Papillary urothelial carcinoma, Grade 2. × 320

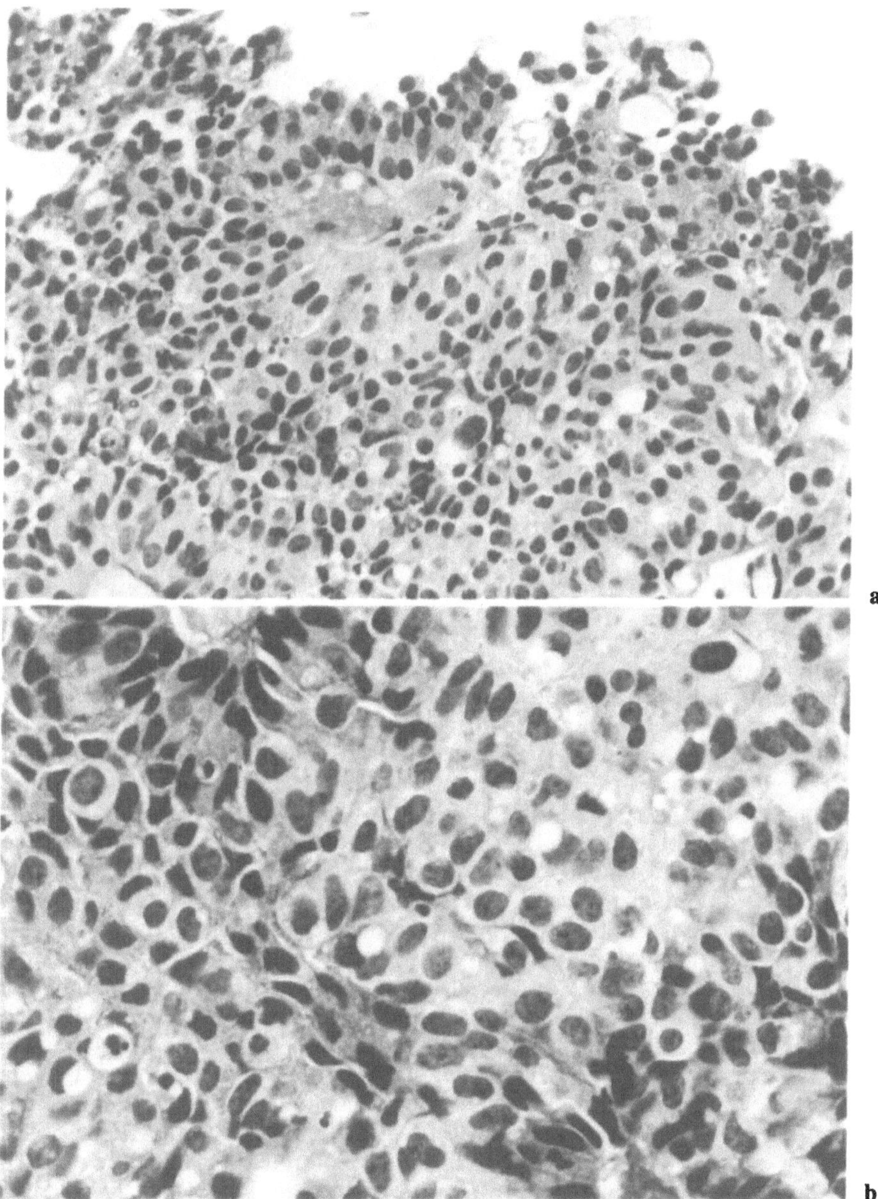

Fig. 2.6a, b. Papillary and solid urothelial carcinoma, Grade 3. **a** × 320; **b** × 500

Grade 3 tumours died of their disease by 5 years. The picture with Grade 1 tumours is very different; only 6% died of the disease at 5 years.

It is rather difficult to assess the relative proportions of urothelial carcinomas falling into these three grades, but recent studies suggest that the three grades of tumour are more or less equally distributed amongst patients with urothelial carcinomas (Chisholm et al. 1980). However, it has to be admitted that the criteria for placing a tumour into a particular grade are somewhat subjective, and even experienced pathologists may have difficulty in allocating a tumour to a particular grade. In practice we rarely make a diagnosis of urothelial papilloma (i.e. a Grade 0 tumour), but others clearly make this diagnosis much more frequently. This is probably an indication that the papillomas of some reports are equivalent to the Grade 1 papillary urothelial carcinomas of others, e.g. see the report of Mäkinen et al. (1978).

Development of Urothelial Carcinoma

Much of the current interest in research into bladder cancer is concerned with the development of these tumours, or their cytogenesis, from the earliest preneoplastic changes to the fully developed invasive carcinoma. This field of research extends back many years, e.g. to the pioneer work of Melicow (1952), who described carcinoma in situ changes associated with bladder cancer, Melamed et al. (1966), who mapped the urinary bladder in a case of carcinoma in situ, the important studies of Koss (Koss et al. 1974, 1977), who extended the work of Melamed, and of Farrow et al. (1976). These authors emphasised the importance of a preneoplastic field change in the urothelium. This field change has also been studied by means of giant sections of whole bladders (Soto et al. 1977) and multiple random mucosal biopsies (Soloway et al. 1978; Wallace et al. 1979).

From the experience gained from these and similar studies a variety of abnormal changes have been described in the bladder urothelium, namely (1) simple hyperplasia, (2) dysplasia—sometimes referred to as atypical hyperplasia —and (3) carcinoma in situ. These are depicted in Figs. 2.7–2.9. Hyperplasia may be defined as urothelium showing an increased number of its component layers but without cellular atypia. Dysplasia, which is customarily classified into mild, moderate or severe types, shows atypia of the epithelial cells with irregularity of shape and size of cells, and hyperchromicity of nuclei with some loss of orientation. Carcinoma in situ, irrespective of the number of cell layers, is a condition in which the epithelial cells have the features of malignancy of high grade, i.e. cytologically it corresponds to a Grade 3 lesion. It is questionable if it is possible to make any clear distinction between severe dysplasia and carcinoma in situ (Murphy and Soloway 1982). For further descriptions of these epithelial changes the reader is referred to the work of Koss (1975, 1979) and the papers by Friedell et al. (1980) and Utz et al. (1980).

There has been an assumption that these epithelial changes represent a progression which leads ultimately to invasive carcinoma. This view seems to be based on a number of observations which may be summarised as follows:

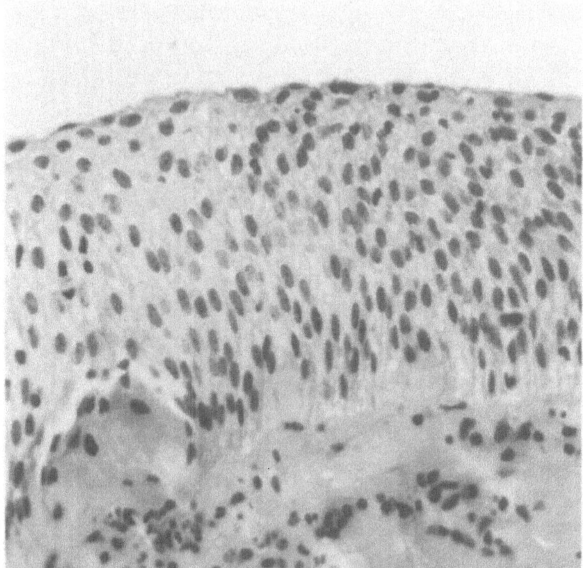

Fig. 2.7. Urothelial hyperplasia (simple). × 320

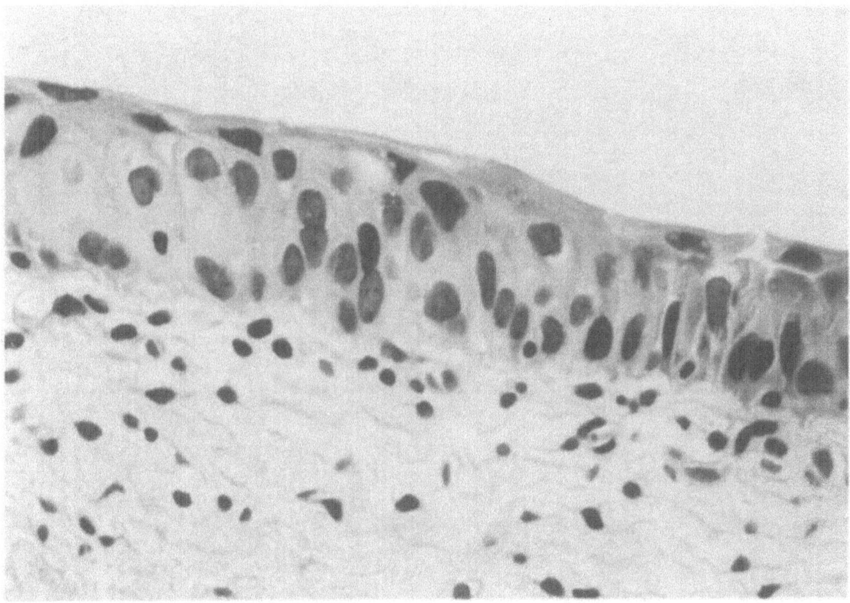

Fig. 2.8. Urothelial dysplasia. × 500

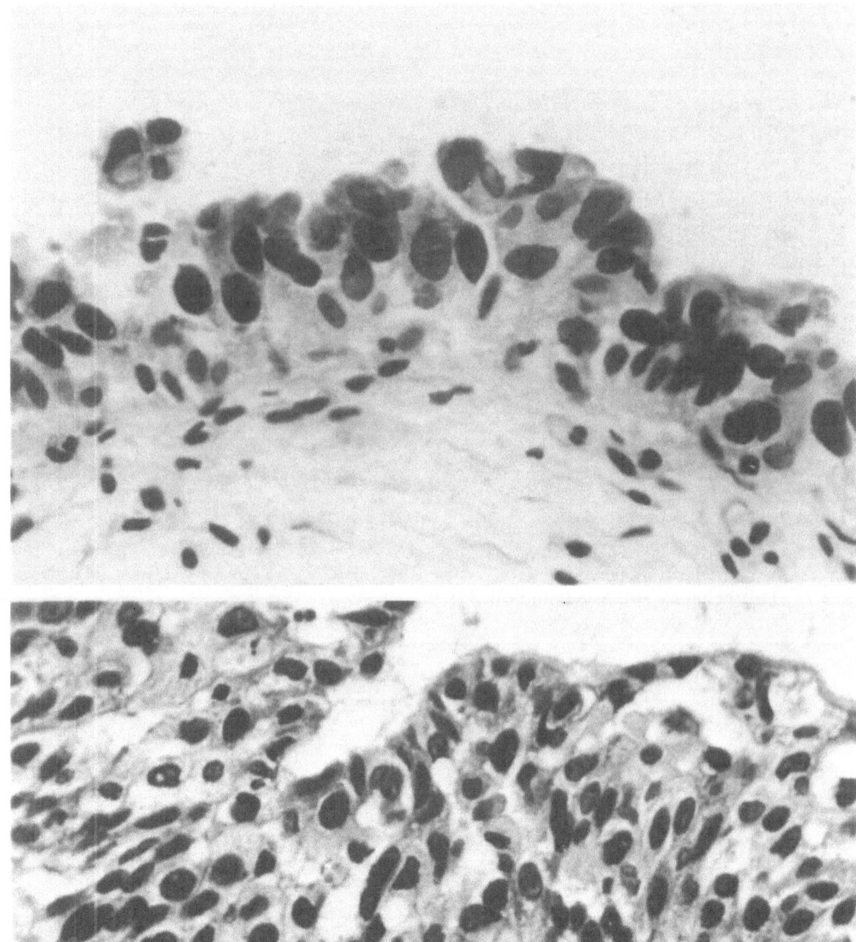

a

b

Fig. 2.9a, b. Urothelium with carcinoma in situ. **a** Reduced number of cell layers; **b** increased number of cell layers. Both × 500

1. All three types of change are frequently present in the same bladder which bears a carcinoma (Koss 1979).
2. There is no sharp distinction between these presumed preneoplastic changes.
3. An analogy has been drawn with the dysplasia/carcinoma in situ sequence in the uterine cervix (Murphy and Soloway 1982).
4. An analysis of the changes in the urothelium of experimentally induced cancers in laboratory animals in which sequential changes in the epithelium have been observed from preneoplastic states to frankly invasive tumours (Murphy and Irving 1981).
5. The same histological and cytological changes have been followed in humans.

Koss and his associates (1969) studied a group of workers exposed to a potent bladder carcinogen (4-aminobiphenyl). These patients were followed over a number of years and it was shown that cancer cells could be detected in the urine before any visible tumour was demonstrable in the bladder. Subsequently it was shown that these patients had the changes of carcinoma in situ, and some of these went on to invasive carcinoma; the duration of carcinoma in situ before invasive carcinoma supervened had a median of 26–33 months, with a maximum of 67 months. Earlier, Eisenberg et al. (1960) had also described abnormal changes in bladder urothelium including hyperplasia and carcinoma in situ in cases of bladder carcinoma. They interpreted their observations with caution and refrained from implying that there was a sequence of progressive changes. Rather they suggested that these various epithelial changes might represent different responses to the initiating agent. In this study three distinct changes were noted in the bladder: (1) atypical hyperplasia, (2) papillary hyperplasia and (3) carcinoma in situ, or intra-epithelial hyperplasia with atypia. They were able to show that patients without these atypical changes made satisfactory progress. In those patients with these abnormal changes it was otherwise, in that they identified a group with epithelial atypia whose average survival was no more than 3 years. In a more recent and somewhat similar study Althausen et al. (1976) showed that in tumours of low grade where the peripheral urothelium was abnormal—dysplasia or carcinoma in situ—the disease was likely to progress to invasive carcinoma within 5 years. If, on the other hand, the peripheral urothelium was normal, a progression to invasive carcinoma was unlikely.

To what extent and at what point any or all of these changes are reversible is a matter of debate at the present time. Recent studies using intravesical cytotoxic drugs in experimentally induced bladder cancer in rodents would seem to show that while the carcinoma in situ of the urothelium may be at least temporarily eradicated there is no evidence to date that they reverse the process (Murphy and Soloway 1980; Murphy et al. 1981). The interest which has been focused on these presumed preneoplastic states and the clear evidence of a field change in the urothelium has provided an explanation for the observation that bladder cancers may be multiple and that they tend to recur or new tumours to develop at new sites. Nevertheless, it might be premature to dismiss wholly the possibility that some bladder carcinomas may form by implantation either at sites of injury or ulceration or even at sites where the urothelium is intact. There is some recent experimental evidence that implantation of tumours—even in intact mucosa — could explain the development of some cases of multiple tumour formation (see Chap. 8, pp. 165–167).

Metaplasia in Bladder Epithelium

In the previous section abnormalities of the urothelium have been described which may be considered to be preneoplastic states and which may ultimately develop into invasive urothelial carcinomas. There is, however, another group of epithelial changes of pathological significance which may be associated with other types of bladder carcinoma. These are the metaplastic changes, which need to be distinguished from normal variant forms of urothelium discussed at the beginning of this chapter (von Brunn's nests, cystitis glandularis, and vaginal-type squamous epithelium).

The metaplastic changes which will be considered are squamous metaplasia, glandular metaplasia and nephrogenic adenoma. These require some words of explanation in order to distinguish them from the normal variants found in the bladder mucosa.

Squamous metaplasia is a change to a keratinising squamous epithelium or epidermoid type of epithelium quite distinct from the glycogen-rich 'vaginal' type of squamous epithelium previously described. This type of metaplasia is commonly found in association with squamous carcinoma. It is typically seen in the bladder carcinoma associated with bilharzial infection (schistosomiasis).

Glandular metaplasia is a metaplastic change in which the normal mucosa is replaced by a mucin-secreting columnar type of epithelium with gland formation resembling that of the large intestine. In the author's opinion it is best to reserve the term glandular metaplasia for this type of mucosa and not to confuse it with cystitis glandularis or cystitis cystica, which, as already described, are normal mucosal variants and not truly metaplastic changes. Glandular metaplasia is seen, perhaps at its most florid, in ectopia vesicae (Abeshouse 1943). Glandular metaplasia is also seen in bilharzial infection of the bladder (Ishak et al. 1967).

The nephrogenic adenoma is a lesion which is almost certainly not truly neoplastic and may well represent a special type of metaplastic change with a reversion to an epithelium which reflects its embryonic origin. In this connection it is relevant to recall the embryological derivation of the bladder, which, although derived from the cloaca of the hindgut, which is of endodermal origin, receives a contribution from the mesonephros which goes to form the trigone (Hamilton et al. 1972). It could well be that the nephrogenic type of epithelium occasionally found in the bladder is a metaplastic reversion to a type of epithelium derived from Wolffian duct or mesonephros. Against this view it might be argued that nephrogenic adenomas are not necessarily confined to the trigone or base of the bladder.

In addition to epithelial metaplasia it is known that the stroma of the bladder is capable of metaplastic change into an osseous or chondroid type of matrix. This has been observed in humans, e.g. the bony metaplasia of the stroma of urothelial carcinomas (Pang 1958), and in experimental conditions in which autografts of bladder epithelium have been shown to induce a bony metaplasia in the adjacent stroma (Constance 1954).

Having described the various pathological forms of metaplasia one may logically proceed to consider those types of bladder carcinoma with which they are commonly associated.

Carcinoma of the Bladder in Schistosomiasis, Ectopia Vesicae and Bladder Diverticula

Schistosomiasis

The pathological changes in the cancerous bladder associated with urinary bilharziasis are well documented. In Egypt, where bladder cancer is the major oncological problem (El-Bolkainy et al. 1981a, b), bilharziasis is endemic, and a clear association between the bladder infestation and bladder cancer is generally accepted. Certain generalisations may be made about these tumours, which differ significantly from bladder cancer in most other countries, e.g. Europe and North America: There is a great preponderance of male patients with a male to female ratio of between 4 and 7 to 1. It tends to affect younger people, with an average age less than 50 years. Squamous carcinoma is the commonest type of cancer. The tumours are often solitary, fungating masses which tend to remain localised to the pelvis. Metaplastic changes in the non-tumourous parts of the mucosa are common. Table 2.3 summarises the findings of the tumour types in bilharzial-infected bladders, taken from a number of reports. These confirm the preponderance of squamous carcinoma.

Table 2.3. Tumour types in bilharzial-infected bladders

References	No. of cases	Tumour types			
		S	U	A	Other
Dimette et al. (1956)	90	50	33	6	1
Ishak et al. (1967)	91	49	35	4	3
El-Bolkainy et al. (1972)	229	152	54	19	4
Khagafy et al. (1972)	86	66	18	2	0
El-Said et al. (1979)	420	286	71	36	27
Total	916	603	211	67	35

S, squamous carcinoma; U, urothelial carcinoma; A, adenocarcinoma

Associated metaplasia is very common in bilharzial-associated bladder cancer. In one report (Ishak et al. 1967) 74 out of 91 cases had metaplastic changes—usually keratinising squamous epithelium. Glandular metaplasia, however, is also common. Squamous carcinoma is associated with metaplasia in the great majority of cases. Transitional cell carcinomas are less commonly associated with metaplastic changes. Khagafy et al. (1972) have analysed these metaplastic changes in a series of 86 cases (Table 2.4).

It has been suggested that the schistosomal infections determine the type of bladder cancer, and El-Bolkainy et al. (1981a) have analysed a series of bladder tumours, first those with schistosomal ova present, and second those without schistosomal ova. Out of 1095 cases 82% had the schistosomal ova present in the bladder. Those patients tended to be younger and there was a greater preponderance of well-differentiated squamous carcinomas. No significant difference in the stage of the tumours could be detected in the two groups.

Table 2.4. Mucosal lesions in relation to type of bladder carcinoma (86 cases) in bilharzial bladder cancer (after Khagafy et al. 1972)

Tumour	No.	Squamous metaplasia	Glandular metaplasia
Squamous carcinoma	66	54	35
Urothelial carcinoma	18	3	8
Adenocarcinoma	2	—	2
Total no.	86	57	45

Although these studies have tended to focus attention on the high incidence of squamous carcinoma, the relative frequency of adenocarcinoma is also particularly noteworthy when one views this against the rarity of adenocarcinomas of the bladder generally. The high incidence of glandular metaplasia in bilharzial bladders may well be a relevant factor in determining the type of bladder tumour. Within the group of squamous carcinomas Egyptian workers have emphasised a verrucous form which is practically never met with in other circumstances (El-Bolkainy et al. 1981b).

Ectopia Vesicae

Ectopia vesicae is a rare congenital malformation predominantly affecting males and characterised by a defect in the anterior abdominal wall, the symphysis pubis and the anterior bladder wall (Ballantyne 1904). The condition may be associated with intestinal openings into the bladder.

The exposed bladder mucosa is subject to trauma and chronic infection and is liable to undergo both squamous and glandular metaplasia. Abeshouse (1943) reviewed the literature of cases of carcinoma associated with ectopia vesicae. He found that tumours usually arose at the apex of the superior aspect of the bladder, with only a few originating in the trigone. The majority of reported cases were adenocarcinomas, in striking contrast to the rarity of adenocarcinomas in the normal population. The other types of tumour were squamous carcinomas. Of Abeshouse's 27 tumour cases 21 were adenocarcinomas.

Bladder Carcinoma and Bladder Diverticula

The association of bladder carcinoma and bladder diverticula has been investigated by Knappenberger et al. (1960) from a series of 1805 adult patients with bladder carcinoma and 425 patients with bladder diverticula. In 18 cases the primary carcinoma arose in the diverticulum (4%). In addition, 11 patients had diverticula and a tumour, the tumour occurring elsewhere in the bladder. Of these 18 cases 14 were urothelial carcinomas. Only two squamous carcinomas were found. This is at some variance with statements that squamous carcinoma is the usual type of carcinoma in bladder diverticula. Kretschmer (1940) made a detailed study of 236 cases of bladder diverticula. He described four cases in which there was an associated bladder carcinoma; three of these were papillary carcinomas and one was squamous.

Other Types of Bladder Carcinoma

The Incidence of Squamous Carcinoma and Adenocarcinoma in Europe and North America

The strikingly high incidence of squamous carcinoma of the bladder in schistosomiasis is in marked contrast to the incidence of this type of bladder cancer in Europe and North America, where the incidence is less than 5% of all tumours. By definition these are purely of squamous type, i.e. they do not have a urothelial or glandular component. There may be associated squamous metaplasia of the urothelium, and the tumour may develop on the basis of long-standing bacterial cystitis or calculus formation (see Chap. 1, p. 8).

The predominance of adenocarcinoma of the bladder in ectopia vesicae is equally striking since they are very rare neoplasms, accounting for less than 1% of bladder cancers in most series. Apart from the association with ectopia vesicae, adenocarcinomas might arise from urachal remnants at the bladder vault, or from foci of cystitis glandularis—usually in the trigone. Although it is possible that such tumours could arise from foci of cystitis glandularis, this is not to imply that these epithelial changes predispose to the neoplastic state. Adenocarcinomas of bladder may be mucin secreting, in which case they may be difficult to distinguish from secondary adenocarcinomas, e.g. of bowel invading the bladder wall. These rare primary bladder tumours may also be difficult to distinguish from secondary spread from ovarian carcinomas. In the male with infiltration of the bladder base one has to distinguish a primary prostatic carcinoma from one arising in bladder

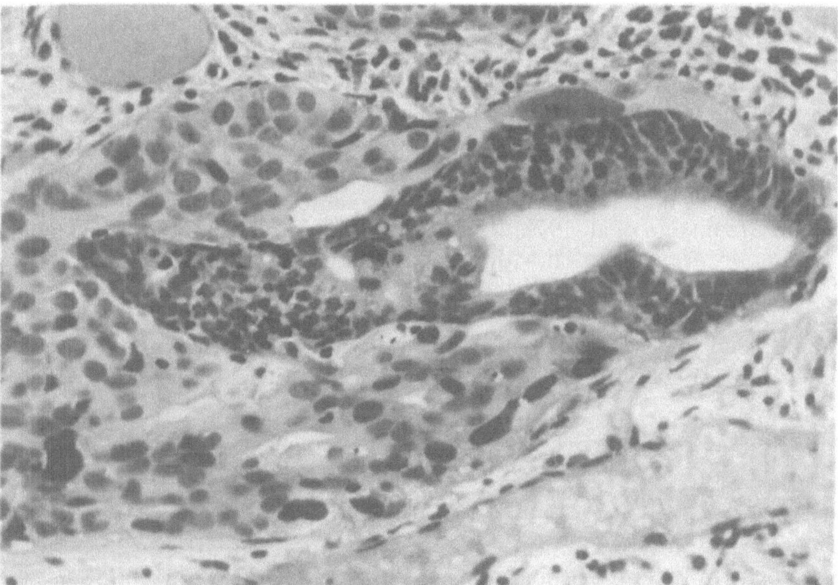

Fig. 2.10. Carcinoma of bladder. Mixed pattern of adenocarcinoma and urothelial carcinoma. Intimately admixed in this field. × 320

mucosa. Points of distinction include the clinical state of the prostate, the serum acid phosphatase and the specific staining of tissue sections for acid phosphatase by the immunoperoxidase method, in order to distinguish a prostatic from a non-prostatic glandular origin (Nadji et al. 1980).

Mixed Types of Carcinoma

1. A combined urothelial and squamous carcinoma is the commonest combination. This may contain fairly extensive areas of squamous differentiation, but more usually it consists of small scattered squamoid foci in a basically urothelial carcinoma.
2. Urothelial and adenocarcinoma—either as distinct areas or intimately admixed (Fig. 2.10). The glandular component often secretes mucin, and may take on a cribriform pattern.
3. Combinations of squamous and adenocarcinoma or all three patterns of carcinoma—urothelial, squamous and glandular. They generally arise at the trigone and are rather uncommon. There has been very little detailed analysis of this group of tumours as regards their grade, behaviour and prognosis.

Undifferentiated Carcinomas

Bladder carcinomas lacking all features of differentiation are rare and probably account for no more than 1% of bladder tumours. Two particular patterns are recognised: (1) a spindle cell structure which may be mistaken for a sarcomatous tumour, unless the particular histological subtype is recognised, and (2) a pleomorphic carcinoma containing bizarre giant cell forms.

A number of reports exist which describe *choriocarcinomas* as arising in the bladder (Weinberg 1939; Ainsworth and Gresham 1960; Civantos and Rywlin 1972; Kawamura et al. 1978). Most of these reports have been in elderly males, and the likelihood of true germ cell tumour arising in the elderly is very improbable; also the illustrations in the reported cases are far from convincing examples of genuine choriocarcinomas. The more likely explanation of these cases is that they represent anaplastic carcinomas with ectopic HCG production. It is perhaps relevant to recall in this connection that carcinomas of bronchus, colon and other organs have been shown to be capable of producing HCG (Rosen et al. 1968; Braunstein et al. 1973; Buckley and Fox 1979). The HCG-producing bladder tumours are associated with gynaecomastia. Recent studies have shown that in these hormone-producing tumours large quantities of HCG can be identified in plasma and urine (Kawamura et al. 1978). The group of anaplastic carcinomas need to be investigated in more detail with regard to their possible hormonal activity.

Sarcomas of the Bladder

In Infancy and Childhood

Embryonal rhabdomyosarcomas or botryoid tumours may arise in the urinary bladder, vagina, prostate or spermatic cord of infants and young children. The great majority of cases arise in the first 3 years of life, and these tumours are very rare after the age of 6 years (Tefft and Jaffe 1973).

Within the bladder they form masses of grape-like vesicular tissue which fill and distend the bladder and invade the bladder wall and neighbouring structures. They are liable to prove fatal unless chemotherapy, supported by surgery and radiotherapy, is instituted. Histologically these tumours consist of primitive strap-like mesenchymal cells set in a myxoid matrix. Special stains reveal that the cytoplasm of a proportion of the tumour cells have the characteristic cross-striations of rhabdomyoblasts. These tumours are presumed to arise from the primitive mesenchyme of the urogenital sinus.

In Adults

Sarcomas are rare tumours in adults, and most of those described have been either leiomyosarcomas or bony or cartilaginous tumours. These latter tumours are of interest and have been reviewed by Pang (1958). They contain an osseous, chondroid or osteochondroid matrix. The various types described include the following:

1. Combined carcinomas and osteo- or chondrosarcomas.
2. Pure osteosarcomas or chondrosarcomas.
3. Rarely a bladder carcinoma may show osseous metaplasia in the stroma and this has to be distinguished from the first type of combined tumour.

The carcinosarcomas of bladder with the osteosarcomatous element are an interesting group of tumours because it has been shown experimentally that implants of urothelium can induce, fairly readily, osseous metaplasia in the adjacent stroma (Constance, 1954). In humans, therefore, it could be that the epithelial component of the tumour determines the type of metaplastic change in these carcinosarcomas. On the other hand, Pang (1958) considers these tumours to be collision tumours, that is two distinct primary neoplasms (epithelial and mesynchymal), the individual components of which have coalesced.

Paragangliomas (Phaeochromocytomas)

Paragangliomas are rare tumours in the bladder and are derived from the chain of aorticosympathetic paraganglia of the autonomic nervous system (Glenner and Grimley 1974). Leestma and Price (1971) have reviewed 58 cases, 24 from the files of the Armed Forces Institute of Pathology and 34 from the literature. Only 5% behaved in a malignant fashion, i.e. metastasised. They arose most commonly from the trigone, and the mean diameter was 3 cm. Haematuria was a common feature and more than half the patients had hypertension. Most cases were shown to secrete catechol amines or their excretion products (VMA). Micturition attacks with headache, shortness of breath, sweating and dizziness were common. The hypertension may be cured by excision of the tumour.

Histologically these tumours are characteristic, forming cell nests supported by a generally delicate vascular stroma. Ultrastructure reveals characteristic cytoplasmic secretory granules. Bladder paragangliomas may give a positive chromaffin reaction (Glenner and Grimley 1974).

Spread of Bladder Carcinoma

The recording of the extent of spread of bladder carcinoma is based on the UICC Tumour Node Metastases (TNM) classification (UICC 1978; see also Table 6.1, p. 119). In many respects this system is superior to other systems of evaluating the degree of spread or stage of a tumour in that it provides more detailed and precise information of the status of the tumour.

Local Spread Within the Bladder

The extent of invasion of bladder carcinoma can be correlated to a great extent with the grade of the tumour. Few Grade 1 urothelial carcinomas are invasive, or if invasive at all appear to push into or compress the underlying lamina propria rather than showing true infiltrating properties. This form of growth with 'pushy' borders is not considered as invasive growth in our practice at the Western General Hospital, Edinburgh. In fact we very rarely recognise invasion in these Grade 1 tumours. On the other hand, the great majority of Grade 3 carcinomas are invasive when first diagnosed. Furthermore, there is seldom any doubt histologically about establishing true invasion in these high-grade tumours. They may be deeply invasive when first seen. As previously mentioned, up to 50% of Grade 2 carcinomas are invasive when first diagnosed (Friedell et al. 1976). It may be possible to demonstrate evidence of lymphatic invasion in biopsy specimens, but this is seen only in a small minority of cases in routinely processed biopsies (personal observation). Whether this finding indicates a greater likelihood of spread beyond the bladder has not been conclusively demonstrated at the present time.

While the TNM system of classification separates those tumours infiltrating superficial muscle only from those infiltrating into deep muscle, it is not possible from examining transurethral resection specimens for the surgical pathologist to state whether it is superficial or deep muscle which is involved. Strictly speaking, a pT category cannot be applied to such cases, and it is only with cystectomy specimens that the extent of invasion can be assessed by the pathologist with any precision.

A further problem in evaluating the extent of disease exists where there is a carcinomatous change in the prostatic urethra or periurethral ducts, since it has been shown in cases of bladder cancer that if the prostatic urethra is routinely biopsied, a urothelial tumour will frequently also be found there, either as a superficial papillary tumour or as a carcinoma involving periurethral ducts (Chibber et al. 1981). It would be incorrect to classify such cases of T4a tumours, as the prognosis is different. On occasions, however, it might be difficult to distinguish between a urothelial carcinoma arising in prostatic ducts from a bladder carcinoma invading prostatic tissues (a genuine T4a tumour).

Lymph Node Secondaries

Information on spread to regional lymph nodes (obturator, external iliac, hypogastric, common iliac and perivesical) has been derived mainly from studies

Table 2.5. Status of 134 cases with lymph node secondaries at 5 years (after Smith and Whitmore 1981)

5-year status	No. of cases
Alive, no disease	9
Dead from tumour	109
Dead from other causes	14
Total	134

Table 2.6. Lymph node involvement and pT category (after Smith and Whitmore 1981)

pT category	No. with lymph node secondaries	Percentage
pTis	0/22	0
pT1	2/37	5
pT2	14/108	13
pT3	71/389	18
pT4	47/106	44
All	134/662	20

analysing the results of radical cystectomy combined with lymphadenectomy. There are two particularly noteworthy and informative studies in this regard: the work of Skinner et al. (1982), in which they record the results of 131 cases, and an even larger series by Smith and Whitmore (1981); (see Tables 2.5 and 2.6). Skinner et al. (1982) showed that 25% of all their cases had lymph node secondaries. As one might anticipate, these were mainly from pT2, pT3 and pT4 tumours. However, it is of interest to note that 2 out of 41 pT1 or pTis tumours, i.e. those which locally only extended into lamina propria, had still metastasised to regional lymph nodes. In the large series of Smith and Whitmore (662 cases) the dismal prognosis of those patients with lymph node secondaries is clearly shown. Of their 134 cases with secondaries (20% of the total) the 5-year survival was only 7%—the great majority of patients dying of their tumour. Not surprisingly, the greater the extent of lymph node secondaries, the worse the prognosis. The long-term survivors were almost exclusively in the N_1 group (single homolateral lymph node). As in the report by Skinner et al., in the patients with pT2 to pT4 tumours there was more likely to be spread to lymph nodes (P2, 30%; P3a, 31%; P3b, 64%). The conclusion from several studies would seem to be that radical surgery has little hope of long-term cure when there are lymph node secondaries (see Chap. 9, pp. 195–196).

Immunological Aspects of Invasive Bladder Carcinoma

In invasive carcinoma of the bladder it is not uncommon to observe an inflammatory cell response in the stroma adjacent to the invasive tumour. This usually takes the form of a lymphocyte infiltrate with a variable admixture of plasma cells. Generally this cellular reaction is only of mild to moderate degree. Occasionally, however, the cellular infiltrate may be very dense. One may sometimes observe a neutrophil leucocyte response; rarely there may be an eosinophil leucocyte infiltrate (Feldsbausch 1900). These various inflammatory cell responses may represent secondary infection as a consequence of ulceration or loss of the integrity of the urothelial layer. However, some observers have suggested that the chronic inflammatory cell response might represent an immune response mounted by the host to the invasive tumour cells. Mostofi and Sesterhenn (1978) investigated the lymphocytic response in relation to urothelial carcinomas and considered that some degree of lymphocyte and plasma cell response could be observed in over 80% of cases; however, the significance of this was obscure. Sarma (1970) has also investigated the lymphocyte response in cases of bladder carcinoma: 73% of 230 unselected cases of bladder cancer had some degree of cellular response. The author claimed that in the absence of cellular response the carcinoma was likely to be more aggressive in its behaviour, whereas with a marked response invasive properties were much less likely to be observed. The precise significance of those findings is somewhat uncertain, as a negative cellular response was more likely to be from tumours of high grade. It may therefore be the grade which is the determining factor of behaviour and not the—perhaps incidental—cellular response.

Nevertheless, immunological aspects of invasive cancer have attracted the attention of a number of investigators, without, it must be admitted, resulting in any concrete conclusions or shedding light on the possible immunological mechanisms involved. The types of investigation have included cellular immunity in patients with bladder cancer, the presence of immune complexes and lymphocyte toxicity testing (UICC 1981). While recent studies have shown an impaired immune response in patients with bladder cancer, the significance of this in relation to the evolution of the disease process is obscure (see Chap. 3, pp. 62–64).

Distant Metastases in Bladder Carcinoma

Data on fatal cases of bladder carcinoma are inevitably highly selective — depending as they do on autopsy studies—but they provide the most reliable source of information on the distribution of distant spread. There would appear to be a consistent pattern in most major studies of this kind. Willis (1967), in 45 autopsy cases, stated that the lymph nodes, liver, lungs and bone were the most frequent sites of metastases. In a study by Fetter et al. (1959) metastases were analysed from a number of reports totalling over 1000 autopsy cases of bladder cancer. Of these, 40% had metastases. In Fetter et al.'s own series of 55 cases 39 (71%) had metastases. In an analysis of 307 cases with metastatic disease, the common sites were lymph nodes, liver, lungs and bone. Similar results were obtained by Cooling (1959), who analysed 77 cases of bladder cancer with metastases. While other organs may be the site of metastases (e.g. skin, adrenal, kidney, pancreas, myocardium), metastases at these latter sites would appear to be distinctly uncommon. In a recent report by Kishi et al. (1981), of 87 autopsy cases, 58 of which had metastases, the findings were remarkably similar, as shown in Table 2.7.

The relationship of metastases to stage of the primary tumour has also been analysed by Kishi et al. (1981) in their autopsy series. All the T3 and T4 tumours had metastases in this admittedly highly selective series. However, it is interesting to note that 2 out of 11 cases of T1 tumours (lamina propria only invaded) had metastatic disease—a finding which has also been demonstrated by Skinner et al. (1982) in their radical cystectomy series.

Table 2.7. Main sites of metastases in 58 out of 87 fatal cases of bladder carcinoma (after Kishi et al. 1981)

Site	Percentage of cases
Lymph nodes	38
Liver	30
Lungs	30
Bone	24

Practical Problems for the Histopathologist

The practical problems facing the histopathologist will be considered under two headings: (1) the reporting of bladder biopsies, including transurethral resection specimens, and (2) radical cystectomy specimens.

Bladder Biopsies and Transurethral Resection of Tumour

The minimum information which should be included in the pathologist's report are, first, the presence or absence of tumour, and, if present, the tumour type, its grade, invasion, e.g. into lamina propria and muscle (whether muscle is present in the specimen or not), and whether or not invasion of lymphatic or vascular channels has occurred. In addition, a clear indication of the changes in the mucosa of any random biopsies should also be given, i.e. whether it is normal or whether the urothelium shows abnormalities such as hyperplasia, dysplasia or carcinoma in situ. With regard to tumour type, this should not present too great a problem—the great majority of tumours are urothelial (transitional cell carcinomas). A few cases show a mixed pattern of histology, e.g. urothelial and squamous or urothelial and adenocarcinoma. Problems may arise in designating a particular grade to the tumour, in that tissue trauma during the resection procedure may obscure cellular detail. However, provided sufficient material is submitted, there will seldom be any problem in identifying areas where cellular morphology is well preserved. Another problem is that the tissue submitted may not be representative of the whole tumour (e.g. if only part of a tumour is submitted for biopsy). Since there may be variations in the grade of a tumour, it is possible that in such circumstances the biopsied portion may be derived from the better differentiated area, in which case the grade allocated by the pathologist would not accurately reflect the true nature of the lesion. It is generally accepted practice to grade tumours according to the least differentiated areas. The placing of a particular urothelial carcinoma into one of the three recognised grades may also present problems. While there is seldom any difficulty about allocating a very well-differentiated tumour and a very poorly differentiated pleomorphic tumour into Grade 1 and Grade 3 categories respectively, there is a continuous spectrum or degree of differentiation between these two extremes. It is therefore not surprising that one will have difficulty on occasions in deciding whether to allocate a tumour to a Grade 1 or Grade 2 category or into Grade 2 or Grade 3. Table 2.2 provides some guidelines as to the various cytological features to be found in each grade, but they are only guidelines and cannot by themselves provide the correct designation in every case. Where partly subjective analysis is concerned there is no substitute for experience in these matters.

Cystectomy Specimens

For an accurate assessment of a cystectomy specimen, the bladder must be sent to the pathologist properly fixed and distended (see Chap. 6, pp. 127–130). When examining a cystectomy specimen the fullest amount of pathological information should be obtained. This means not only sectioning any identifiable tumour but taking representative blocks from all areas of bladder, i.e. lateral walls, trigone, vault, anterior and posterior walls, also the ureters; if the urethra is included this should be sampled at regular intervals (e.g. 5 mm) over its entire length. Abnormalities in the urothelium from all of these areas should be accurately recorded. A pT category, according to the UICC rules, should also be recorded for the bladder tumour or tumours. In examining lymph nodes included with the cystectomy specimen it is necessary to appreciate the problems of identification of small, perhaps microscopic, deposits in the node. Clearly, if the entire node is replaced by tumour, one block from the bisected node will contain tumour. However, if there is only a microscopic deposit—or at any rate a very small deposit—a section from the two cut surfaces of a bisected node will, in all probability, not contain the tumour. The problem and probability of identifying very small secondary deposits in lymph nodes has received detailed analysis in the paper by Wilkinson and Hause (1974). One can therefore either block two halves of the node and step section these blocks or take four blocks of the node and section these. In this way one ought not to miss the presence of very small secondary tumour deposits.

Blood Group Isoantigens and Bladder Cancer

Introduction

One of the problems in the management of patients with bladder cancer—perhaps the main problem—is the difficulty in predicting the behaviour of a bladder tumour in an individual case. If there were some means of identifying those tumours most likely to go on to invasion, and conversely those least likely to do so, one could institute the most appropriate form of therapy at a much earlier stage.

The histological grading of bladder carcinoma is a well-established means by which one classifies the tumours into groups which, broadly speaking, differ in their modes of behaviour. This subject has already been considered in some detail. Nevertheless, ideally one requires some more precise way of identifying those superficial tumours (Ta and T1 tumours for the purposes of this discussion) which are likely to pursue an aggressive course with deep invasion and perhaps metastasise. It is against this background that there has been a resurgence of interest in the identification of specific antigens in the urothelium and in particular the demonstration of blood group isoantigens (BGIs).

BGI Deletion

Coombs et al. (1956) had originally demonstrated the presence of BGIs on the cell surface of normal epithelium. This was followed by a paper by Kay and Wallace (1961) in which they showed that these antigens were lacking in exfoliated bladder cancer cells. Kovarik et al. (1968) applied the technique to paraffin sections of both normal and malignant epithelium by using the specific red cell adherence test (SRCAT), which demonstrates A, B and O (H) antigen in the cell by a sandwich technique in which specific antisera are applied to de-paraffinised histological sections. Red cells of the appropriate group are then applied to the sections and these adhere to the sites where antigen is present—the antibody having been fixed to the section. De Cenzo et al. (1975), using the SRCAT, reported recurrence with invasion of bladder tumours in eight out of nine isoantigen negative bladder tumours, but no such recurrences in 13 tumours which were isoantigen positive. Since then there have been a spate of papers which have confirmed these findings, e.g. Lange et al. (1978), Bergman and Javadpour (1978), Emmott et al. (1979), Young et al. (1979), Johnson and Lamm (1980), Ritchie et al. (1980) and Newman et al. (1980), in that deeply invasive tumours, tumour metastases and carcinoma in situ are isoantigen negative.

Superficial tumours and tumours of low grade are usually isoantigen positive. Normal urothelium invariably contains the antigen. Also initially superficial tumours which are BGI positive are unlikely to proceed to invasion, whereas BGI-negative cases probably will do so. On the face of it this would seem to be a considerable advance in helping to predict how a tumour is likely to behave. Theoretically it might of course be anticipated that loss of differentiation or increasing anaplasia would be associated with loss of surface antigen present on the normal cell. The clear demonstration of the loss of such an antigen might reasonably be considered to be a more objective and accurate indicator of loss of differentiation (and, by implication, potential for invasive growth) than the rather subjective and crude means of histological grading.

Technical Problems

There are, nevertheless, a number of drawbacks to the widespread acceptance of the SRCAT as a routine procedure. These are mainly technical and may be summarised as follows: The test requires skill and experience to obtain reliable results. The precise point at which the test can be said to be positive is somewhat uncertain. Should frozen sections be used instead of paraffin sections? A recent study suggests that there is considerable loss of isoantigen as a result of paraffin embedding and hence some false negative results will occur (Limas and Lange 1982). Blood group O isoantigen is weak and may remain undetected. It has been shown that radiotherapy results in restoration of the BGI. In this regard this may in some ways be analogous to the observation that poorly differentiated squamous carcinomas may become better differentiated and keratinising growths after radiotherapy. Then one has to consider whether the tissue being analysed for BGI is representative of the urothelium as a whole. The great problem in bladder cancer is the development of new tumours which may be at a different site or less well differentiated than the original tumour. Nevertheless, in spite of these reservations, recent reports have been encouraging in predicting likely subsequent behaviour of a tumour.

Prediction of Subsequent Invasion

A valuable recent review of the subject is given by Catalona (1981). This author analysed the SRCAT as an indicator of prognostic importance, based on the study of several large series of cases, in order to define more clearly the proper role of the test in clinical practice. Catalona concluded that normal urothelium is virtually always BGI positive, that nearly 60% of superficial tumours are positive, but that invasive tumours, metastases and carcinoma in situ are negative. The majority of low-grade tumours are positive. The reverse is the case with high-grade tumours. This is summarised in Table 2.8.

Table 2.8. Positive SRCAT results (after Catalona 1981)

	Normal urothelium	Superficial carcinoma	Invasive carcinoma	Metastatic carcinoma	CIS	Grade of tumour	
						High	Low
No. of cases	363/369	300/515	9/77	0/39	2/18	36/159	320/510
Percentage	98	58	12	0	11	23	63

CIS, carcinoma in situ

The BGI-negative tumours are more likely to recur, but since nearly 50% of BGI-positive tumours develop recurrences also, as a predictor of recurrence the test is of little value. On the other hand, as a predictor of invasion its usefulness is borne out by the fact that nearly 70% of BGI-negative cases went on to invasion within 5 years, whereas only 4% of positive cases did so (see Table 2.9).

Table 2.9. Clinical course in relation to SRCAT results (after Catalona 1981)

SRCAT	Recurrence		Invasion within 5 years	
	Negative	Positive	Negative	Positive
Totals	172/191	125/274	130/196	12/294
Percentage	90	46	66	4

If the SRCAT is analysed in relation to grade of tumour and its subsquent behaviour, BGI-positive tumours are unlikely to go on to invasion whatever their grade, whereas antigen-negative tumours will progress to invasion in the majority of cases—again regardless of grade (see Table 2.10).

If one restricts the test to superficial tumours of high grade, Catalona estimates that of 100 such tumours approximately 23% will be positive and 77% negative. If one takes these negative cases, approximately 65 of the 77 would go on to invasion (derived from Table 2.10), still leaving a significant number of cases which might be subjected to an unnecessary cystectomy if based on the results of this test. On the other hand, of the high-grade tumours which retain their BGI, very few will go

Table 2.10. Subsequent invasion as function of grade and SRCAT results (after Catalona 1981)

SRCAT	Low grade		High grade	
	Negative	Positive	Negative	Positive
Totals	89/122	11/243	31/37	2/31
Percentage invasion	73	4.5	83.8	6.5

on to invasion and hence this group might be selected for more conservative treatment than would otherwise be the case.

A useful recent paper on the subject by Jakse and Hofstädter (1983) reviews the results of 143 patients with superficial bladder cancer (pTa and pT1 tumours). These authors applied the SRCAT not only to the tumour but also to random mucosal biopsies from each case (two to four biopsies per patient). They found that 50% of their Grade 1 tumours were BGI positive, whereas none of the Grade 3 tumours were positive. In line with other workers they found that in the great majority of cases normal urothelium was BGI positive, whereas carcinoma in situ was negative. There were, however, a surprisingly high figure of negative results in association with mucosal inflammation (42%). BGI-negative tumours were more likely to be associated with abnormal random mucosal biopsy, i.e. urothelial dysplasia or carcinoma in situ. Their Table V (Table 2.11) is also revealing, in that it demonstrates that the 'normal' urothelium is much more likely to be BGI negative when associated with a BGI-negative tumour, than is the case with a BGI-positive tumour. It may be that the loss of BGI could represent the earliest recognisable alteration in a potentially neoplastic urothelium, which may ultimately proceed to an aggressive or invasive growth. Whether or not this BGI-negative neoplastic urothelium possesses properties fundamentally different (at the molecular level) from BGI-positive neoplastic growths it is not possible to say at the present time.

Table 2.11. Comparison of tumour antigenicity and BGI content of microscopically normal urothelium (after Jakse and Hofstädter 1983)

Tumour	Normal urothelium	
	Positive	Negative
Positive	93%	7%
Negative	76%	24%

Looking to the future one can anticipate attempts to identify BGI in histological sections by a simpler method, e.g. the immunoperoxidase technique, which also has the advantage of providing a permanent record of the result. Provided specific antibody of guaranteed purity and strength can be obtained, this technique offers considerable advantages over the SRCAT and could be applied routinely in histological laboratories. The only drawback one might foresee is that since the BGI O (H) is a weak one this might remain undetected by the immunoperoxidase method. This would be a serious drawback, particularly where a large proportion of the population are of blood group O. This would result in many false negative results and thus invalidate the method as a routine test.

Conclusion

The problem with bladder carcinoma is that the whole of the urothelium has the potential for undergoing neoplastic change. The testing of a single tumour at the outset for surface antigen may not therefore be wholly adequate in predicting subsequent developments. Recurrences of bladder tumours are very often not true recurrences in the strict sense but represent the development of new tumours—either close to the original one or at some distance from it. These new tumours may not resemble the original growth (Brawn 1982). Ideally, therefore, one would need to know the antigen status over a wide area—or at least in representative tissue from a wide area. Such studies need to be correlated with critical morphological studies using standard classifications, together with the adoption of an acceptably reliable technique for identifying BGI. While reports to date indicate this to be a valuable method in predicting tumour behaviour, it is still too early to say what role the test is likely to play in routine urological practice.

References

Abeshouse BS (1943) Exstrophy of the bladder complicated by adenocarcinoma of the bladder and renal calculi. J Urol 49: 259–289

Ainsworth RW, Gresham GA (1960) Primary choriocarcinoma of the urinary bladder in a male. J Pathol Bacteriol 79: 185–192

Althausen AF, Prout GR, Daly JJ (1976) Non-invasive papillary carcinoma of bladder associated with carcinoma in situ. J Urol 116: 575–579

Ballantyne JW (1904) Manual of antenatal pathology and hygiene. The embryo. Green, Edinburgh, p 539

Bergman S, Javadpour N (1978) The cell surface antigen A, B or O (H) as an indicator of malignant potential in stage A bladder carcinoma: preliminary report. J Urol 119: 49–51

Braunstein GD, Vaitukaitis JL, Carbone PP, Ross GT (1973) Ectopic production of human chorionic gonadotrophin by neoplasms. Ann Intern Med 78: 39–45

Brawn PN (1982) The origin of invasive carcinoma of the bladder. Cancer 50: 515–519

Buckley CH, Fox H (1979) An immunohistochemical study of the significance of HCG secretion by large bowel adenocarcinomata. J Clin Pathol 32: 368–372

Catalona WJ (1981) Practical utility of specific red cell adherence test in bladder cancer. Urology 18: 113–117

Chibber PJ, McIntyre MA, Hindmarsh JR, Hargreave TB, Newsam JE, Chisholm GD (1981) Transitional cell carcinoma involving the prostate. Br J Urol 53: 605–609

Chisholm GD, Hindmarsh JR, Howatson AG, Webb JN, Busuttil A, Hargreave TB, Newsam JE (1980) TNM (1978) in bladder cancer. Use and abuse. Br J Urol 52: 500–505

Civantos F, Rywlin AM (1972) Carcinomas with trophoblastic differentiation and secretion of chorionic gonadotrophins. Cancer 29: 789–797

Constance TJ (1954) Localised myositis ossificans. J Pathol Bacteriol 68: 381–385

Cooling CI (1959) Review of 150 post-mortems of carcinoma of the urinary bladder. In: Wallace DM (ed) Tumours of the bladder. Monographs on neoplastic disease, vol 2. Livingstone, Edinburgh, pp 171–186

Coombs RA, Bedford D, Rouillard MM (1956) A and B blood group antigens on human epidermal cells. Demonstrated by mixed agglutination. Lancet I: 461–463

De Cenzo JM, Howard P, Irish CE (1975) Antigenic deletion and prognosis of patients with stage A transitional cell bladder carcinoma. J Urol 114: 874–878

Dimmette RM, Sproat HF, Sayegh ES (1956) The classification of carcinoma of the urinary bladder associated with schistosomiasis and metaplasia. J Urol 75: 680–686

Eisenberg RB, Roth RB, Schweinberg MH (1960) Bladder tumors associated with proliferative mucosal lesions. J Urol 84: 544–550

El-Bolkainy MN, Chu EW, (eds) (1981) Detection of bladder cancer associated with schistosomiasis. The National Cancer Institute, Cairo University. Al-Ahram Press, Cairo
El-Bolkainy MN, Ghoneim MA, Mansour MA (1972) Carcinoma of the bilharzial bladder in Egypt: clinical and pathological features. Br J Urol 44: 561–570
El-Bolkainy MN, Tawfik HN, Kamel IA (1981a) Histopathologic classification of carcinomas in the schistosomal bladder. In: El-Bolkainy and Chu (1981) pp 106–123
El-Bolkainy MN, Mokhtar MN, Ghoneim MA, Hussein MH (1981b) The impact of schistosomiasis on the pathology of bladder carcinoma. Cancer 48: 2643–2648
El-Said A, Omar S, Ibrahim S, Tawfik H, Eissa S, Ali I, Demerdash S, Badawi S, Medbed H, Manieh M (1979) Bilharzial bladder cancer in Egypt. A review of 420 cases of radical cystectomy. Jpn J Clin Oncol 9: 117–122
El-Sebai T (1981) Bladder cancer in Egypt: current clinical experience. In: El-Bolkainy and Chu (1981), pp 9–18
Emmott RC, Javadpour N, Bergman SM, Soares T (1979) Correlation of the cell surface antigens with stage and grade in cancer of the bladder. J Urol 121: 37–39
Farrow GM, Utz DC, Rife CC (1976) Morphological and clinical observations of patients with early bladder cancer treated with total cystectomy. Cancer Res 36: 2495–2501
Feldsbausch F (1900) Über das Vorkommen von eosinophilen Leucocyten in Tumoren. Virchows Arch Pathol Anat Physiol Klin Med 161: 1–18
Fetter TH, Bogaev JH, McCuskey B, Seres JL (1959) Carcinoma of the bladder: sites of metastases. J Urol 81: 746–748
Foulds L (1975) Neoplastic development 2. Academic, London
Friedell GH, Bell JR, Burney SW, Soto EA, Tiltman AJ (1976) Histopathology and classification of urinary bladder carcinomas. Urol Clin North Am 3: 53–70
Friedell GH, Parija GC, Nagy GK, Soto EA (1980) The pathology of human bladder cancer. Cancer 45: 1823–1831
Gilbert HA, Logan JL, Kagan AR, Friedman HA, Cove JK, Fox M, Muldoon TM, Lonni YW, Rowe JH, Cooper JF, Nussbaum H, Chan P, Rao A, Starr A (1978) The natural history of papillary transitional cell carcinoma of the bladder and its treatment in an unselected population on the basis of histological grading. J Urol 119: 488–492
Glenner GG, Grimley PM (1974) Tumors of the extra-adrenal paraganglion system (including chemoreceptors). Atlas of tumour pathology, fascicle 9, 2nd ser. Armed Forces Institute of Pathology, Washington DC
Hamilton WJ, Boyd JD, Mossman HW (1972) Human embryology, 4th edn. Heffer, Williams and Wilkins, Cambridge, Mass
Hattori M, Yashimoto Y, Matsukura S, Fujita T (1980) Qualitative and quantitative analyses of human chorionic gonadotrophin and its subunits produced by malignant tumors. Cancer 46: 355–361
Hicks RM, Chowaniec J (1978) Experimental induction, histology and ultra-structure of hyperplasia and neoplasia of the urinary bladder epithelium. In: Richter GW and Epstein MA (eds) International review of experimental pathology, 18. Academic, London, pp 199–280
Ishak KG, le Golvan PC, El-Sebai I (1967) Malignant bladder tumors associated with bilharziasis: a gross and microscopic study. In: Mostofi FK (ed) Bilharziasis. Springer, Berlin Heidelberg New York
Jakse G, Hofstädter F (1983) Investigation of ABH antigenicity of random mocosal biopsies and transitional cell carcinoma of the urinary bladder. Eur Urol 9: 97–101
Johnson JD, Lamm DL (1980) Prediction of bladder tumour invasion with mixed cell agglutination test. J Urol 123: 25–28
Kawamura J, Machida S, Yoshida O, Oseko F, Imura H, Hattori M (1978) Bladder carcinoma associated with ectopic production of gonadotrophin. Cancer 42: 2773–2780
Kay HEM, Wallace DM (1961) A and B antigens of tumors arising from urinary epithelium. J Natl Cancer Inst 26: 1349–1365
Khagafy M, El-Bolkainy MN, Mansour MA (1972) Carcinoma of the bilharzial urinary bladder: A study of the associated mucosal lesions in 86 cases. Cancer 30: 150–159
Kishi K, Hirota T, Matsumoto K, Kakizoe T, Murase T, Fujita J (1981) Carcinoma of the bladder: A clinical and pathological analysis of 87 autopsy cases. J Urol 125: 36–39
Knappenberger ST, Uson AC, Melicow MM (1960) Primary neoplasms occurring in vesical diverticula: a report of 18 cases. J Urol 83: 153–159
Koss LG (1975) Tumors of the urinary bladder. Atlas of tumor pathology, fascicle 11, 2nd ser. Armed Forces Institute of Pathology, Washington DC

Koss LG (1979) Mapping of the urinary bladder. Its impact on the concepts of bladder cancer. Human Pathol 10: 533–548

Koss LG, Melamed MR, Kelly RE (1969) Further cytologic and histologic studies of bladder lesions in workers exposed to *para*-aminodiphenyl. Progress report. J Natl Cancer Inst 43: 233

Koss LG, Tiamson EM, Robbins MA (1974) Mapping cancerous and precancerous bladder changes: a study of the urothelium in 10 surgically removed bladders. JAMA 227: 281–286

Koss LG, Nakanishi I, Freed SZ (1977) Non-papillary carcinoma in situ and atypical hyperplasia in cancerous bladders. Further studies of surgically removed bladders by mapping. Urology 9: 422–455

Kovarik S, Davidson I, Stejskal R (1968) ABO antigens in cancer. Detection with the mixed cell agglutination reaction. Arch Pathol 86: 12–21

Kretschmer HL (1940) Diverticula of the urinary bladder: a clinical study of 236 cases. Surg Gynecol Obstet 71: 491–503

Lange PH, Limas C, Fraley EE (1978) Tissue blood group antigens and prognosis in low stage transitional cell carcinoma of the bladder. J Urol 119: 52–55

Leestma JE, Price EB (1971) Paragangliomas of the urinary bladder. Cancer 28: 1063–1073

Limas C, Lange P (1982) A, B, H antigen detectability in normal and neoplastic urothelium. Influence of methodologic factors. Cancer 49: 2476–2484

Mäkinen J, Collan Y, Heikkinen A (1978) Transitional cell tumours of the urinary bladder. The histological grade (WHO) and clinical stage (UICC). Eur Urol 4: 176–181

Melamed MR, Grabstald H, Whitmore WF (1966) Carcinoma in situ of bladder: clinico-pathologic study of case with suggested approach to detection. J Urol 96: 466–471

Melicow MM (1952) Histological study of vesical urothelium intervening between gross tumours in total cystectomy. J Urol 68: 261–279

Mostofi FK, Sesterhenn I (1978) Lymphocytic infiltration in relationship to urologic tumours. Natl Cancer Inst Monogr 49: 133–141

Mostofi FK, Sorbin LH, Torloni H (1973) Histological typing of urinary bladder tumours. International classification of tumours, No. 10. WHO, Geneva

Murphy WM, Irving CC (1981) The cellular features of developing carcinoma in murine urinary bladder. Cancer 47: 514–522

Murphy WM, Soloway MS (1980) The effect of thio-tepa on developing and established mammalian bladder tumors. Cancer 45: 870–875

Murphy WM, Soloway MS (1982) Urothelial dysplasia. J Urol 127: 849–854

Murphy WM, Soloway MS, Finebaum S (1981) Pathological changes associated with topical chemotherapy for superficial bladder cancer. J Urol 126: 461–463

Nadji M, Tabei SZ, Castro A, Chu TM, Morales AR (1980) Prostatic origin of tumours. An immunohistochemical study. Am J Clin Pathol 73: 735–739

Newman AJ Jr, Carlton CE Jr, Johnson S (1980) Cell surface A, B or O (H) blood group antigens as an indicator of malignant potential in stage A bladder carcinoma. J Urol 124: 27–29

Pang LSC (1958) Bony and cartilaginous tumours of the urinary bladder. J Pathol Bacteriol 76: 357–377

Ritchie JP, Blute RD, Waisman J (1980) Immunologic indicators of prognosis in bladder cancer: The importance of cell surface antigens. J Urol 123: 22–24

Rosen SW, Becker CE, Schlaff S, Easton J, Gluck MC (1968) Ectopic gonadotrophin production before clinical recognition of bronchogenic carcinoma. N Engl J Med 279: 640–641

Sarma KP (1970) The role of lymphoid reaction in bladder cancer. J Urol 104: 843–849

Skinner DG, Tift JP, Kaufman JJ (1982) High dose, short course pre-operative radiation therapy and immediate single stage radical cystectomy with pelvic lymph node dissection in the management of bladder cancer. J Urol 127: 671–674

Smith JA, Whitmore WF (1981) Regional lymph node metastasis from bladder cancer. J Urol 126: 591–593

Soloway MS, Murphy W, Rav MK, Cox C (1978) Serial multiple-site biopsies in patients with bladder cancer. J Urol 120: 57–59

Soto EA, Friedell GH, Tiltman AJ (1977) Bladder cancer as seen in giant histologic sections. Cancer 39: 447–455

Tefft M, Jaffe M (1973) Sarcoma of the bladder and prostate in children. Cancer 32: 1161–1177

UICC (1978) TNM classification of malignant tumours. UICC, Geneva

UICC (1981) Skrabanek P, Walsh A (eds) Bladder cancer. UICC Technical Report Series, vol. 60. Workshop on the Biology of Human Cancer, Report no. 13. UICC, Geneva

Utz DC, Farrow GM, Rife CC, Sequra JW, Zincke H (1980) Carcinoma in situ of the bladder. Cancer 45: 1842–1848

Wallace DMA, Hindmarsh JR, Webb JN, Busuttil A, Hargreave TB, Newsam JE, Chisholm GD (1979) The role of multiple biopsies in the management of patients with bladder cancer. Br J Urol 51: 535–540

Weinberg T (1939) Primary chorioepithelioma of the urinary bladder in a male. Am J Pathol 15: 783–795

Wiener DP, Koss LG, Sablay B, Freed SZ (1979) The prevalence and significance of Brunn's nests, cystitis cystica and squamous metaplasia in normal bladders. J Urol 122: 317–321

Wilkinson EJ, Hause L (1974) The probability in lymph node sectioning. Cancer 33: 1269–1274

Willis RA (1967) Pathology of tumours, 4th edn. Butterworths, London, pp 480–481

Young AK, Hammand E, Middleton AW Jr (1979) The prognostic value of cell surface antigens in low grade, non-invasive transition cell carcinoma of the bladder. J Urol 122: 462–464

Chapter 3

Immunological Aspects of Bladder Cancer

R. Ackermann

Basic Principles in Tumour Immunology

The hypothesis that the immune system may not only be responsible for the elimination of bacteria, parasites and viruses but also for the defence of the cellular integrity of the organism was postulated as early as 1909 by Paul Ehrlich. It is based on the assumption that tumour cells in an organism arise continuously, and, were it not for the immune mechanisms, '*Karzinome würden entstehen in einer geradezu ungeheuerlichen Frequenz*' (cancer would occur with appalling frequency). This hypothesis was restated, but with some modifications, by Thomas (1959) and Burnet (1971), who both regarded the elimination of malignant cells to be one of the major functions of the immune system. This concept is known as the immunosurveillance theory (IS).

When this theory was repostulated, observations obtained from experimentally induced animal tumours indicated the presence of tumour-associated transplantation antigens on the membranes of tumour cells. In transplantation experiments with experimentally induced tumours in highly inbred animal strains, it could be demonstrated that immunisation of the animals with such tumours evoked a rejection-geared immune response which resulted in the elimination of a subsequent tumour graft of the same type (Gross 1943; Foley 1953; Prehn and Main 1957).

With the rapid progress in the field of immunology, regulatory and effector mechanisms have been identified by which the immune system may act against aberrant cells in the organism. In general, two distinct immunological effector mechanisms specifically eliminate or neutralise an immunogen like a tumour cell, which is recognised as 'non-self' by the organism. The humoral immune response is mediated by antibody-producing B-lymphocytes. The effector mechanisms of the cellular immunity comprise T-lymphocytes, K-cells, natural killer cells (NK-cells), and macrophages. Both arms of the immune system depend on each other, in as much as antibodies may inhibit or amplify cell-mediated immune reactions. In addition, antibodies may also be essential for the recognition of tumour cells by certain cellular effector mechanisms.

A description of the basic principles of antitumour immune reactions and their possible relevance in host defence is presented in the following part of this chapter.

Tumour Cell Lysis Mediated by T-Cells

Thymus-dependent mononuclear cells, referred to as T-lymphocytes, represent one cell population which is responsible for surveillance against tumours induced by oncogenic viruses and chemical carcinogens. Fig. 3.1 demonstrates the mode of action of T-cells against tumour cells and their possible suppression by T-suppressor cells. In addition, T-cell cytotoxicity may also be inhibited by circulating or cell-bound antigen-antibody complexes as shown in Fig. 3.3. Many experiments, such as have been reported by Allison and Taylor (1967), demonstrate the participation of T-cells in IS. These authors have shown that T-cell deficiency in neonatal animals, obtained by thymectomy or treatment with antilymphocyte serum (ALS), will result in a high tumour incidence following induction with polyoma or SV 40 viruses. This in turn can be prevented either by thymus grafting or inoculation of syngeneic mature lymphocytes. Similar findings have been obtained in a variety of, but not all, chemically induced tumours (Balner and Dersjant 1969; Cerilli and Treat 1969; Rabbat and Jeejeebhoy 1970). The increased tumour incidence of 3%–6% in humans under immunosuppression, e.g. in renal transplant recipients, has been used as evidence to support

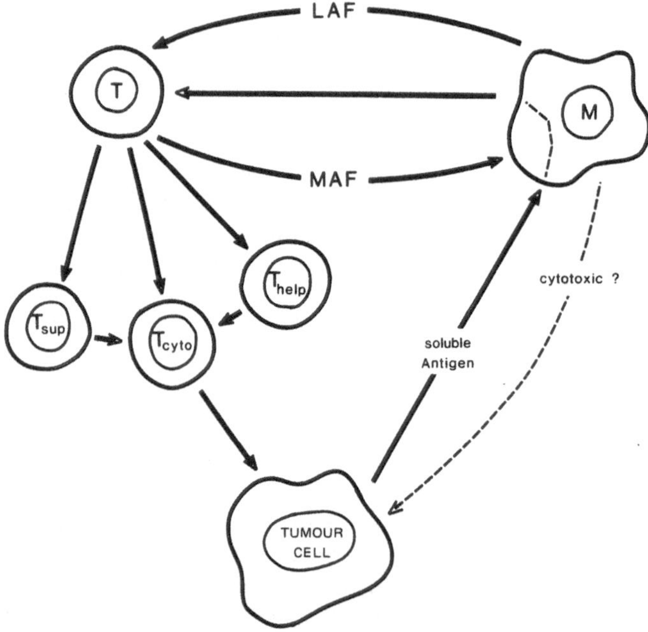

Fig. 3.1. Regulatory pathways of T-lymphocyte-mediated tumour cell lysis. *T*, T-lymphocyte; *M*, macrophage; T_{help}, T helper cell; T_{cyto}, cytotoxic T-lymphocyte; T_{sup}, T suppressor cell; *LAF*, lymphocyte arming factor; *MAF*, macrophage arming factor

the view that immune surveillance is mediated by T-lymphocytes (Hoover and Fraumeni 1973; Sterioff et al. 1975; Vollenweider et al. 1982). The observation that most of the tumours that develop under immunosuppression originate from the reticuloendothelial system cannot be explained by the suppression of the immunosurveillance mechanisms.

Chronic anigenic stimulation by the histo-incompatible renal transplant, in combination with the immunosuppressive treatment, are experimentally proven factors responsible for the high frequency of mesenchymal malignancies in renal transplant recipients (Krüger et al. 1971). Since the above-mentioned experiments, as well as tumour transplantation experiments, are not possible to repeat in humans, attempts have been made to demonstrate tumour-specific T-cell reactions against human tumours in vitro. However, clear evidence for T-cell-mediated tumour cell lysis in man has only been obtained in Burkitt's lymphoma, a tumour which appears to express viral antigenic determinants (Jondal et al. 1975).

Numerous reports have been published in the past decade on tumour-specific immune reaction against a variety of human malignancies (e.g. renal cell carcinoma, breast cancer, ovarian carcinoma etc.) which were interpreted as T-cell responses to tumour-associated transplantation antigens (Hellström et al. 1968; Bubenik et al. 1971; Disala et al. 1971; Hellström et al. 1971; Baldwin et al. 1973). The first evidence that false conclusions may have been drawn from these studies was produced by Takasugi et al. (1973), who demonstrated that the reactivity of lymphocytes from normal persons against a variety of cultured human tumour cells was significantly stronger than that of lymphocytes obtained from patients with a malignant disease of the same histological type. It is now well established that the tumour cell destruction observed in these earlier studies is mediated mainly by a subpopulation of lymphocytes referred to as natural killer cells (NK-cells). The observation that spontaneous tumour development rarely occurs in nude mice which are T-cell-deficient because of their thymus dysplasia is used as an additional argument against the T-cell as an all-encompassing surveillance mechanism. In a study of 15 700 nude mice, no spontaneous tumour development was observed (Castro 1978). Although the low incidence of spontaneous tumours in nude mice may merely be due to the short life span of these animals, it is likely that the natural killer cell system of these animals may be the powerful surveillance mechanism. Despite the fact that there is little evidence that the immunosurveillance mediated by T-lymphocytes plays a major role in the development and growth of spontaneously arising tumours in man, it is still important to make this system work in the defence against malignant tumours. The possible low immunogenicity resulting from the multistep progression of spontaneously developing malignancies, as has been observed by several investigators in rodents (Baldwin 1966; Hewitt et al. 1976; Prehn 1976), may be the critical factor responsible for the lack of T-cell response against human tumours. Increasing the immunogenicity of spontaneously arising tumours is one approach currently under investigation.

Spontaneous Cell-Mediated Cytotoxicity

The lack of evidence that T-cells form a powerful immunosurveillance mechanism has led to a rapidly growing interest in NK-cells as the mediators of spontaneous

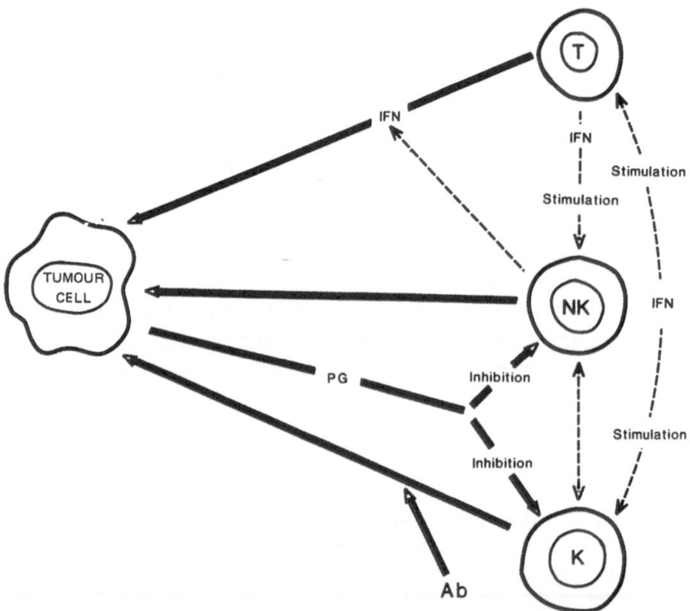

Fig. 3.2. Stimulatory and inhibitory regulation of natural killer cells and K-cells. *T*, T-lymphocyte; *NK*, natural killer cell; *K*, K-cell; *IFN*, interferon; *PG*, prostaglandin; *Ab*, antibody

cell-mediated cytotoxicity. NK-cells represent a subpopulation of mononuclear cells which differs from other types of lymphocytes and macrophages. Most notably, the cytotoxicity mediated by NK-cells takes place without deliberate sensitisation against the target structures of malignant cells, as shown in Fig. 3.2.

Although little is known about the in vivo relevance of NK-cells in man, there is some experimental evidence obtained from the murine system which supports the theory that NK-cells may act as the 'first line of defence' against the development of tumours. Haller et al. (1977) inoculated semisyngeneic tumours cells into F1 hybrids of mice exhibiting a low NK-cell activity and into mice with high NK-cell activity. Tumour development was observed only in animals with low NK-cell activity. Similar experiments have been reported by other investigators (Kasai et al. 1979; Cheever et al. 1980). Furthermore, Talmadge et al. (1980) have observed that the inoculation of melanoma B16 in NK-cell-deficient 'beige' mice has resulted in a significantly higher incidence of tumours and metastases as compared with the inoculation of the same tumour in syngeneic heterozygous C 57 BL/6 mice which possess normal NK-cell activity.

Most of the in vitro cell-mediated cytotoxicity directed against a variety of human tumour cells has been found to be mediated by NK-cells. In addition, it can be demonstrated for some tumours, such as carcinoma of the prostate, that the degree of spontaneous cell-mediated cytotoxicity correlates well with the extent of the disease, and is significantly reduced in patients with tumours of advanced stage (Okabe et al. 1979). Studies of NK-activity in tumour-draining lymph nodes of patients with breast cancer and carcinoma of the prostate has yielded contradictory results. NK-cell activity in tumour-draining lymph nodes has been found to be impaired in some studies (Vose et al. 1977; Wirth et al. 1983), whereas no alteration of natural cell-mediated immunity was observed in other studies (Eremin 1980). Furthermore, tumour cells of the same histological type may differ in their NK-cell susceptibility, although certain types of tumour cells, e.g. T-lymphoma, tend to be highly sensitive for NK-cells (Klein 1980).

Investigations on the specificity of NK-cell reactions with a variety of methods, e.g. immunoabsorption and cold inhibition assay, were unsuccessful in indicating any pattern of reactivity. Many of the human tumour cell lines used in such experiments appeared to possess a common target structure, whereas other cell lines seemed to express additional target structures which are recognised by different NK-cell subsets.

Despite considerable efforts, the nature of the target structure on the tumour cell membrane for NK-cells has not been discovered. Differences in the membrane glycolipid profiles have been detected between NK-cell susceptible and unsusceptible target cell clones indicating that NK-cells may recognise membrane glycoconjugates (Durdik et al. 1980).

Compared with the limited knowledge concerning the specificity of NK-cell reactions, more information is available on the regulatory mechanisms of the NK-cell system. Augmentation of spontaneous cell-mediated cytotoxicity by interferons was first described by Trinchieri and Santoli (1978; Fig. 3.2). Several other agents which have also been found to augment NK-cell activity, e.g. polyinosinic and polycytidylic acids (poly I:C), *Corynebacterium parvum*, bacille Calmette-Guérin (BCG), have in common the ability to induce the production of interferons. The effect of interferons on NK-cells is time and dose dependent and can be measured after both in vivo and in vitro administration of interferons. The regulatory potential of interferons on the NK-cell system appears to be mainly in the transformation of precursors of NK-cells into mature cytotoxic NK-cells (Hayakawa et al. 1984), although evidence exists that interferons may also act by augmenting the cytotoxicity of mature NK-cells.

It is not clear whether the growth inhibition or tumour regression, documented in a number of patients during interferon treatment, is due to the activation of the NK-cell system, or the result of the direct cytolytic potential of interferons. The observation that human tumours are hardly, if at all, infiltrated by NK-cells has been used as an argument in favour for the latter. However, the findings of NK-cell infiltration in some types of mouse tumours points towards an alternative explanation. If NK-cells act only at the early stage of the disease, they may not be detectable in clinically overt cancers. Although NK-cells may play a role in tumour defence, it remains unresolved whether they can be definitely regarded as the first barrier against tumour growth in man.

Antibody-Dependent Cell-Mediated Cytotoxicity

Apart from the tumour cell lysis mediated by the T-lymphocytes or NK-cells, additional effector mechanisms have been elaborated by which the immune systems may act against tumour cells. It has been demonstrated that certain immune sera in experimental animal tumour systems are capable of mediating the cytotoxicity of lymphoid cells from non-immune syngeneic donors (Pollack et al. 1972; Pollack 1973). Further studies provided evidence that this arming of

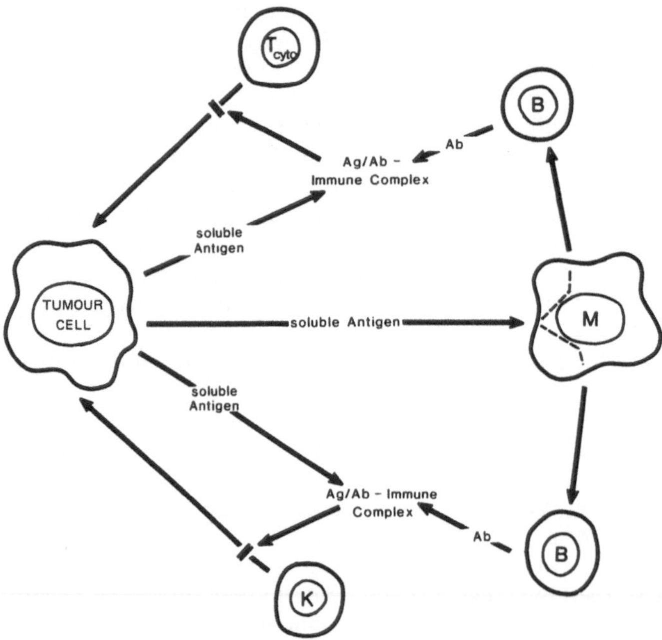

Fig. 3.3. Inhibition of cell-mediated cytotoxicity by antibodies. *B*, B-lymphocyte; *M*, macrophage; *K*, K-cell; T_{cyto}, cytotoxic T-lymphocyte; *Ab*, antibody; *Ag/Ab-Immune Complex*, antigen-antibody immune complex

lymphoid cells may be explained by another cytotoxic phenomenon described as antibody-dependent cell-mediated cytotoxicity (ADCC), which is mediated by a subpopulation of mononuclear cells, referred to as K-cells (MacLennan 1972; Perlmann et al. 1972). The cytotoxic capacity of K-cells depends on the presence of IgG antibodies on the surface of the target cells (Fig. 3.2). The intriguing observation that, in experiments in which the K-cells were removed from the effector cell suspension, both ADCC and spontaneous cell-mediated cytotoxicity were also removed has suggested strong similarities between NK-cells and K-cells. Both cell types have been found to possess common surface markers; they both belong to the large granular lymphocytes, and their activity can be boosted by interferons and inhibited by prostaglandins E1 and E2 (Herberman 1980; Fig. 3.2). Circulating antigen-antibody immune complexes may also prevent K-cells from exerting their activity (Fig. 3.3). Although K-cells may well be involved in host defence mechanisms against tumours (Hahn et al. 1976; Peter et al. 1976), there is no information available on the relevance of this system in vivo. Any participation of K-cells in antitumoural immune reactions would be indicative of tumour-directed IgG antibody formation, implying the expression of antigens on the tumour cell surface which are recognised by the host as 'non-self'. However, such antigens have not yet been detected in spontaneously arising human tumours.

Natural Cytotoxicity of Human Monocytes and Macrophages

The importance of mononuclear phagocytes in antimicrobial host defence and tissue repair is well established. In the past decade evidence has accumulated that cells of the macrophage lineage exhibit additional functional properties, among those being the ability to destroy other cells, in particular tumour cells (Alexander and Evans 1971). It is now generally accepted that the cytolytic potential of macrophages is expressed spontaneously following activation by lymphokines, interferons or lipopolysaccharides, or through specific activation with antibodies, or with a specific macrophage arming factor. Apart from the observation that tumour cell lysis mediated by macrophages may be favoured by intimate cell-to-cell contact, macrophages may also act by releasing soluble factors (e.g. cytotoxic oxidants, proteases, the third component of complement, arginase and interferon) which possess lytic activity (see Fig. 3.1). Several substances, e.g. BCG and *Corynebacterium parvum*, which are used in the treatment of carcinoma of the bladder have been shown to be effective macrophage activators in vivo under certain conditions (Woodruff and Boak 1966). Experiments with the DMBA-12 fibrosarcoma demonstrated that the enhancement of the host resistance obtained by *C. parvum* depends markedly on the timing of the administration of these substances. Furthermore, the efficiency of this system appears to be restricted because spontaneous macrophage-mediated cytotoxicity may only be operative in the earliest phase of tumour growth, whereas immunospecifically armed macrophages may actively interfere with tumour growth in a later phase (Keller 1980). However, this system can be suppressed with a variety of agents, e.g. fetal tissues, resulting in enhanced tumour growth (Keller 1979). Macrophages have been found to suppress immune reactions (Kilburn et al. 1974); they may also inhibit NK-cell activity via the production of prostaglandins (Myatt et al. 1975; Humes et al. 1977).

Although it appears to be difficult to differentiate between the various pathways by which macrophages can interact with tumour cells and other effector cell systems, it is believed that cells of the macrophage lineage, together with NK-cells, may constitute the first barrier against neoplastic growth.

Experimental Evidence for Immunological Interactions in Carcinoma of the Bladder

It is generally accepted that experimental tumours induced by chemical carcinogens express rather weak tumour-associated transplantation antigens which are unique for each individual tumour. In contrast, virally induced tumours have been found to express common transplantation antigens. Since bladder cancer is generally regarded as being induced by chemical carcinogens it can be assumed that this type of tumour will express individual and weak antigens. Despite this presumed limitation human bladder tumours have been used for the investigation of various aspects of tumour immunology.

Bubenik et al. (1970a) demonstrated that leucocytes from bladder cancer patients were capable of killing bladder cancer cells obtained from tissue cultures.

These investigators demonstrated that the same leucocytes were not cytotoxic for target cells derived from other tumours, normal urothelium or fibroblasts, which indicated a specific destruction of bladder cancer cells. In addition, they were able to demonstrate that sera from 8 out of 13 bladder cancer patients exhibited complement-dependent humoral cytotoxicity against bladder carcinoma cells (Bubenik et al. 1970b). This humoral cytotoxicity was not consistently detectable in all samples taken from the same patients within a period of 8 months. Sera from four out of nine patients inhibited the cytotoxicity of leucocytes from bladder cancer patients which was attributed to 'blocking' antibodies (probably IgM). Contrary to the findings with chemically induced experimental tumours, the specific humoral and cellular cytotoxicity of bladder cancer patients was interpreted as an immunological response to the presence of a tumour type-specific transplantation antigen on all of the 11 individual bladder cancer cells tested in this study (Bubenik et al. 1970b).

These findings were subsequently confirmed by other investigators (Bean et al. 1974; Hakala et al. 1974a, b; Troye et al. 1977), except that the cell-mediated reactions were not as tumour specific as suggested by the results of Bubenik et al. (1970b). In the study reported by Bloom et al. (1974), lymphocytes from patients with bladder cancer were more cytotoxic than those from healthy donors, but were not significantly more cytotoxic than lymphocytes from patients with non-maligant disorders of the genitourinary tract. The degree of lymphocyte-mediated cytotoxicity of bladder cancer patients correlated inversely with the stage of the disease, confirming earlier results (O'Toole et al. 1972). Several investigators have found that lymphocytes from healthy donors occasionally exhibited the same degree of cytotoxicity as those from bladder cancer patients. Due to the discrepancies in the literature the reproducibility and comparability of the results obtained by leading research groups were re-evaluated in a workshop. Using the same blood donors and target cells the participating investigators were unable to find clear-cut answers as to whether or not cell-mediated cytotoxicity, as seen in bladder cancer patients, reflects a tumour-specific immune response. However, the pattern of reactivity as determined by the various groups suggested that some disease-related cytotoxicity may exist (Bean et al. 1975). This assumption has not yet been proven. By testing lymphocytes from 2094 cancer patients and healthy controls for their cytotoxicity against 45 target cells lines, including a number of bladder carcinoma cell lines, Takasugi et al. (1973) clearly demonstrated that effector cells from normal donors were as reactive as those from patients with malignant disease, even when the target cells were of the same histological type as the patient's tumour. Lack of tumour specificity was also observed by Catalona et al. (1977) in their study measuring the cytotoxicity of lymphocytes from 25 bladder cancer patients, 19 patients with non-transitional cell carcinoma and 9 patients with benign conditions against the bladder tumour cell line T24. In order to understand the biological meaning of cell-mediated cytotoxicity in carcinoma of the bladder, as determined by a variety of in vitro assays, interest has been focused on the identification and characterisation of the effector cells responsible for the tumour cell killing in vitro.

O'Toole et al. (1974) demonstrated that after removal of a subpopulation of lymphocytes which form spontaneous rosettes with sheep erythrocytes, and which are known to be T-cells, cytotoxicity was exhibited by the non-rosette forming cell fraction. The enrichment of the effector cells obtained by this separation procedure resulted in an enhanced antibody-dependent and independent cell-mediated cytotoxicity. Thus, this experiment gave evidence that cell-mediated tumour cell lysis does not require T-lymphocytes. The fact that allogeneic cultured tumour cells may lack HLA antigens further supports the finding that target cell lysis in vitro is not mediated by T-lymphocytes, as T-cells can act only if they share at least one major histocompatibility determinant with the target cell (Zinkernagel and Doherty 1975).

The observation that sera obtained from patients with transitional cell carcinoma occasionally contained a factor which induced lymphocytes from most donors, with or without bladder carcinoma, to become cytotoxic against bladder carcinoma cells, further indicates that most if not all cell-mediated killing of bladder tumour cells in vitro is of non-T-cell nature (Hakala and Lange 1974). This active serum factor has been identified as an IgG immunoglobulin and induces cytotoxicity only in the presence of K-cells (Hakala et al. 1974b, c).

Using a murine bladder tumour model, Droller and Remington (1975a) provided evidence that macrophages, activated with *Toxoplasma gondii* or *Besnoitia jellisoni*, were able to inhibit tumour cell growth both in vivo and in vitro. These authors reported a significant reduction of adenyl cyclase activity of spleen and peritoneal lymphocytes of chronically *Toxoplasma*-infected animals in which the growth of the isogeneic bladder tumours was inhibited (Droller and Remington 1975b). Apart from K-cells and macrophages, NK-cells have been found to constitute the major cell type responsible for the non-selective in vitro killing of bladder carcinoma cells. It has been demonstrated that natural cytotoxicity can be enhanced in a non-specific manner by various types of interferons and that interferons, although not as effective, may also enhance antibody-dependent K-cell activity (Droller et al. 1979a). By contrast, both antibody-dependent and natural cytotoxicity can be inhibited by exposure of lymphoctyes to prostaglandins E1 and E2 (Droller et al. 1978). These findings appear to be important because human bladder tumour cell lines have been found to produce prostaglandin E2 in tissue culture, which can be inhibited by prostaglandin synthetase inhibitors, e.g. indomethacin. Furthermore, addition of peripheral mononuclear cells from healthy human donors to confluent monolayers of human bladder carcinoma cell lines gave rise to an enhanced prostaglandin production by the tumour cells (Droller et al. 1979b). Identical observations were made using cell lines from carcinogen-induced bladder and mammary tumours in Fisher rats, indicating that prostaglandin E2 production may be a response of bladder carcinoma cells to being attacked by effector cells. It is conceivable that by using this mechanism bladder tumour cells are able to subvert a cell-mediated immune response directed against them (Owen et al. 1980).

Despite the considerable progress which has been made in the past decade in dissecting and analysing the mechanisms by which the immune system may act against bladder cancer, it appears that there are even more questions that remain unanswered. Pertinent problems such as the nature and antigenic properties of the target structures on the tumour cells which enable the different types of effector cells to attack tumour cells are still to be resolved. Even if this can be accomplished, we need to search for ways to manipulate this system so that it may work more efficiently in vivo. Although most of the experimental work contributes little to the management of carcinoma of the bladder, recent attempts have been made to obtain more immunological information in these patients.

Clinical Considerations

Immunological Contributions to Evaluating the Clinical Stage and Prognosis

On the assumption that the immune system of the patient may act against tumours, it has been postulated that lymphocytic and/or plasmacytic infiltration of a bladder carcinoma reflects a tumour-related immune response mounted against it. Several studies have been undertaken to determine the prognostic value of granulomatous reactions and/or lymphocytic infiltration in carcinomas of the bladder based on the observation that the 5-year mortality is lower in seminoma patients with lymphocytic infiltration than in those in whom tumour infiltration with mononuclear cells is absent. Looking at the histological slides of some 400 bladder tumours Mostofi and Sesterhenn (1978) were able to detect lymphocytic and plasmacytic infiltration of varying degrees in 81% of the cases, which is similar to the 73% reported by Sarma (1970). He claimed that the survival time of patients with lymphocytic clusters was longer. In contrast to these findings, Tanaka et al. (1970) reviewed 1000 biopsy specimens from 762 patients with bladder cancer. It was impossible to find any difference in the survival of patients with and without mononuclear cell infiltrations. Although absence of lymphocytic infiltration appeared to be associated with a poorer prognosis in the series of 128 total cystectomy specimens reported by Pomerance (1972), extensive mononuclear cell infiltration did not indicate a more favourable prognosis. Cell-mediated cytotoxicity in bladder cancer patients also does not correlate with lymphocytic tumour infiltrations (Jones and O'Toole 1977). The assumption that mononuclear cell infiltration of bladder tumours indicates a better prognosis is further questioned by experimental observations. Elimination of the intense lymphocytic reactions, which are commonly observed in FANFT-induced mouse bladder tumours (see Chap. 1, p. 13) by immunosuppressive treatment with cyclophosphamide, did not influence the induction time and tumour incidence when compared with animals receiving the carcinogen alone (Soloway et al. 1974). Since the biological meaning of such cellular infiltrates are not yet understood, it is certainly not justified to draw any conclusion with regard to the prognosis from this finding. It may well indicate a favourable immune response (Catalona et al. 1975a), but lymphocytic tumour infiltration may also induce an increased prostaglandin production and secretion. This may in turn inhibit an otherwise efficient antitumoural response, as has already been described (see p. 59). It is also likely that the infiltrating mononuclear cells exhibit suppressor cell activity. Further characterisation of these cells, and of the factors which may lead to the infiltration, are needed before this immunological reaction can be used for the evaluation of bladder carcinomas.

Changes in the histological pattern of regional lymph nodes have been described in bladder cancer patients and correlated with the extent of the disease. A markedly improved 5-year survival has been noted in patients whose regional lymph nodes appeared to be stimulated, as compared with patients with either unstimulated or cell-depleted lymph nodes. Furthermore, lymph node metastases have been found less frequently in patients whose regional lymph nodes have been regarded as stimulated with prominent germinal centres and expansion of the deep cortex (Herr et al. 1976a). Since the status of the regional lymph nodes does not correspond in every case with the outcome of the disease, it is likely that the histological pattern of the lymph node does not entirely reflect the actual state of the immune defence of the patient.

Apart from the evaluation of morphological changes in the regional lymph nodes, various approaches have been used to correlate the stage and prognosis of carcinoma of the bladder with a variety of immune parameters. They fall into three categories:

1. In vivo tests which are designated to evaluate the host immunocompetence
2. In vitro assays which measure the responsiveness of T-cells and B-cells against histoincompatible allogeneic cells and against a variety of mitogens such as phytohaemagglutin and concanavalin A
3. Quantification of the various types of mononuclear cells in peripheral blood

Catalona et al. (1974c), analysing blood samples from 21 patients with bladder carcinoma, found a significant reduction of the T-cell level in these patients as compared with that of 83 healthy control subjects. T-cell deficiency was more pronounced in patients with pathological stage P3 and P4 tumours, but T-cell levels did not differ from those of healthy individuals in stage P1 and P2 lesions. An additional reduction in total lymphocyte counts and T-cells was noted in patients who received radiation therapy for bladder carcinoma (Catalona et al. 1974a; Amin and Lich 1974). Blomgren et al. (1974), however, were unable to demonstrate a decrease in circulating T-cells in bladder cancer patients receiving radiotherapy, although total lymphocyte count decreased significantly. In their study, radiation therapy appeared to reduce both the number and percentage of circulating B-cells.

It has been suggested that the reduction of T-cells in bladder cancer patients may be in part responsible for the impaired proliferative response of lymphocytes to mitogens such as phytohaemagglutinin (PHA) or to allogeneic cells. A significant inhibition of PHA-induced blastogenesis has been observed in bladder cancer patients with pathological stage P3 and P4 tumours. Lymphocyte response to PHA or allogeneic cells in patients with P1 and P2 lesions did not differ from that of healthy subjects (Catalona et al. 1974b). Merrin and Han (1974) were able to detect a reduced lymphocytic reaction in 4 out of 10 patients, all of whom died within 1 year. These hyporesponsive lymphocytes were found to suppress the proliferative response of normal reacting lymphocytes. The suppressive activity may be mediated by monocytes (Herr 1980). Although a diminished blastogenesis to PHA was observed by other investigators, which did not return to normal following cystectomy, impaired lymphocyte response did not correlate with the extent of the disease (McLaughlin et al. 1974). In contrast to these observations, Blomgren et al. (1974) documented an unchanged blastogenesis following PHA-stimulation. Herr et al. (1976b) observed impaired blastogenesis in only 9 out of 55 patients with bladder carcinoma, while lymphocytes of these patients when used as stimulator cells in one-way mixed leucocyte cultures (MLC) exhibited a subnormal stimulator activity in 31 out of 55 cases. Since stimulatory activity returned to normal in 12 out of 15 patients after complete tumour removal, it has been suggested that reduced stimulatory activity may be a sensitive marker for tumour burden in patients with carcinoma of the bladder (Herr et al. 1976b). Significant discrepancies exist as to whether the reduced PHA-induced lymphocyte response in bladder cancer patients is mainly due to an intrinsic defect of the lymphocytes (Catalona et al. 1974b) in addition to suppressor cell activity, or caused by serum factors which may inhibit the mitogen-induced blast transformation (McLaughlin and Brooks 1974). The controversial results obtained in the various studies mentioned above clearly demonstrate that the in vitro responsiveness of peripheral lymphocytes to various mitogens or allogeneic cells appears to be of little help in the clinical evaluation of malignant diseases of the urinary bladder.

More general information on non-tumour-specific host immunocompetence is obtained from in vivo stimulation of bladder cancer patients with a variety of recall antigens—*Candida*, streptokinase-streptodornase, purified protein derivative (PPD) and mumps—and other antigens such as keyhole limpet haemocyanin (KLH) or dinitrochlorobenzene (DNCB). Olson et al. (1972) initially studied the responsiveness of bladder cancer patients to a battery of recall antigens and KLH. Impaired delayed cutaneous hypersensitivity reaction to KLH was observed in 63% of the 35 patients studied in this series. Unreactivity was even more notable in patients with active disease at the time skin testing was performed. This observation has been confirmed by other investigators using DNCB or 2, 4-dinitrofluorobenzene (DNFB). Catalona and Chretien (1973) were able to demonstrate among 25 patients a significant relationship between impaired immunocompetence and the extent of the disease and the histological grade of the malignant lesions. Impaired hypersensitivity reactions have been found in 100% of patients with T3 and T4 Grade 4 tumours, as compared with 33% in T2 tumours and 25% in Grade 2 tumours. A similar correlation between tumour stage and responsiveness to DNCB has been observed by Adolphs and Steffens (1977) and by Brosman et al. (1979). The incidence of impaired hypersensitivity appeared to correlate also with the extent of the disease when streptokinase-streptodornase was used as the antigen. Although negative skin test responses to DNCB returned to normal following therapy of the bladder tumours, this improvement was notably seen in patients with superficial tumours. A significant change has not been observed in patients with stage D disease, in whom the tumour load has been reduced. The value of the DNCB skin test in predicting tumour recurrences following transurethral resection of stage O and A lesions, or following cystectomy for invasive cancer, appears to be limited, since no difference in the incidence of tumour recurrence was detectable in patients with and without positive DNCB skin tests approximately 2 years after therapy. A positive delayed cutaneous hypersensitivity reaction to DNCB does not seem to indicate a better prognosis with regard to the survival of stage B and C tumours, although the chance of surviving the first year following therapy is greater for those patients who respond to DNCB. Differences in the survival of DNCB responders and non-responders among bladder tumour patients have also been reported by Catalona et al. (1975b), but the follow-up was only 1 year.

In view of the results of the various studies presented above, host immunocompetence as measured by skin tests, in particular with DNCB, appears to correlate with the stage of the bladder cancer, but impaired hypersensitivity reactions may well be observed in the presence of low-stage lesions. On the other hand, a positive response to DNCB may occur even in disseminated cancers. Since immunocompetence does not seem to predict reliably the outcome of the disease these skin tests cannot be used for making therapeutic decisions.

Carcinoembryonic Antigen

In 1965, Gold and Freedman described a glycoprotein with a molecular weight of 180 000–200 000 daltons which was isolated from colorectal neoplasms and fetal entodermal tissue. As it was not detectable on normal colon at that time it was regarded as a tumour-specific antigen. The antigenic properties of this material have enabled a variety of sensitive immunological methods to be developed by which concentrations of carcinoembryonic antigen (CEA) and CEA-like substances can be measured in various body fluids. Extensive investigations have shown elevated CEA plasma levels not only in patients with malignant disease of the gastrointestinal tract, but also in patients with a variety of other tumours and even in smokers who were free of malignant disease.

The reported incidence of elevated plasma CEA levels in patients with bladder cancer has varied from 41% to 85%. This wide range of elevated CEA levels in these studies is due to several factors, such as the use of different test kits, which may differ with regard to the specificity of the anti-CEA antibody, the heterogeneity of the patients tested and the different upper limits of normal. There is agreement that plasma CEA is elevated particularly in patients with advanced tumours, and it is therefore not useful as a screening test for early detection of bladder tumours. In most cases with low-stage bladder tumours CEA plasma concentrations are only slightly elevated, which may also be seen in smokers and patients with inflammatory disease of the gastrointestinal tract. Considering the many factors which give false negative and false positive results, the determination of plasma CEA levels appears to be of little value in the diagnosis and follow-up of bladder tumours (Fraser et al. 1975).

Elevated urinary CEA (U-CEA) levels have been found in 40%–100% of tumour-free patients with urinary tract infection (Guinan et al. 1975; Zimmermann et al. 1976; Turner et al. 1977). This interference has to be taken into consideration when U-CEA is used in the evaluation and follow-up of transitional cell carcinomas. Several studies have shown that the incidence of elevated U-CEA levels increases with the extent of the disease (Zimmermann et al. 1976; Fleischer et al. 1977; Wahren et al. 1982), but there is no difference according to the grade of the tumour (Hering et al. 1976; Wahren et al. 1982). No correlation appears to exist between plasma and U-CEA levels, and therefore renal filtration cannot account for the CEA in the urine of bladder cancer patients (Guinan et al. 1974). Since no substances which possibly cross-react with CEA have been discovered in bacterial cultures from patients with urinary infections, it can be assumed that U-CEA is shed from the urothelium into the urine (Wahren et al. 1982).

Wahren et al. (1982) investigated 425 patients who were free of urinary infection and were able to demonstrate that patients with U-CEA levels less than 30 μg/ml prior to therapy had a significantly better survival than those with levels of more than 30 μg/ml. Patients with T3 and T4 tumours with decreasing U-CEA levels had a significantly better symptom-free survival than those with increasing levels following therapy: 201 patients were followed up for more than 1 year after radiotherapy and those with initial U-CEA levels less than 50 μg/ml remained tumour-free significantly more often than those whose pre-treatment levels were above 50 μg/ml. Urinary CEA appears to be an independent prognostic factor, as patients with initial low U-CEA levels had a better survival than those with high U-CEA, regardless of the stage and grade of the disease. It may therefore be a suitable test for selecting high-risk patients. Patients with ileal or colonic urinary diversions after cystectomy may have high levels of U-CEA in the absence of tumour recurrence or metastases, and it is therefore not a reliable test in these circumstances (Klippel et al. 1983).

Clinical Significance of ABO(H) Isoantigens

In 1968, Kovarik et al. reported on the ubiquitous expression of blood group isoantigens (BGIs) on human endothelial and epithelial tissues, which were frequently not detectable on the corresponding carcinomas. In addition to the expression of new antigens on malignant cells (which remains to be proven for spontaneously arising human neoplasms) and the re-expression of fetal antigens, the loss of BGIs represents another alteration of the tumour cell membrane. These isoantigens can be detected on fixed or frozen tissue sections with the specific red cell adherence test (SRCAT; see also Chap. 2, p. 45) or with the more practical and reliable immunoperoxidase staining technique (Hsu et al. 1981, see Fig. 3.4).

Davidsohn et al. (1973) observed the loss of BGIs in the majority of high-grade bladder tumours and concluded that the SRCAT may be of additional help in the histological grading of bladder tumours. Decenzo et al. (1975) however, noted that the results of the SRCAT did not necessarily correlate with the grade of

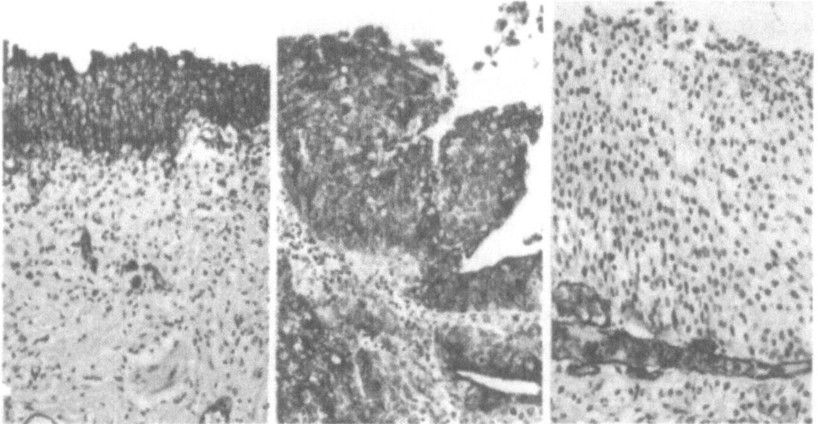

Fig. 3.4. *Left*: Normal urothelium—antigen-positive immunoperoxidase staining. *Centre*: Transitional cell carcinoma Grade 2—antigen-positive immunoperoxidase staining. *Right*: Transitional cell carcinoma Grade 2 without expression of BGIs. *Note*: antigen presence in normal endothelium in the lamina propria. H&E, blood group A, ×100

tumour, as lack of isoantigenicity was observed in 4 low-grade tumours out of 22 patients studied. This observation was later confirmed (Newman et al. 1980; D'Elia et al. 1982; Jakse and Hofstädter 1983). Decenzo et al. (1975) were able to compare the results of the initial SRCAT with the eventual outcome of the disease by following those patients with stage A disease for an average of 7 years (range 1–14 years). Seven out of nine patients with a negative SRCAT developed invasive cancer within a period of 3–14 years, regardless of the histological grade of the initial tumour. Another patient with an SRCAT-negative Grade 3 tumour died of metastatic disease within 1 year of treatment. None of the 13 patients whose initial tumours were positive developed invasive cancer, although there were recurrences in 11 of these patients. The impression of this study was that the alteration in A, B, O-antigenicity of bladder tumours may be a prognostic factor indicating the aggressiveness of the tumour that is not otherwise detectable. This has subsequently been confirmed. Lange et al. (1978) were able to predict invasive tumour growth in 81% of 37 patients with low-stage bladder tumours, and Newman et al. (1980) found invasive tumour growth in 88% of patients with isoantigen deletion in their initial tumours.

Although the loss of BGIs has been considered as a pre-existing event in the course of cellular de-differentiation (Decenzo et al. 1975) there are two reasons why this may not always be the case. Not all patients with initial SRCAT- negative superficial bladder tumours will develop invasive recurrence, and Jakse and Hofstädter (1983) were able to demonstrate that carcinoma in situ and urothelial dysplasia are significantly more often associated with antigen-negative superficial tumours than with antigen-positive lesions. Since preneoplastic alterations of the urothelium and carcinoma in situ have been found to be associated with a poor prognosis, the likelihood of subsequent invasive tumour growth indicated by the antigen deletion may at least in part be due to unrecognised dysplasia or carcinoma in situ elsewhere in the bladder. This assumption may also account for the observation of changes in the SRCAT from positive to negative in sequential tumours in three patients who later developed invasive tumours (D'Elia et al. 1982). It would appear reasonable from this assumption that random biopsies of the bladder mucosa should be taken more frequently from those patients with initial antigen-negative low-stage tumours.

Although a lack of BGIs on low-stage bladder tumours seems to predict a poor prognosis and the presence of these antigens indicate a low risk of developing invasion, it is certainly not justified at this time to argue for or against more agressive treatment of low-stage bladder tumours on the basis of the ABO-antigenicity of the initial lesion. Further investigations are needed to explain why some antigen-negative tumours will not recur with invasive growth, whereas the majority of these tumours will. The higher rate of antigen-negative tumours among patients with blood group O appears to be another problem (Weinstein et al. 1981). Askari et al. (1981) detected antigen-negative tumours in 91% of patients with blood group O. The weak antigenicity of the H-antigen in these patients and the use of the Ulex Europeus preparation, which has been mostly applied in the SRCAT for the H-antigen, contribute considerably to the high rate of false negative results. Evidence has recently been provided that the refinement of the methodology, as with the immunoperoxidase techniques and probably with the use of anti-H-antibody from patients with Bombay blood (a rare blood type without A, B or H antigens), will improve the reliability of this test among blood group O patients.

Immunotherapy of Bladder Tumours

The treatment of metastatic bladder cancer, the limited efficacy of cystectomy in locally advanced tumours and the high rate of recurrences in superficial papillary bladder tumours must be regarded as the major problems in the management of carcinoma of the bladder. In the search for new therapeutic modalities interest has focused on various forms of immunotherapy, particularly in preventing recurrent disease in low-stage bladder tumours.

The work by Zbar et al. (1971) has provided evidence that non-tumour-specific stimulation of the immune system can effectively suppress tumour growth. In their experiments BCG was injected into tumour nodules 7 days following subcutaneous inoculation of 10^6 cells of a carcinogen-induced hepatoma into guinea pigs. This resulted in a 60% survival of the animals, while all untreated controls died within 60–80 days. They were also able to demonstrate regression of metastatic lesions in some instances. Although the mode of action of BCG is still not completely understood, its therapeutic effect is attributed to a stimulation of the immune system, in particular of macrophages, and does not seem to be due to the toxicity of BCG.

The first clinical trial designed to evaluate the effectiveness of active non-tumour-specific immunostimulation in carcinoma of the bladder was performed by Olson et al. (1974). Nine patients were treated subcutaneously with the immunogen keyhole limpet haemocyanin following transurethral resection of papillary bladder tumours of stage O-B1. This resulted in a significant reduction of tumour recurrences, as compared with an unstimulated group of 10 patients. The 9 patients had 1 recurrence in 204 patient-months, while 7 of the 10 untreated patients developed 7 recurrences within 228 patient-months of follow-up. These promising observations were then confirmed in a small prospective randomised trial (Klippel 1982).

BCG Therapy

Morales and associates (1976) initially reported on their experience with BCG as a non-specific stimulant in Ta and T1 bladder tumours. In their study BCG was given intradermally at a dosage of 5 mg and intravesically at a dosage of 120 mg at weekly intervals for 6 weeks. The 9 patients who received the regimen had had a total of 22 recurrences within 77 patient-months before treatment, while only 1 recurrence developed within 41 patient-months following immunostimulation. Although this difference did not show statistical significance because of the disparity in the observation time, a significantly reduced recurrence rate following BCG therapy could be demonstrated in a later study in which 16 patients had 53 recurrences within 163 patient-months prior to therapy. Following immunostimulation with BCG, only 7 recurrences were noted within 222 patient-months (Morales 1978). In a prospective randomised trial using the same regimen, Lamm et al. (1981) were able to confirm essentially the results reported by Morales (1978). In this study, 28 patients who received BCG following transurethral resection developed 6 recurrences within a 12-month period of observation, while 13 recurrences were seen in 26 patients not treated with adjuvant immunotherapy.

In a prospective, randomised study Brosman (1982), using the Tice strain of BCG, did not observe tumour recurrence in the BCG-treated group of 27 patients, as compared with 9 recurrences in the group of 22 patients who were treated with thiotepa. In addition, 12 patients who had previously not responded to treatment with thiotepa were treated with BCG and did not develop tumour recurrence within the minimal observation period of 24 months. The combination of cyclophosphamide and BCG (Adolphs and Bastian 1983) also seems to be effective in reducing the recurrence rate in patients with superficial bladder tumours, but this was not a randomised trial so it is not possible to draw conclusions about the synergistic effect of these two treatments.

Despite the encouraging results which were demonstrable using immunotherapy with BCG, it is unfortunately associated with a high incidence of side effects. Although transitory symptoms such as bladder irritability, low-grade fever and malaise were commonly noted in most studies (Morales 1978; Lamm et al. 1981), severe systemic side effects with arthralgia, prolonged episodes of fever, chills, anorexia and severe bladder irritability were also reported (Brosman 1982). Some of these patients required hospitalisation and isoniazide or triple drug treatment, which resulted in amelioration of the symptoms. Treatment with a reduced BCG dosage of 60 or 120 mg, administered by one or two intravesical instillations, caused less side effects, but was not effective in controlling the recurrence of papillary bladder tumours following transurethral resection (Flamm and Grof, 1981).

Apart from the dosage, the mode of administration of BCG appears to be another important factor which determines the effect of adjuvant immunotherapy. Martinez-Piñeiro and Muntañola (1977) were unable to detect tumour regression in three patients in whom BCG was given intradermally, while partial tumour regression was observed in two patients after intralesional BCG administration. Tumour regression in four out of six patients following intralesional BCG injection was also observed by Douville et al. (1978). However, tumour regression may also be achieved by intravesical instillation of BCG, as observed in 59% of 17 patients with incompletely resected superficial tumours (Morales et al. 1981).

Intracavitary BCG instillation has yielded promising results in five out of seven patients with carcinoma in situ of the urinary bladder. Using the regimen described on p. 68 (Morales et al. 1976), patients with carcinoma in situ remained free of tumour with follow-up periods ranging from 12 to 33 months. Complete resolution of carcinoma in situ was also observed in 65% of 17 patients treated by Herr et al. (1982), and in five out of seven patients reported by Brosman (1982). In contrast to the promising results obtained with BCG in preventing recurrent disease in superficial bladder cancer including carcinoma in situ, objective responses in patients with metastatic disease appear to occur rarely, if at all (Morales and Ersil 1979).

Several other agents, which are thought to stimulate the immune system in a non-specific manner, have been used in the treatment of bladder cancer patients. Levamisole has been shown to be ineffective even in controlling minimal residual disease in patients with superficial bladder tumours (Smith et al. 1978). Disappointing results have also been obtained in a prospective randomised trial with transfer factor (Tarkkanen et al. 1981). Miller and Hollinshead (1980) reported on attempts to treat three patients who had superficial bladder tumours with active specific immunotherapy. The antigen preparation, which was administered three times with complete Freund's adjuvant at monthly intervals, was isolated from a bladder tumour specimen and chemically characterised as a polypeptide with a molecular weight of 40 000 daltons. Although all three patients showed beneficial alterations of their recurrence pattern within a follow-up period of 18 months, further clinical evaluation of this therapeutic modality is needed.

Human Leucocyte Interferon

A limited number of patients with carcinoma of the bladder have been treated with human leucocyte interferon (IFN-α). The rationale for this type of treatment is based on the observation that various types of human interferon possess direct cytotoxic potentials against a variety of human tumour cells. The cytotoxic activity of human fibroblast interferons (IFN-α) against T24 bladder tumour cells is shown in Fig. 3.5, and demonstrates a significant growth inhibition of these cells in the presence of 100 and 1000 IU IFN-α/ml culture medium, as compared with the growth of untreated T24 cells. Furthermore, interferons may act against tumour cells by augmentation of the activity of NK-cells, although the definite pathways by which interferons may exert their antiproliferative potential remains unclear.

Christophersen and associates (1978) reported on their initial experience with IFN-α in the treatment of superficial papillary bladder tumours. Two of three patients received a total of 1.1×10^{10} IU IFN-α within a period of 7 months, whereas a total of 4.6×10^{9} IU were given to the remaining patients within 18 months. Tumours with a diameter less than 1 cm completely regressed, while lesions with a diameter of more than 1 cm remained stable. Ikĭc et al. (1981) have treated eight patients with superficial papillary bladder tumours. Unpurified IFN-α was injected intralesionally through a cystoscope. Four of these eight patients received additional IFN-α by daily intramuscular injection. A total dosage of IFN-α ranging from 4.2×10^{7} to 1.2×10^{8} IU was given systemically. All

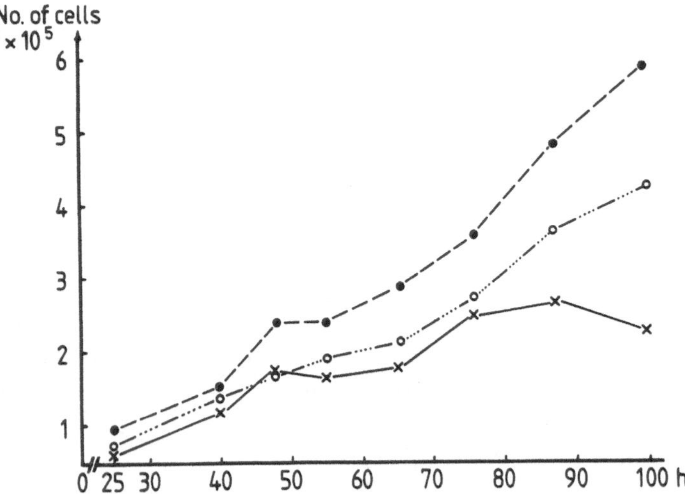

Fig. 3.5. Inhibition of growth of T24 cell cultures with IFN-β. ×——×, 1000 IU IFN-β/ml culture medium; ○——○, 100 IU IFN-β/ml culture medium; ●——●, untreated T24 cells

tumours treated with intralesional injections regressed within 3 months. Untreatable tumour recurrence was noted in one of these patients at 4 months. Complete tumour regression was observed in two out of four patients who received IFN-α both intralesionally and systemically. Tumours of the remaining two patients showed partial regression facilitating complete transurethral resection. Although the promising observations may be due to the effect of IFN-α, it is also conceivable that toxic material other than IFN-α contained in the crude preparation may be responsible. It remains to be shown whether or not additional systemic IFN-treatment is needed apart from the intralesional administration. Complete regression of tumours in two patients following intravenous administration of a total of 1.89×10^8 IU IFN-α indicates that systemic treatment may be as effective as local IFN administration (Hill et al. 1981). This however, may not always be the case, as complete tumour regression was noted in only one out of five patients, with a partial response in another patient, following systemic IFN-treatment with a total of 9×10^7 IU IFN-α (Scorticatti et al. 1981).

In this context it may be of interest that systemic treatment with in vivo- induced IFN, obtained by treatment with poly I:C, which are known to be interferon inducers, did not result in a significant decrease of recurrences in 14 patients with carcinoma in situ or stage O Grade I or II tumours, as compared with 12 untreated patients. A significant increase in survival rate, however, was observed: four patients of the control group died within 76 months, while all poly I:C-treated patients were still alive after 170 months (Kemeny et al. 1981).

Conclusion

It is obvious from this overview on immunotherapy of bladder cancer that metastatic disease continues to present a major problem. Non-specific immunostimulation, in particular with BCG administered intravesically, is effective in preventing local recurrence after transurethral resection of superficial bladder tumours, and BCG instillation may be an alternative approach in the management of carcinoma in situ of the urinary bladder. Although it remains unclear as to whether BCG may act in a non-specific manner by inducing an inflammatory response, or gives rise to an efficient tumour-specific immune response, BCG instillation can be recommended as adjuvant therapy in patients with recurrent superficial bladder tumours. In spite of some promising results obtained with interferons, further experimental and clinical studies are definitely needed before IFN can be regarded as an alternative therapeutic modality for carcinoma of the bladder. Since large amounts of recombinant interferons are now available, further evaluation of interferons can be expected in the near future.

References

Adolphs HD, Bastian HP (1983) Chemoimmune prophylaxis in superficial bladder cancer. J Urol 129: 29–32

Adolphs HD, Steffens L (1977) Correlation between tumour stage, tumour grade and immunocompetence in patients with carcinoma of the bladder and prostate. Eur Urol 3: 23–25

Alexander P, Evans R (1971) Endotoxin and double stranded RNA render macrophages cytotoxic. Nature 232: 76–78

Allison AC, Taylor RB (1967) Observations on thymectomy and carcinogenesis. Cancer Res 27: 703–707

Amin M, Lich R Jr (1974) Lymphocytes and bladder cancer. J Urol 111: 165–169

Askari A, Colmenares E, Saberi A, Jarman WD (1981) Red cell surface antigen and its relationship to survival of patients with transitional cell carcinoma of the bladder. J Urol 125: 182–184

Baldwin RW (1966) Tumour-specific immunity against spontaneous rat tumours. Int J Cancer 1: 257–264

Baldwin RW, Embleton MJ, Jones JSP, Langman MJS (1973) Cell-mediated and humoral immune reactions to human tumours. Int J Cancer 12: 73–83

Balner H, Dersjant H (1969) Increased oncogenic effect of methylcholanthrene after treatment with anti-lymphocyte serum. Nature 224: 376–378

Bean M, Pees H, Fogh JE, Grabstald H, Oettgen HF (1974) Cytotoxicity of lymphocytes from patients with cancer of the urinary bladder: detection by a ^{3}H-proline microcytotoxicity test. Int J Cancer 14: 186–197

Bean MA, Bloom BR, Herberman RB, Old LJ, Oettgen HF, Klein G, Terry WD (1975) Cell-mediated cytotoxicity of bladder carcinoma: evaluation of a workshop. Cancer Res 35: 2902–2913

Blomgren H, Wasserman J, Littbrand B (1974) Blood lymphocytes after radiation therapy of carcinoma of prostate and urinary bladder. Acta Radiol [Ther] (Stockh) 13: 357–367

Bloom ET, Ossorio RC, Brosman SA (1974) Cell-mediated cytotoxicity against human bladder cancer. Int J Cancer 14: 326–334

Brosman SA (1982) Experience with bacillus Calmette-Guérin in patients with superficial bladder carcinoma. J Urol 128: 27–30

Brosman SA, Elhilali M, Vescera C, Fahey J (1979) Immune response in bladder cancer patients. J Urol 121: 162–169

Bubenik J, Perlmann P, Helmstein K, Moberger G (1970a) Immune response to urinary bladder tumours in man. Int J Cancer 5: 39–46

Bubenik J, Perlmann P, Helmstein K, Moberger G (1970b) Cellular and humoral immune responses to human urinary bladder carcinomas. Int J Cancer 5: 310–319

Bubenik J, Jakoubkova J, Krakora P, Baresowa M, Helbich P, Viklicky V, Malaskova V (1971) Cellular immunity to renal carcinomas in man. Int J Cancer 8: 503–513

Burnet FM (1971) Immunological surveillance in neoplasia. Transplant Rev 7: 3–25

Castro JE (1978) Immunological aspects of cancer. MTP Press, Lancaster, p 212

Catalona WJ, Chretien PB (1973) Correlation among host immunocompetence and tumor stage, tumor grade and vascular permeation in transitional carcinoma. J Urol 110: 526–528

Catalona WJ, Potvin C, Chretien PB (1974a) Effect of radiation therapy for urologic cancer on circulating thymus-derived lymphocytes. J Urol 112: 261–267

Catalona WJ, Tarpley JL, Chretien PB, Castle JR (1974b) Lymphocyte stimulation in urologic cancer patients. J Urol 112: 373–377

Catalona WJ, Potvin C, Chretien PB (1974c) T-lymphocytes in bladder and prostatic cancer patients. J Urol 112: 378–382

Catalona WJ, Mann R, Nime F, Potvin C, Harty JI, Gomolka D, Eggleston JC (1975a) Identification of complement-receptor lymphocytes (B-cells) in lymph nodes and tumor infiltrates. J Urol 114: 915–921

Catalona WJ, Smolev JK, Harty JI (1975b) Prognostic value of host immunocompetence in urologic cancer patients. J Urol 114: 922–926

Catalona WJ, Oldham RK, Herberman RB, Dieu JY, Cannon GB (1977) Lack of specificity of lymphocyte-mediated cytotoxicity against the bladder cancer cell line T 24. J Urol 118: 254–257

Cerilli GJ, Treat RCH (1969) The effect of antilymphocyte serum on the induction and growth of tumour in the adult mouse. Transplantation 8: 774–781

Cheever MA, Greenberg PD, Fefer A (1980) Therapy of leukemia by nonimmune syngeneic spleen cells. J Immunol 124: 2137–2142

Christophersen IS, Jondal R, Osther K, Lindenberg J, Pedersen PH, Berg K (1978) Interferon therapy in neoplastic disease. Acta Med Scand 204: 471–476

Davidsohn I, Stejskal R, Lill P (1973) The loss of isoantigens A, B and H in carcinoma of the urinary bladder. Lab Invest 28: 382

Decenzo JM, Howard P, Irish CE (1975) Antigenic deletion and prognosis of patients with stage A transitional cell bladder carcinoma. J Urol 114: 874–878

D'Elia FL, Cooper HS, Mulholland SG (1982) ABH isoantigens in stage O papillary transitional cell carcinoma of the bladder: correlation with the biological behavior. J Urol 127: 665–667

Disala PJ, Rutledge FN, Smith JP, Sinkovics JG (1971) Cell-mediated immune reaction to two gynecologic malignant tumors. Cancer 28: 1129–1137

Douville Y, Pelouze G, Roy R, Charrois R, Kibrite A, Martin M, Dionne L, Coulonval L, Robinson J (1978) Recurrent bladder papillomata treated with bacillus Calmette-Guérin: A preliminary report (phase 1 trial). Cancer Treat Rep 62: 551–552

Droller MJ, Remington JS (1975a) A role for the macrophage in in vivo and in vitro resistance to murine bladder tumor cell growth. Cancer Res 35: 49–53

Droller MJ, Remington JS (1975b) Lymphocyte and macrophage adenyl cyclase activity in animals with enhanced cell-mediated resistance to infection and tumors. Cell Immunol 19: 349–355

Droller MJ, Schneider MU, Perlmann P (1978) A possible role of prostaglandins in the inhibition of natural and antibody-dependent cell-mediated cytotoxicity against tumor cells. Cell Immunol 39: 165–177

Droller MJ, Borg H, Perlmann P (1979a) In vitro enhancement of natural and antibody-dependent lymphocyte-mediated cytotoxicity against tumor target cells by interferon. Cell Immunol 47: 248–260

Droller MJ, Lindgren JA, Claessen HE, Perlmann P (1979b) Production of prostaglandin E_2 by bladder tumor cells in tissue culture and a possible mechanism of lymphocyte inhibition. Cell Immunol 47: 261–273

Durdik JM, Beck BN, Henney CS (1980) The use of lymphoma cell variants differing in their susceptibility to NK-cell mediated lysis to analyse NK-cell–target cell interactions. In: Herberman RB (ed) Natural cell-mediated immunity against tumors. Academic, New York, pp 805–817

Ehrlich P (1909) Über den jetzigen Stand der Karzinomforschung. Ned Tijdschr Geneeskd 35: 273–290

Eremin O (1980) NK-cell activity in the blood, tumor-draining lymph nodes and primary tumors of women with mammary carcinoma. In: Herberman RB (ed) Natural cell-mediated immunity against tumors. Academic, New York, pp 1011–1029

Flamm J, Grof F (1981) Adjuvant local immunotherapy with bacillus Calmette-Guérin (BCG) in treatment of urothelial carcinoma of the urinary bladder. Wien Med Wochenschr 131: 501–506

Fleischer M, Grabstald H, Whitmore WF, Pinsky CM, Oettgen HF, Schwartz MK (1977) The clinical utility of plasma and urinary carcinoembryonic antigen in patients with genitourinary disease. J Urol 117: 635–637

Foley EJ (1953) Antigenic properties of methylcholanthrene induced tumors in mice of the strain of origin. Cancer Res 13: 835–837

Fraser RA, Ravry MJ, Segura JW, Go VLW (1975) Clinical evaluation of urinary and serum carcinoembryonic antigen in bladder cancer. J Urol 114: 226–229

Gold P, Freedman SO (1965) Demonstration of tumorspecific antigens in human colonic carcinomata by immunological tolerance and absorption techniques. J Exp Med 121: 439–462

Gross L (1943) Intradermal immunization of C3 H mice against a sarcoma that originated in an animal of the same line. Cancer Res 3: 326–333

Guinan P, Ablin RJ, Sadoughi N, Bush I (1974) Carcinoembryonic-like antigen in the urine of patients with carcinoma of the bladder and normal controls. J Surg Oncol 6: 127–131

Guinan P, Dubin A, Bush I, Alsheik H, Ablin RJ (1975) The CEA test in urologic cancer: an evaluation and a review. Oncology 32: 158–168

Hahn WV, Hatlen LE, Kagnoff MF (1976) Antibody-dependent cell-mediated cytotoxicity of human colon cancer. (Abstract). Gastroenterology 70: 892

Hakala TR, Lange PH (1974) Serum induced lymphoid cell mediated cytotoxicity to human transitional cell carcinomas of the genitourinary tract. Science 184: 795–797

Hakala TR, Lange PH, Castro A, Elliott A, Fraley EE (1974a) Cell-mediated cytotoxicity against human transitional cell carcinomas of the genitourinary tract. Cancer 34: 1929–1934

Hakala TR, Castro AE, Elliott AY, Fraley EE (1974b) Humoral cytotoxicity in human transitional cell carcinoma. J Urol 111: 382–385

Hakala TR, Lange PH, Castro AE, Elliott AY, Fraley EE (1974c) Antibody induction of lymphocyte-mediated cytotoxicity against human transitional cell carcinomas of the urinary tract. N Engl J Med 291: 637–641

Hakala TR, Lange PH, Castro AE, Elliott AY, Fraley EE (1975) Lymphocyte antibody interaction in cytotoxicity against human transitional cell carcinoma. J Urol 113: 663–667

Haller O, Hanson M, Kiessling R, Wigzell H (1977) Role of non-conventional natural killer cells in resistance against syngeneic tumor cells in vivo. Nature 270: 609–611

Hayakawa M, Schmitz-Dräger BJ, Ackermann R (1984) Studies on human natural killer (NK-cell) activity against cell lines derived from malignant urinary tract tumors. Part I: Effects of human interferon-β on augmentation of NK-cell activity and its mechanism. Jpn J Urol 75: 32–41

Hellström I, Hellström KE, Pierce GE, Yang JPS (1968) Cellular and humoral immunity to different types of human neoplasms. Nature 220: 1353–1354

Hellström I, Hellström KE, Sjörgen HO, Warner GA (1971) Demonstration of cell-mediated immunity to human neoplasms of various histologic types. Int J Cancer 7: 1–16

Herberman RB (1980) Natural cell-mediated immunity against tumors. Academic, New York, p 392

Hering H, Hering FJ, Weidner W (1976) Die Bedeutung des carcinoembryonalen Antigens (CEA) im Urin und Plasma bei Patienten mit Karzinomen der Harnblase. Med Welt 27: 920–922

Herr HW (1980) Suppressor cells in immunodepressed bladder and prostate cancer patients. J Urol 123: 635–639

Herr HW, Bean MA, Whitmore WF (1976a) Prognostic significance of regional lymph node histology in cancer of the bladder. J Urol 115: 264–267

Herr HW, Bean MA, Whitmore WF (1976b) Decreased ability of blood leukocytes from patients with tumors of the urinary bladder to act as stimulator cells in mixed leukocyte culture. Cancer Res 36: 2754–2760

Herr HW, Pinsky CM, Whitmore WF, Oettgen HF, Melamed MR (1982) Effect of intravesical bacillus Calmette-Guérin (BCG) on carcinoma in situ of the bladder. Cancer 51: 1323–1326

Hewitt HB, Blake ER, Walder AS (1976) A critique of the evidence for active host defence against cancer based on personal studies of 27 murine tumours of spontaneous origin. Br J Cancer 33: 241–259

Hill NO, Pardue A, Khan A, Aleman C, Dorn G, Hill JM (1981) Phase-I human leukocyte interferon trials in leukemia and cancer. J Clin Hematol Oncol 11: 23–35

Hoover R, Fraumeni JF (1973) Risk of cancer in renal-transplant recipients. Lancet II: 55–57

Hsu SM, Raine L, Fanger H (1981) The use of avidin-biotin peroxidase complex (ABC) in immunoperoxidase techniques. A comparison between ABC and unlabeled antibody (PAP) procedures. J Histochem 29: 577–580

Humes JL, Bonney RJ, Pelus L, Dahlgreen ME, Sadowski SJ, Kuehl FA, Davis P (1977) Macrophages synthesise and release prostaglandins in response to inflammatory stimuli. Nature 269: 149–151

Ikïk D, Maričič Z, Oresič V, Rode B, Nola P, Smudj K, Kneževič M, Jušič D, Sooš Ě (1981) Application of human leucocyte interferon in patients with urinary bladder papillomatosis, breast cancer and melanoma. Lancet I: 1022–1024

Jakse G, Hofstädter F (1983) Investigation of ABH antigenicity of random mucosal biopsies and transitional cell carcinoma of the urinary bladder. Eur Urol 9: 97–101

Jondal M, Svedmyr E, Klein E, Singh S (1975) Killer T-cells in a Burkitt's lymphoma biopsy. Nature 255: 405–407

Jones LW, O'Toole C (1977) Lymphocyte response to transitional cell carcinoma peripheral cytotoxicity and local tumour infiltration. J Urol 118: 974–977

Kasai M, Leclerc JC, McVay-Boudreau L, Shen FW, Cantor H (1979) Direct evidence that natural killer cells in nonimmune spleen cell populations prevent tumor growth in vivo. J Exp Med 149: 1260–1264

Keller R (1979) Competition between foetal tissue and macrophage-dependent natural tumour resistance. Br J Cancer 40: 417–423

Keller R (1980) Regulatory capacities of mononuclear phagocytes with particular reference to natural immunity against tumors. In: Herberman RB (ed) Natural cell-mediated immunity against tumors. Academic, New York, pp 1219–1269

Kemeny N, Yagoda A, Wang Y, Field K, Wrobleski H, Whitmore W (1981) Randomized trial of standard therapy with or without poly I:C in patients with superficial bladder cancer. Cancer 48: 2154–2157

Kilburn DG, Smith JB, Gorczynksi RM (1974) Nonspecific suppression of T-lymphocyte responses in mice carrying progressively growing tumors. Eur J Immunol 4: 784–788

Klein G (1980) Tumor immunology. In: Fougereau M, Dausset J (eds) Immunology 80. Academic, New York, pp 680–687

Klippel KF (1982) Tumorimmunologie. In: Hohenfellner R, Zingg EJ (eds) Urologie in Klinik und Praxis. Thieme, Stuttgart, p 477

Klippel KF, Ax D, Schärfe T, Preiss J, Alves De Oliveira CR (1983) Intestinal urinary diversion raises CEA-values. Onkologie 6: 126–131

Kovarik S, Davidsohn I, Stejskal R (1968) ABO-antigens in cancer. Detection with the mixed cell agglutination reaction. Arch Pathol 86: 12–16

Krüger GR, Malmgren RA, Berard CW (1971) Malignant lymphomas and plasmacytosis in mice under prolonged immunosuppression and persistent antigenic stimulation. Transplantation 11: 138–144

Lamm DL, Thor DE, Winters WD, Stogdill VD, Radwin HM (1981) BCG immunotherapy of bladder cancer: inhibition of recurrence and associated immune responses. Cancer 48: 82–88
Lange PH, Limas C, Fraley EE (1978) Tissue blood-group antigens and prognosis in low stage transitional cell carcinoma of the bladder. J Urol 119: 52–55
MacLennan ICM (1972) Antibody in the induction and inhibition of lymphocyte reactivity. Transplant Rev 13: 67–90
Martinez-Piñeiro JA, Muntañola P (1977) Nonspecific immunotherapy with BCG vaccine in bladder tumours. Eur Urol 3: 11–22
McLaughlin AP, Brooks JD (1974) A plasma factor inhibiting lymphocyte reactivity in urologic cancer patients. J Urol 112: 366–372
McLaughlin AP, Kessler WO, Triman K, Gittes RF (1974) Immunologic competence in patients with urologic cancer. J Urol 111: 233–237
Merrin C, Han T (1974) Immune response in bladder cancer. J Urol 111: 170–172
Miller HC, Hollinshead AC (1980) Specific active immunotherapy of bladder cancer. Abstracts of the 75th Annual Meeting of the American Urological Association, San Francisco, Calif, 1980. No 127, p 106. Obtainable from Williams & Wilkins, Baltimore
Morales A (1978) Adjuvant immunotherapy in superficial bladder cancer. Natl Cancer Inst Monogr 49: 315–319
Morales A, Ersil A (1979) Prophylaxis of recurrent bladder cancer with bacillus Calmette-Guérin. In: Johnson DE, Samuels ML (eds) Cancer of the genito-urinary tract. Raven, New York, p 131
Morales A, Eidinger D, Bruce AW (1976) Intracavitary bacillus Calmette-Guérin in the treatment of superficial bladder tumors. J Urol 116: 180–183
Morales A, Ottenhof P, Emerson L (1981) Treatment of residual non-infiltrating bladder cancer with bacillus Calmette-Guérin. J Urol 125: 649–651
Mostofi FK, Sesterhenn I (1978) Lymphocytic infiltration in relationship to urologic tumors. Natl Cancer Inst Monogr 49: 133–141
Myatt L, Bray MA, Gordon D, Morley J (1975) Macrophages on intrauterine contraceptive devices produce prostaglandin. Nature 257: 227–228
Newman AJ, Carlton CE, Johnson S (1980) Cell surface A, B or O (H) blood group antigens as an indicator of malignant potential in stage A bladder carcinoma. J Urol 124: 27–29
Okabe T, Ackermann R, Wirth M, Frohmüller HGW (1979) Cell-mediated cytotoxicity in patients with cancer of the prostate. J Urol 122: 628–632
Olson, CA, Rao CN, Menzoian JO, Byrd WE (1972) Immunologic unreactivity in bladder cancer patients. J Urol 107: 607–609
Olson CA, Chute R, Rao CN (1974) Immunologic reduction of bladder cancer recurrence rate. J Urol 111: 173–176
O'Toole C, Perlmann P, Unsgaard B, Moberger G, Edsmyr F (1972) Cellular immunity to human urinary bladder carcinoma. I. Correlation to clinical stage and radiotherapy. Int J Cancer 10: 77–91
O'Toole C, Stejskal V, Perlmann P, Karlsson M (1974) Lymphoid cells mediating tumor-specific cytotoxicity to carcinoma of the urinary bladder. J Exp Med 139: 457–466
Owen K, Gomolka D, Droller MJ (1980) Production of prostaglandin E_2 by tumor cells in vitro. Cancer Res 40: 3167–3171
Perlmann P, Perlmann H, Wigzell H (1972) Lymphocyte mediated cytotoxicity in vitro. Induction and inhibition by humoral antibody and nature of effector cells. Transplant Rev 13: 91–114
Peter HH, Knoop F, Kalden JR (1976) Spontaneous and antibody-dependent cellular cytotoxicity in melanoma patients and healthy control persons. Z Immunitaetsforsch 151: 263–281
Pollack S, Heppner G, Brawn RJ, Nelson K (1972) Specific killing of tumor cells in vitro in the presence of normal lymphoid cells and sera from hosts immune to the tumor antigen. Int J Cancer 9: 316–323
Pollack S (1973) Specific 'arming' of normal lymph node cells by sera from tumor-bearing mice. Int J Cancer 11: 138–142
Pomerance A (1972) Pathology and prognosis following total cystectomy for carcinoma of bladder. Br J Urol 44: 451–458
Prehn RT (1976) Tumor progression and homeostasis. Adv Cancer Res 23: 203–236
Prehn RT, Main JM (1957) Immunity of methylcholanthrene-induced sarcomas. J Natl Cancer Inst 18: 769–778
Rabbat AG, Jeejeebhoy HF (1970) Heterologous antilymphocyte serum (ALS) hastens the appearance of methylcholanthrene-induced tumours in mice. Transplantation 9: 164–165
Sarma KP (1970) The role of lymphoid tissue in bladder cancer. J. Urol. 104: 843–849

Scorticatti CH, de la Peña NC, Bellora OG, Mariotto RA, Casabe AR, Comolli R (1981) Systemic IFN-α treatment of multiple bladder papilloma grade I or II patients—pilot study. In: Proceedings of the Second Annual International Congress for Interferon Research, San Francisco, 1981

Smith RB, deKernion J, Lincoln B, Skinner DG, Kaufman JJ (1978) Preliminary report of the use of levamisole in the treatment of bladder cancer. Cancer Treat Rep 62: 1709–1714

Soloway MS, Myers GH, Krueger G (1974) Lymphocytic reaction associated with bladder cancer. Urology 3: 437–443

Sterioff S, Rios CN, Zachary JB, Williams GM (1975) Neoplasia in kidney transplant recipients. Am J Surg 130: 622–626

Takasugi M, Mickey MR, Terasaki PI (1973) Reactivity of lymphocytes from normal persons on cultured tumor cells. Cancer Res 33: 2898–2902

Talmadge JE, Meyers KM, Prieur DJ, Starkey JR (1980) Role of NK cells in tumor growth and metastasis in beige mice. Nature 284: 622–624

Tanaka T, Cooper EH, Anderson CK (1970) Lymphocyte infiltration in bladder carcinoma. Rev Eur Etud Clin Biol Res 15: 1084–1089

Tarkkanen J, Gröhn P, Heinonen E, Alfthan O, Pyrhönen S (1981) Transfer factor immunotherapy of recurrent non-infiltrative papillary bladder tumors. Cancer Immunol Immunother 10: 251–255

Thomas L (1959) Discussion In: Lawrence HS (ed) Cellular and humoral aspects of the hypersensitive states. Hoeber-Harper, New York, pp 529–532

Trinchieri G, Santoli D (1978) Anti-viral activity induced by culturing lymphocytes with tumor-derived or virus transformed cells. J Exp Med 147: 1314–1333

Troye M, Perlmann P, Larsson A, Blomgren H, Johansson B (1977) Cellular cytotoxicity in vitro in transitional cell carcinoma of the human urinary bladder: ^{51}Cr-release assay. Int J Cancer 20: 188–198

Turner AG, Carter S, Higgins E, Glashan RW, Neville AM (1977) The clinical diagnostic value of the carcinoembryonic antigen (CEA) in hematuria. Br J Urol 49: 61–66

Vollenweider A, Largiadèr F, Uhlschmid G, Binswanger U, Briner R (1982) Maligne Tumoren bei Nierentransplantatempfängern unter immunsuppressiver Therapie. Schweiz Med Wochenschr 112: 102–111

Vose BM, Vanky F, Argov S, Klein E (1977) Natural cytotoxicity in man: activity of lymph node and tumor infiltrating lymphocytes. Eur J Immunol 7: 753–757

Wahren B, Nilsson B, Zimmermann R (1982) Urinary CEA for prediction of survival time and recurrence in bladder cancer. Cancer 50: 139–145

Weinstein RS, Coon J, Alroy J, Davidsohn I (1981) Detection and significance of tissue associated blood group antigens ABH (O) in human carcinomas. In: Dellelis RA, Sternberg SS (eds) Diagnostic immunology, vol 2. Masson, New York, pp 239–261

Wirth M, Schmitz-Dräger BJ, Ackermann R (1983) Functional properties of NK-cells in carcinoma of the prostate. J Urol (accepted for publication).

Woodruff MFA, Boak JL (1966) Inhibitory effect of injection of '*Corynebacterium parvum*' on the growth of tumour transplants in isogenic hosts. Br J Cancer 20: 345–355

Zbar B, Bernstein D, Rapp HJ (1971) Suppression of tumor growth at the site of infection with living bacillus Calmette-Guérin. J Natl Cancer Inst 46: 831–839

Zimmermann R, Wahren B, Edsmyr F (1976) Measurement of urinary CEA-like substance. An aid in management of patients with bladder carcinoma. Bull Cancer 63: 563–573

Zinkernagel RM, Doherty PC (1975) H-2 compatibility requirements for T-cell-mediated lysis of target cells infected with lymphocytic choriomeningitis virus. J Exp Med 141: 1427–1436

Chapter 4

Symptomatology

D. M. A. Wallace

Introduction

In over 90% of cases of bladder cancer it is the symptoms that lead to the diagnosis and treatment; relatively few cases are detected incidentally or by routine screening methods. The period of time that a tumour is symptomatic is relatively short, compared with the total life span of the tumour, and the period when the tumour is symptomatic and curable (i.e. is localised) varies with the biological characteristics of the tumour. When breakthrough of the basement membrane occurs and the tumour becomes invasive, then the prognosis decreases sharply with each stage of invasion. This is clearly shown in the 3-year survival figures for each depth of infiltration (Table 4.1) reported by Pryor (1973). Assuming that both the depth of invasion and the development of metastases are functions of time, then every delay in instituting treatment may have a marked effect on the survival. Conversely, there may be little consequence in delaying treatment for a non-invasive papillary tumour, but the risks of leaving such tumours untreated have not, for obvious reasons, been established. Even so, there is clearly an appreciable risk of invasion and metastases, and therefore the low malignant potential of most papillary tumours cannot be used as an excuse for any lack of urgency in instituting treatment.

Table 4.1. The 3-year survival according to the depth of invasion of the bladder tumour (Pryor 1973)

Depth of invasion	UICC histopathological category	3-Year survival
Non-invasive	PIS	88%
Tumour cores (P1a)	P1	77%
Lamina propria (P1b)	P1	64%
Superficial muscle	P2	52%
Deep muscle	P3	24%

Haematuria

The presentation of bladder cancer is clearly dominated by haematuria. Microscopic haematuria should not be regarded as a completely separate entity from macroscopic haematuria, and therefore these two subjects will be discussed in succession.

Macroscopic Haematuria

The proportion of cases with bladder cancer presenting with haematuria varies from 68% to 97.5% (Massey et al. 1965; Wallace and Harris 1965; Hendry et al. 1981). Haematuria is a common symptom in clinical practice, and the correct appreciation of its significance is an essential part of undergraduate medical teaching. Malignant disease of the urinary tract is diagnosed in 11.3%–22% of patients with haematuria (Lee and Davis 1953; Burkholder et al. 1969; Turner et al. 1977; Hendry et al. 1981). The majority of these malignancies are carcinomas of the bladder. The management of patients with macroscopic haematuria is therefore primarily directed towards the rapid diagnosis or exclusion of urological malignancies.

Any patient who passes 'red' urine must be assumed to have haematuria. This can easily be verified by microscopy or with a simple 'stick test'. This symptom may be intermittent; the patient's own observations must not be dismissed, nor much time wasted in its verification. Other causes of passing discoloured urine that may be mistaken for haematuria are rare and include drugs (Pyridium, rifampicin), patent medicines, porphyria, bile pigments and vegetable dyes, such as are found in beetroot, which some 10% of the population cannot metabolise and excrete unchanged in the urine. Some women may be poor witnesses or may be too embarrassed to describe clearly to the doctor the exact nature of their bleeding. Thus haematuria can be misinterpreted as vaginal bleeding or even as normal menstruation. The history must therefore be taken with care and when the description is not precise then all possibilities must be considered. Useful information about the origin of the haematuria can be obtained by ascertaining if the haematuria is initial, total or terminal. When the haematuria is initial the lesion is likely to be below the bladder neck, when total anywhere above the bladder neck, and when terminal the lesion may be in the bladder or prostatic urethra. Worm-like clots will have come from the upper tracts; the presence of clots is a useful indicator of the severity of the bleeding and the need for urgent action.

Microscopic Haematuria

With improving medical care and increasing use of 'stick tests' for haematuria more patients are being detected with asymptomatic microscopic haematuria. These cases pose a problem for the clinician as to how they should be investigated. When, if ever, can red cells in the urine be dismissed as normal? Must the same significance be attached to microscopic as to macroscopic haematuria?

Table 4.2. Red cells in the urine in routinely screened males and females (Alwall and Lohi 1973)

RBC/HPF	Men	Women
> 3	3.9%	5.7%
> 7	1.0%	2.3%
>11	0.6%	1.4%

Addis (1926) demonstrated with a technique using blood counting chambers that red blood cells could be detected in 40 out of 64 healthy medical students, and that the excretion rate varied between 0 and 425 000 red blood cells per 12 h. Wright (1959), using the standard and less laborious technique of microscoping the centrifuged deposit of a sample of urine, found that 21.6% of males attending life insurance examinations had more than 10 red blood cells per high power field (rbc/hpf). Using more careful methods of the centrifugation technique, Sanders (1963) found red cells in 74.4% of employees aged 16–70 years. Both Sanders and Wright calculated that 1 rbc/hpf is equivalent to approximately 2300 rbc/ml of urine using the centrifugation technique. Alwall and Lohi (1973) found red cells present at 3, 7 and 11 rbc/hpf in 3.9%, 1.0% and 0.6% respectively of routinely screened males and in 5.7%, 2.3% and 1.4% of females (Table 4.2). Strom (1975) also found that 1% of males and 4% of females had more than 12 rbc/hpf.

All of the above investigations used the standard techniques of centrifuging 10–15 ml of urine and examining the deposit as a wet preparation. Freni et al. (1977) adapted urine cytology techniques to examine the whole deposit from 40 ml of urine which was transferred to albumen-coated slides and stained with the Papanicolaou method. They showed that while the standard examination of urine can demonstrate red cells when there are more than 500 rbc/ml, the use of cytological techniques could detect as few as 50 rbc/ml. In screening 446 men over 50 years of age red cells were detected in every urine sample by using the cytological technique. The authors tentatively suggested that if a line exists at all between physiological values and abnormal values it should be drawn at 20 000 rbc/ml. This figure corresponds to 8 rbc/hpf using the standard techniques and 40 rbc/hpf using cytological techniques. In none of these studies was it reported that the patients with microscopic haematuria were investigated for a cause of their haematuria or were followed up.

The clinical significance of microscopic haematuria was reported on by Carson et al. (1979), who investigated 200 consecutive patients with asymptomatic microscopic haematuria detected by routine laboratory screening of urine samples at the Mayo Clinic. Urine cultures, cytology, urography and cystoscopy were carried out for each patient. Carcinoma of the bladder was found in 22 patients (11%); in 9 of these patients the cytological results were positive, and 5 of these had carcinoma in situ. Thirty-eight patients who had no cause diagnosed initially for their microscopic haematuria were followed up for 2 years. Six of these patients were later found to have significant lesions, of which one was a bladder cancer. One of the findings of this study was that the grade of haematuria did not correlate with the severity of the pathological findings, as four of the patients with bladder cancer had between 1 and 8 rbc/hpf.

The results of another study by Golin and Howard (1980) are remarkably similar. They investigated 246 patients with microscopic haematuria and found 10% to have urological neoplasms. They also found no relationship between the severity of the haematuria and the significance of the lesion, with cases of bladder cancer being detected with less than 8 rbc/hpf.

In a much earlier study from the Mayo Clinic Greene et al. (1956) had investigated 500 patients with microscopic haematuria and found only 9 bladder neoplasms. In none of these patients, however, had investigation with urine cytology been carried out, and no cases with carcinoma in situ were found. The explanation for the much higher detection of malignancy in the second series is likely to be the use of urine cytology and mucosal biopsies to detect carcinoma in situ rather than a real increase in the incidence of bladder cancer (Greene 1980).

The findings of more than 1 rbc/hpf on routine screening of urine samples by the standard technique, which is usually performed by the most junior and inexperienced laboratory technician, cannot therefore be dismissed as normal. However, the full investigation of every patient with 1 rbc/hpf is clearly impracticable, but for these patients a repeat urinalysis and urine cytology should be carried out. Urography and cystoscopy are indicated when persistent microscopic haematuria is confirmed, and referral to a nephrologist should be made if red cell casts or albuminuria are present. If a 'stick' method of testing gives positive results, then it should be assumed that at least 20 000–50 000 rbc/ml of urine are present (Sacre 1969), and these cases should then be investigated in the same manner as cases with macroscopic haematuria.

An important new development which may separate those patients whose urine contains red cells which have come through the glomerulus from those in whom the bleeding is from elsewhere in the urinary tract is the study of the red cell morphology by phase-contrast microscopy. Red cells that have passed through the glomerulus are distorted or fragmented, whereas those that have not come via the glomerulus retain their normal shape (Birch and Fairly 1979). Urine samples from 376 healthy individuals were examined and showed that 95% had up to 8000 rbc/ml; in each case the erythrocytes exhibited the dysmorphic pattern suggesting that the erythrocytes in healthy individuals enter the urine via the glomerulus. Dysmorphic cells were also found in 86 of 87 patients subsequently shown to have glomerular lesions (Birch et al. 1983). Fassett et al. (1982) also showed that 115 of 120 patients with glomerular bleeding as judged by phase-contrast microscopy had glomerulonephritis; 100 of 105 patients with non-glomerular bleeding had lesions in the lower urinary tract, and 5 had glomerulonephritis. Phase-contrast microscopy is therefore likely to be useful in separating those patients with microscopic haematuria who need urological investigation from those who can be reassured or who need nephrological assessment.

Symptoms of Bladder Irritation

Some 20%–25% of patients with bladder cancer will present with symptoms of bladder irritation. These symptoms may be caused by a variety of pathological processes:

1. *Secondary infection of the urine*: 39%–41% of patients presenting with bladder cancers also had urinary infections (Cox et al. 1969; Turner et al. 1977). Appell et al. (1980) demonstrated that bacteria could be cultured from resected

bladder tumours in 65.5% of cases, even though the urine was sterile before transurethral resection (TUR). Malignant disease of the bladder makes a breach in the bladder's defences against infection and thus becomes a privileged site for bacterial growth. The tumour then acts like a foreign body and prevents the eradication of the infection.

2. *A reduction in bladder capacity* may be caused by infiltration of the bladder wall or by the filling of the lumen with exophytic growth.
3. *Outflow obstruction* may be caused by the tumour obstructing or infiltrating the bladder neck or prostate.
4. *Pain* may be due to direct infiltration beyond the wall of the bladder. Pain is also a feature of carcinoma in situ (see below).
5. *Necrosis of tumour* within the bladder may cause a non-specific inflammatory reaction.
6. *The presence of carcinoma in situ.* A symptom complex that must now be recognised is that which occurs in association with widespread carcinoma in situ. Not all patients with carcinoma in situ have symptoms, but, when symptoms do occur, the prognosis is usually worse (Riddle et al. 1976). The main symptoms are dysuria, frequency and urgency, with occasional urge incontinence (Farrow et al. 1977). In addition, these patients may have a pain which is quite characteristic; it is a constant pain in the suprapubic, penile or perineal region. These symptoms may be due to chemical irritation by the urine but are more likely to be due to the in situ carcinoma. A striking feature is the rapid relief of symptoms within 48 h of receiving effective chemotherapy, as reported by England et al. (1981).

Symptoms of Advanced Disease

The symptoms of locally advanced or metastatic disease may be very non-specific and their pathogenesis is complex. When fully investigated it is frequently revealed that the causes of these symptoms are not the direct effects of advanced cancer but are systemic disturbances that can be treated, such as anaemia, infection, hypercalcaemia (see Chap. 5, p. 93) and renal failure. Hypercalcaemia may be a non-specific effect that can also result in renal failure.

Patients with locally advanced bladder cancer will nearly always have haematuria or pyuria, so that the diagnosis of the primary tumour in such cases is seldom a problem. Pain in the groin may be caused by obstruction and pain in the leg is likely to be caused by pelvic nerve involvement. Lymphoedema may be the result of nodal metastases. Urinary leakage may be caused by a vesicovaginal fistula when the tumour necroses.

Causes of Delay in the Diagnosis of Bladder Cancer

While it is accepted that enormous efforts will have to be made in the screening and early diagnosis of bladder cancer to make any improvement in the overall survival, the failure of early diagnosis and treatment in individual patients is a not infrequent occurrence in everyday clinical practice. Does delay in diagnosis and treatment have an adverse effect on the prognosis? This must be carefully examined and the causes for delay analysed.

Payne (1959) studied 1420 patients with bladder cancer and analysed them according to age, sex, history, tumour type and survival. He found that when the length of history was less than 2 months from the onset of symptoms to the first examination in hospital then the crude 3-year survival was 57%; this fell to 37% if the history was 3–8 months but rose again to 44% for those with histories of 9–24 months. Wallace and Harris (1965) showed that when infiltrating tumours were treated within 1 month of the onset of symptoms the crude 3-year survival was 60% whereas when a delay of 1–6 months had occurred then the prognosis was less than half as good, with a 3-year survival of only 25%. Richie et al. (1975) reported that for patients treated by total cystectomy when the history was less than 6 months the 5-year survival was 44.5%; this dropped to 28.6% if the history was longer than 6 months. In this study patients with dysuria not associated with urinary infection had a poorer survival. Cox et al. (1969), however, found no correlation between length of history and survival in a 26-year review of 371 patients with bladder cancer. Mommsen et al. (1983) studied 212 consecutive cases of bladder cancer to elucidate the causes of delay in the diagnosis and treatment. They found that the length of delay did not influence the survival of

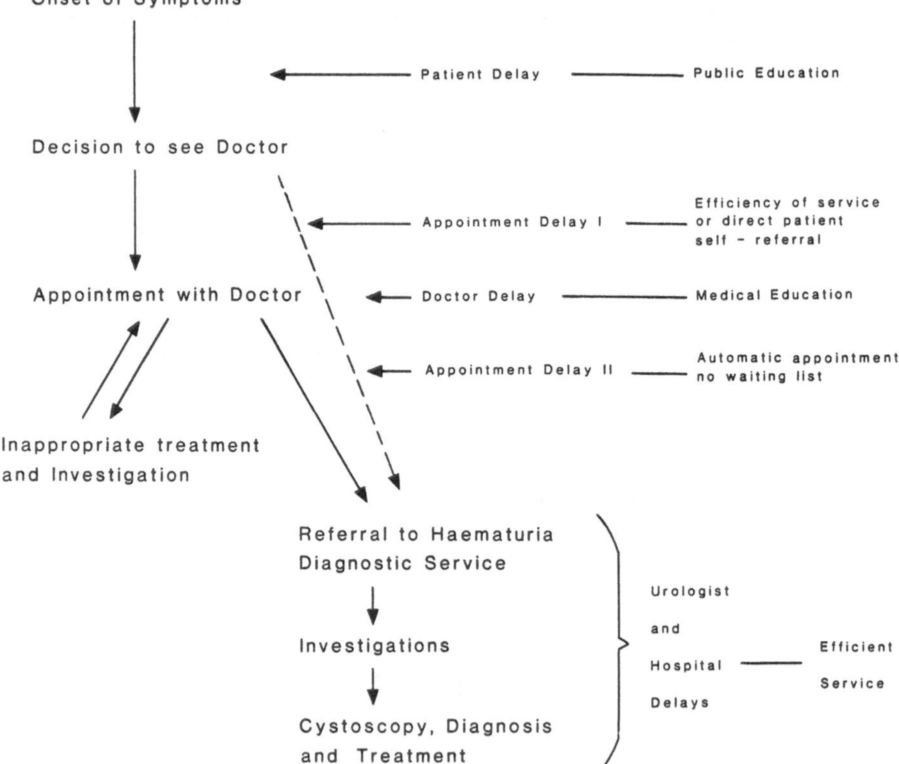

Fig. 4.1. Delays in the diagnosis and treatment of patients with bladder cancer

those with T3 or T4 tumours, but there was a tendency to better survival when the delay was shorter with the T1 and T2 tumours. Of those that presented with haematuria the crude 3-year survival was 55% when the history was less than 1 month and 35% when there was a delay of 1–6 months.

From these results it seems possible that if we could achieve the ideal of treating all patients within 1 month of the onset of their symptoms then the crude survival would be 10%–20% better. When we fail to start treatment within 6 months then the prognosis is at least 10% worse. We must now carefully examine the pathways that patients must follow to reach the point of diagnosis and treatment. It is the total time between the onset of symptoms and the initiation of treatment that is important and this is made up of many delay periods, which are set out in Fig. 4.1.

Patient Delay

The term 'patient delay' refers to the interval between the onset of symptoms and the point when the patient seeks advice. Wallace and Harris (1965) reported that this was not a major cause of delay, as half of the patients reported to their doctors within 1 week. Delays were more frequently found in women patients, to whom the occurrence of genitourinary bleeding may be less frightening. Mommsen et al. (1983) found that half the patients consulted their doctors within 1 week of the onset of their symptoms, but also found that 19% of males and 13% of females delayed for more than 13 weeks. Efforts at public education must continue to maintain this patient response, but increased efforts here are not likely to bring about a significant improvement.

Appointment Delay I

Usually a patient will be seen immediately by a doctor only in an emergency. The degree of urgency attached to haematuria and thus the speed with which the patient sees a doctor is variable but should always be less than 1 week. An alternative is direct self-referral to a haematuria diagnostic service.

Doctor Delays

In the study by Mommsen et al. (1983) 82% of men and 62% of women were referred within 12 weeks of consulting their general practitioner. Of the patients with haematuria 13% of the men but 35% of the women were referred to hospital after 13 weeks or more. When cystitis was the presenting symptom, referral was significantly later than when haematuria was present. It is appropriate here to enumerate some of the main pitfalls which may cause doctors to delay in referring patients for investigation when bladder cancer is a possibility:

1. *The haematuria is due to infection.* As shown earlier, infection is frequently present with bladder tumours, but haematuria must not be attributed to the infection until a bladder tumour has been excluded. Relapsing urinary infections in the absence of frank haematuria may also be due to a bladder tumour.

2. *The haematuria is due to benign prostatic enlargement.* This is a diagnosis of exclusion only. Most large prostates look as if they could cause some bleeding, and a coincidental bladder tumour must not be overlooked.
3. *The haematuria is caused by anticoagulants.* Anticoagulants may make urinary tract bleeding more pronounced but they must not be regarded as the cause until all other possibilities have been excluded. They must therefore be fully investigated.
4. *The bleeding is gynaecological.* In the case of a female patient who is not a good witness, both the doctor and the patient may make the wrong assumption that the haematuria is vaginal bleeding.
5. *Lower urinary tract symptoms without haematuria.* Haematuria is so clearly associated with bladder cancer that when lower tract symptoms are present without haematuria the diagnosis of bladder cancer may not be considered. This is particularly true in men with carcinoma in situ where the symptoms are often attributed to prostatic obstruction and no urine cytology or bladder biopsies are performed. In elderly women the symptoms may be attributed to urinary infections without a urine culture being performed.

Appointment Delay II

Patients may have to wait up to several weeks for a hospital appointment if the urgency of the situation is not made clear. The hospital system should allow for patients with the key symptom of haematuria to have an automatic urgent appointment without having to be placed on any waiting list. This is the essential feature of the haematuria diagnostic service as reported by Turner et al. (1977) and Hendry et al. (1981).

Urologist and Hospital Delays

All too often the speed and efficiency with which the patient with bladder cancer is investigated and diagnosed breaks down in the hospital system. This is the area of the urologist's responsibility, and he and the hospital administration must ensure that there are no unnecessary delays between clinic appointment, investigation and admission for treatment.

Conclusion

The symptoms of bladder cancer are common in general clinical practice. It is only by a thorough basic medical training and the running of an efficient diagnostic service that we can maintain the highest standards of care for the patient with bladder cancer. The first essential is the rapid diagnosis of all cases in which bladder cancer is a possibility. If we can thereby improve the prognosis by only a small amount then we will have achieved our objective. Therapeutic nihilism must never allow us to lower the standards of investigation of patients with lower tract symptoms where bladder cancer is suspected.

References

Addis T (1926) The number of formed elements in the urinary sediment of normal individuals. J Clin Invest 2: 409–415

Alwall N, Lohi A (1973) A population study on renal and urinary tract diseases. Acta Med Scand 194: 529–535

Appell RA, Flynn JT, Paris AMI, Blandy JP (1980) Occult bacterial colonisation of bladder tumours. J Urol 124: 345–346

Birch DF, Fairley KF (1979) Haematuria—glomerular or non-glomerular? Lancet II: 845–846

Birch DF, Fairley KF, Whitworth JA, Forbes IK, Fairley JK, Cheshire GR, Ryan GB (1983) Urinary erythrocyte morphology in the diagnosis of glomerular haematuria. Clin Nephrol 20: 78–84

Burkholder GV, Dotin LN, Thomason WB, Beach PD (1969) Unexplained hematuria. JAMA 210: 1729–1733

Carson CC, Segura JW, Greene LF (1979) Clinical importance of microhematuria. JAMA 241: 149–150

Cox CE, Cass AS, Boyce WH (1969) Bladder cancer: A 26 year review. J Urol 101: 550–558

England HR, Molland EA, Oliver RTD, Blandy JP (1981) Systemic cyclophosphamide in flat carcinoma in situ of the bladder. In: Oliver RTD, Hendry WF, Bloom HJG (eds) Bladder cancer: principles of combination therapy. Butterworths, London, pp 97–105

Farrow GM, Utz DC, Rife CC, Greene LF (1977) Clinical observations on sixty-nine cases of in situ carcinoma of the urinary bladder. Cancer Res 37: 2749–2798

Fassett RG, Horgan BA, Mathew TH (1982) Detection of glomerular bleeding by phase-contrast microscopy. Lancet II: 1432–1434

Freni SC, Heedrik GJ, Hol C (1977) Centrifugation techniques and reagent strips in the assessment of microhaematuria. J Clin Pathol 30: 336–340

Golin AL, Howard RS (1980) Asymptomatic microscopic hematuria. J Urol 124: 389–391

Greene LF (1980) Editorial comment. J Urol 124: 391

Greene LF, O'Shaughnessy EJ, Hendricks ED (1956) Study of five hundred patients with asymptomatic microhematuria. JAMA 161: 610–613

Hendry WF, Manning N, Perry NM, Whitfield HN, Wickham JEA (1981) The effects of a haematuria service on the early diagnosis of bladder cancer. In: Oliver RTD, Hendry WF, Bloom HJG (eds) Bladder cancer: principles of combination therapy. Butterworths, London, pp 19–25

Lee LW, Davis E (1953) Gross urinary hemorrhage: A symptom not a disease. JAMA 153: 781–784

Massey BD, Nation EF, Gallup CA, Hendricks ED (1965) Carcinoma of the bladder: 20 years experience in private practice. J Urol 93: 212–216

Mommsen S, Aagard J, Sell A (1983) Presenting symptoms, treatment delay and survival in bladder cancer. Scand J Urol Nephrol 17: 163–167

Payne P (1959) Sex, age, history, tumour type and survival. In: Wallace DM (ed) Tumours of the bladder. Livingstone, Edinburgh, pp 285–386

Pryor JP (1973) Factors influencing the survival of patients with transitional cell tumours of the urinary bladder. Br J Urol 45: 586–592

Richie JP, Skinner DG, Kaufman JJ (1975) Radical cystectomy for carcinoma of the bladder: 16 years of experience. J Urol 113: 186–189

Riddle PR, Chisholm GD, Trott PA, Pugh RCB (1976) Flat carcinoma in situ of bladder. Br J Urol 47: 829–833

Sacre MH (1970) An assessment of the Labstix strip test. J Med Lab Technol 27: 213–217

Sanders C (1963) Clinical urine examination and the incidence of microscopic haematuria in apparently normal males. Practitioner 191: 192–197

Strom J (1975) Cellular elements in the urine in health and in acute infectious diseases, especially with respect to the presence of haematuria. Scand J Infect Dis 7: 97–102

Turner AG, Hendry WF, Williams GB, Wallace DM (1977) A haematuria diagnostic service. Br Med J 2: 29–31

Wallace DM, Harris DL (1965) Delay in treating bladder tumours. Lancet II: 332–334

Wright WT (1959) Cell counts in urine. Arch Int Med 103: 76–78

Chapter 5

Diagnostic Procedures

M. C. Bishop

Introduction

The techniques described in this chapter are applicable both to the diagnosis of new tumours and the assessment of recurrent ones. Their efficiency in staging the tumour is central to this discussion. The practicality of using such techniques for screening groups of patients at special risk will also be considered.

The diagnosis of bladder cancer will be suspect in any patient with painless haematuria and in the clinical circumstances outlined in Chapter 4. Virtually any symptom of urinary tract disorder can be associated with a bladder tumour (Fig. 5.1). Recently, with increasing popularity of the health check, microscopic haematuria has become a significant entity requiring further investigation. Routine urinalysis for blood may prove to be among the most cost effective of the screening investigations of a general population, whilst exfoliative cytology

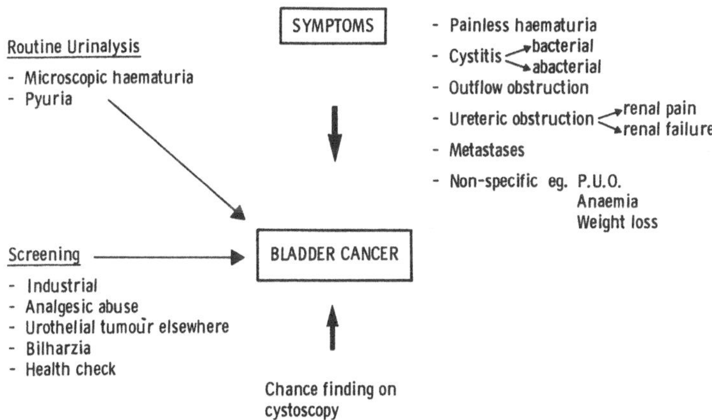

Fig. 5.1. The origins of a diagnosis of bladder cancer

should still be reserved for groups at risk. As with all forms of cancer, the application of these screening procedures may be costly and liable to introduce widespread fear of the disease. These must ultimately be justified by improved results of treatment. Proof that prompt diagnosis of early disease prevents death from advanced tumour growth is so hard to achieve that the problem becomes almost philosophical. The reorganisation of a urological clinic or outpatient department necessary to deal with the referrals for haematuria should also be justified (see Chap. 4, pp. 82–83).

The advantages of early diagnosis may be summed up thus:

1. Small superficial growths are more easily dealt with by local means before they become extensive.
2. Superficial tumours can be treated before they become invasive.
3. Invasive tumours can be treated before they have metastasised and become incurable.

The key distinctions in terms of prognosis for bladder cancer are shown in Fig. 5.2 (Jewett and Strong 1946; Marshall 1956; Schmidt and Weinstein 1976; Murphy 1978). The two thresholds usually define a change of treatment plan, although completely hard and fast rules cannot be drawn. Indeed, it may eventually be shown that T1 tumours, as opposed to Ta tumours, may be most effectively treated by radical surgery. On the other hand, some urologists regard complete endoscopic resection of a small T2 tumour as adequate treatment. Similarly, the threshold between the T3b and T4 tumour is often indistinct, and the optimistic surgeon may feel obliged to embark on a cystectomy on the off chance that the tumour has not advanced beyond the limits of resectability.

An efficient system for classification and staging ought to be capable of demonstrating down-staging of the invasive tumour after radiotherapy, since it is clear that the best results from radical surgery are obtained in patients responding to preoperative radiotherapy. Eventually it may be shown that these are the patients for whom cystectomy is unnecessary (van der Werf-Messing 1973).

Staging methods must also be capable of detecting regional lymph node metastases by demonstrating enlargement and distortion of the architecture of the regional and juxtaregional lymph nodes. The search for distant metastases should

Ca in situ	Tis	
Papillary non-invasive	TA	Local resection
Infiltration of lamina propria	T1	Instillation
Infiltration of superficial muscle	T2	
Infiltration of deep muscle	T3a	Radical
Infiltration through bladder wall	T3b	
Invasion of prostate, uterus, vagina	T4a	Palliative
Fixed to pelvic or abdominal wall	T4b	

Fig. 5.2. Carcinoma of the bladder: UICC 'T' classification. The critical limits determining local, radical and palliative therapy are shown

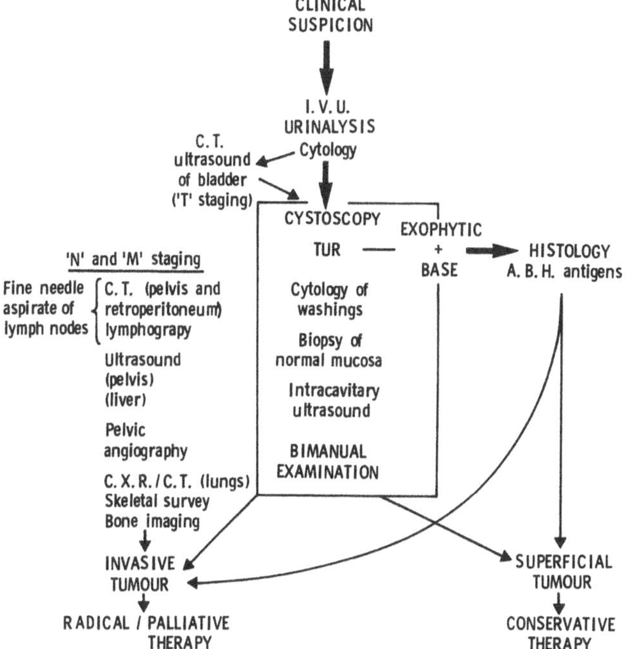

Fig. 5.3. Flow chart of diagnosis and treatment of bladder cancer. This emphasises (1) that assessment of T category by CT and ultrasound must be done before cystoscopy and (2) that decisions on treatment of invasive tumours are made on the results of investigations for nodal and distant metastases

also, within reason, be as comprehensive as possible. The demonstration of nodal or distant metastases means that radical local therapy is unlikely to be curative.

Most of the available methods used in diagnosis and staging of bladder cancer which are discussed in this chapter are shown as a flow chart between 'clinical suspicion' and 'treatment' (Fig. 5.3). They will be taken in the order of urine tests, tumour markers, radiology and endoscopic assessment. This is done to emphasise the importance of making a complete assessment before biopsy and transurethral resection of the tumour.

Urine Examination

Urinalysis

Following history taking and physical examination, the first and simplest investigation is the routine urinalysis. The most obvious abnormality indicative of urothelial malignancy is macro- or microscopic haematuria. The circumstances in which this is sought and discovered are dealt with more fully in the section on screening (see p. 108) and in Chapter 4 (see p. 78).

Pyuria is common in bladder cancer. In the absence of additional bacteriologically proven infection, a diligent search for the cause of the leucocytes in the urine should always be made. The differential diagnosis includes urinary tract calculi, tuberculosis, chronic cystitis and incompletely controlled bacterial infection. However, proof of infection on bacterial culture should not detract from a diagnosis of bladder cancer as, like any foreign body, a tumour predisposes to bacterial colonisation (Appell et al. 1980).

Simple microscopy of individual cells in the urinary sediment can also be undertaken, with special emphasis on the epithelial elements (de Voogt et al. 1977). This can be distinguished from formal cytological examination of urine and bladder washings. The technique is easily learned and can be carried out by the urologist as an office procedure. Light microscopy with phase-contrast separation is used to evaluate the cytological detail of the epithelial cells, and atypical or frankly malignant cells can be distinguished. Minimal preparation of the specimen is required, and at best the sensitivity approaches that of cytology after the more complicated processes of cell concentration and special staining. The method has disadvantages in that permanent preparations cannot be made, and the precision is obviously determined by the experience of the observer. The cells cannot be graded, and the diagnosis of carcinoma is all that is possible. The presence of large numbers of cells when urine is contaminated with blood or an infection will always cause problems.

Exfoliative Cytology

The urinary tract is lined with urothelium from the tip of the renal papilla to the fossa navicularis, and these urothelial cells exfoliate into the urine. There they can be recovered from the sediment or trapped on a millipore filter and, after suitable fixation, stained by the Papanicolaou method for examination of the cytological detail. The sampling, preparation and staining of the cells are crucial to the accuracy of the diagnosis that the cytologist can make.

Technique

Samples of urothelial cells may be obtained from the voided urine, from bladder washings (by saline barbotage), from the upper tracts by ureteric catheterisation or ureteric brushing and from the urethra by irrigation with saline or swabbing with soluble swabs. For purposes of screening for bladder tumours voided urine is adequate, but where the index of suspicion is high then the more invasive methods of sampling are justified. Urothelial cells degenerate in urine, which is seldom isotonic. The early morning sample of urine is therefore not suitable for cytological examination. The specimen for urine cytology should preferably be sent to the laboratory for immediate processing; otherwise it should either be fixed or refrigerated until it can be examined.

The recovery of urothelial cells can be improved and the cellular detail better preserved if bladder washings are taken. After evacuation of the residual urine, 50 ml physiological saline are introduced through the catheter or cystoscope; the saline is injected and withdrawn several times and then sent immediately to the laboratory (Esposti et al. 1970; Harris et al. 1971; Esposti and Zajicek 1972; Frable et al. 1977). It is essential for the cytologist to know certain clinical details in order to interpret the specimen. The most important are whether there was prior use of intravesical or systemic cytotoxic therapy or radiotherapy, where the specimen has come from and how it has been taken (e.g. ileal loop urine or ureteric brushings).

After fixation in alcohol or an alcohol-acetic acid mixture, the cells are recovered on filters, or alternatively processed in a centrifuged pellet, stained and examined by microscopy. Other types of analysis can be undertaken on cells rather than tissue. These include the A, B, and H antigen expression, scanning and transmission electron microscopy, and flow cytometry for the DNA and RNA content.

Cytology in the Diagnosis and Treatment of Urothelial Cancer

Whilst the definitive diagnosis of a bladder tumour must be by histological examination of a tissue biopsy, cytology of voided urine or bladder washings is less invasive and more readily performed. Many urologists use urine cytology as a complementary technique in the early diagnosis of urothelial cancer and also to follow the response to treatment (Lewis et al. 1976; Esposti 1981). Others have been less enthusiastic in view of the unsatisfactory rates of diagnostic accuracy reported. These can be highly variable and suggest that case selection and the skill of the cytologist may have been inconsistent (de Voogt et al. 1977). It may be impossible to distinguish cells of a low-grade tumour from the normal urothelium. The sensitivity, however, increases with the degree of de-differentiation of the tumour, and the correlation between histological and cytological diagnosis for Grades 2 and 3 tumours approaches 90%. On the other hand, sensitivity can be as low as 45%, particularly where the tumour is necrotic or severe coexisting inflammation or haemorrhage mask the malignant cells (de Voogt et al. 1977; Frable et al. 1977; El-Bolkainy 1980). A positive result from urine cytology in a patient showing no tumour on cystoscopy and mucosal biopsies is regarded as a false positive. However, during prolonged follow-up a urothelial carcinoma usually appears, and thus the initial false positive rate of up to 15% steadily decreases (Allegra et al. 1972; Frable et al. 1977; Heney et al. 1977). In such patients special attention should be paid to early diagnosis of upper tract tumours by urography, cytological sampling of urine and washings from the renal pelvis and ureter (Leistenschneider and Nagel 1980) and perhaps now also by direct ureteropyeloscopy.

After radiotherapy or chemotherapy exfoliated cells will usually show signs of acute injury. These changes will lead to difficulties in interpretation for the inexperienced cytologist. However, disappearance of malignant cells from the urine after radiotherapy or intravesical chemotherapy is a reliable sign of a satisfactory response to treatment. This may reduce the need for repeat cystoscopic examinations. Conversely, the reappearance of malignant cells in the urine and bladder washings is a signal that greater vigilance is required (Esposti et al. 1978; Esposti 1981).

Flow Cytometry

The dye acridine orange has a strong affinity for nucleic acids and fluoresces in ultraviolet light with a different colour according to the form of nucleic acid to which it has bound. This property has been used in automated flow cytometry in which the cellular contents of DNA and RNA and also the nuclear size can be measured. Objective measurements can be rapidly made on a large number of cells from a single urine sample. Bladder tumours are characterised by an increase in the proportion of cells with more than diploid DNA content and secondly by aneuploid cell peaks (Tribukait et al. 1979; Klein et al. 1982a, b; Tribukait et al. 1982). The flow cytometer is, however, a very expensive piece of apparatus, and this will certainly preclude its general use in the immediate future.

Summary of Indications for Exfoliative Cytology

1. In screening populations at risk of developing urothelial malignancy, e.g. workers who have been exposed to carcinogens and individuals with a history of analgesic abuse (see section on screening, p. 108).
2. In patients in whom a diagnosis of carcinoma in situ is suspected. In these patients cytology is best supplemented by random mucosal biopsies, since maximum sensitivity is achieved with a combination of both techniques.
3. Urine cytology is useful in the investigation of a patient with a bladder diverticulum, where the isthmus is too narrow to admit the cystoscope and the wall of the diverticulum is usually too thin to be biopsied safely.
4. To replace the review cystoscopy in the follow-up of patients with previously treated bladder tumours in whom the risk of recurrent tumour is low or multiple anaesthetics is high.
5. Exfoliated cells from tumours of the upper tracts also appear in the urine, especially during a diuresis with frusemide; therefore urine cytology can be used for their surveillance after treatment of a bladder carcinoma. This may also be performed after a cystectomy, when ileal loop urine can be used.
6. After a total cystectomy when the urethra has been left in situ, urethral washings or soluble urethral swabs should be used for regular cytological examinations to detect recurrent tumour in the urethra.

Tumour Markers

A marker substance present in the blood or urine should be easily measured and reliably indicate the existence and extent of the tumour for the purpose of initial diagnosis or detection of recurrent growth. The marker substance may be derived from the tumour itself or from surrounding tissue whose metabolism is influenced by the tumour. The established role of alpha-fetoprotein and beta-HCG in the management of testicular cancer and of carcinoembryonic antigen (CEA) in colorectal cancer have stimulated much interest and research into the detection of marker substances for many other tumours.

Carcinoembryonic Antigen

CEA, an oncofetal protein, was originally identified in malignant and fetal digestive tract tissue and its derivatives. It is now regarded as virtually a tumour-specific antigen in colorectal carcinoma. However, it is found in cells of a variety of tumours, including transitional cell carcinoma (Shevchuk et al. 1981). It can also be measured in elevated concentrations in the plasma and urine (Wahren et al. 1975; Colleen et al. 1979). Although the tests lacked both specificity and sensitivity in the initial diagnosis of bladder cancer, it was hoped that it might be a useful aid to prognosis and the detection of recurrence since a fall and later elevation of urine CEA were shown to occur with resection and subsequent regrowth respectively (Hall et al. 1973). It later became apparent that elevated levels related to the presence of inflammatory reactions in either acute or chronic cystitis (Colleen et al. 1979). Urinary infection and non-specific inflammatory changes commonly coexist with bladder tumours, and it is their activity rather than that of the tumour itself which is reflected in the urinary levels of CEA. However, there may yet be some value in the measurement, particularly for the enthusiast, since a recent study suggests that higher levels in bacteria-free urine reflect adversely on the prognosis (Wahren et al. 1982).

Enzymes, Proteins and Mucopolysaccharides

Several substances have been investigated as possible markers of tumour activity in the urinary tract but none of them has found a useful role in the management of patients with bladder cancer (Lessing 1978). Amongst those investigated have been urinary lactate dehydrogenase, creatinine phosphokinase, alkaline phosphatase (Lessing 1978; Motomiya et al. 1979), beta-glucuronidase (Cooper et al. 1973), collagenase (Chowaniec and Hicks 1977; Kunit et al. 1980), urinary protein excretion (Hemmingsen et al. 1981), glycosoaminoglycans (Hennessey et al. 1981) and fibrinogen degradation products (Martinez-Piñeiro et al. 1977; Alsabti 1979). In general they have all been found to lack specificity and sensitivity and many are complex and expensive tests to perform.

Paraneoplastic Endocrinopathies

The paraneoplastic endocrinopathies are of considerable interest and importance both to the basic scientist, who would wish to explain how a non-endocrine cell apparently acquires hormone-secreting potential, and to the clinician, who can use measurements of hormone levels and their target effects as markers. Recognition of these phenomena is important since they can be confused with the manifestations of advanced metastatic disease and thereby the patient may be regarded as a hopeless prospect for curative therapy.

Inappropriate secretion of parathyroid hormone, catecholamines, serotonin, anterior pituitary trophic hormones, gonadal hormones, erythropoietin and insulin-like substances have all been described in urological tumours (Altaffer 1982). However, such endocrinopathies are unusual in urothelial cancer. Hypercalcaemia is occasionally found and is not necessarily due to osteolytic bone metastases. A parathyroid hormone-like substance secreted by the primary tumour may be the cause, although for these particular tumours prostaglandins are most likely to be responsible (McKay et al. 1978; Droller 1981). In this case a fall in the level of serum calcium can provide useful evidence of response of the primary tumour to treatment. The contribution of sodium depletion and dehydration as factors that exacerbate the hypercalcaemia in patients with malignancy should not be underestimated. These factors can of course be corrected without any change in the state of the tumour and will result in a considerable improvement in the wellbeing of the patient (Stewart 1983). In these circumstances the plasma calcium will be an unreliable marker.

Radiology

Intravenous Urography

The principal reason for intravenous urography (IVU) in the adult patient with haematuria—the bladder tumour suspect—is to diagnose disease in the upper urinary tracts (Lang 1969; Sherwood et al. 1980). A second lesion in the upper tract of a patient with bladder cancer is not uncommon and can have an important bearing on treatment. IVU may also give useful information about the lower urinary tract and of the tumour itself. However, IVU alone lacks precision in either diagnosis or staging of bladder tumour and should always be followed by cystoscopy in a patient with haematuria or if there is any doubt that the patient could have a urothelial cancer. A normal IVU appearance does not exclude a bladder tumour, as up to 30% of bladder tumours may not be apparent as filling defects in the bladder.

Upper Tracts

In order to exclude disease in the upper tracts in the patient with haematuria it is essential that the IVU film is of the highest quality. The renal outlines must be clearly demonstrated and the whole of the collecting system should be visualised. This may require tomography and delayed films and a high dose of contrast. If the quality of the IVU film is substandard, then either IVU should be repeated or consideration given to obtaining an ascending ureteropyelogram.

A diligent search must be made of the whole collecting system for filling defects which may indicate a second urothelial tumour. It is important to establish if the upper tracts are normal at the time of first presentation as these patients must be regarded as being at risk of developing upper tract tumours throughout the period of their follow-up. Panurothelial disease will be particularly familiar to urologists working in localities where analgesic abuse is common or potent environmental factors operate (see section on screening, p. 110). Elsewhere, it is much less common to find coexisting renal and bladder tumours either simultaneously or serially. The value of routine urography during bladder tumour follow-up is therefore doubtful (Walzer and Soloway 1983). Urographic review should be undertaken only where frequent recurrences are found (Booth and Kellett 1981).

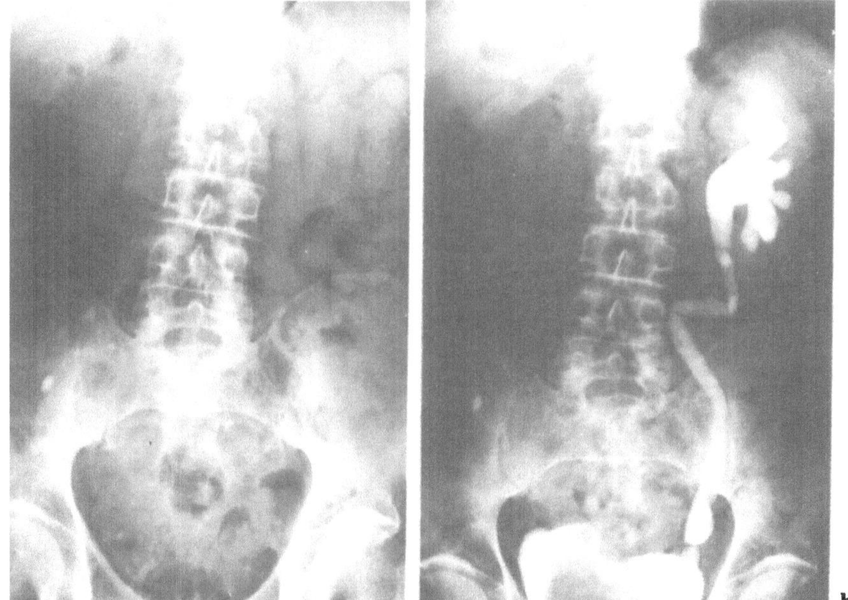

Fig. 5.4a,b. Intravenous urography in bladder cancer. **a** Calcification in the tumour (T3b). **b** Contrast film shows large space-occupying lesion in the bladder with bilateral obstructive nephropathy, severe on the right. (Courtesy of Dr. P. Davies, Nottingham City Hospital)

Dilatation of one or both upper urinary tracts is a most important sign since this usually indicates that the tumour in the bladder is invasive (Lang 1969; Fig. 5.4). A rare exception is the superficial papillary tumour involving the intramural segment of the ureter. When the kidney is non-functioning or the excretion of contrast is so poor that the upper tracts cannot be visualised, as in cases of phenacetin nephropathy, a second tumour in the renal pelvis or ureter cannot be excluded. An accurate diagnosis in these circumstances has important therapeutic consequences in that a nephroureterectomy may be required in addition to radical treatment of the bladder tumour. Renal ultrasound or computed tomography (CT) can identify the hydronephrotic kidney, and it may even be possible to demonstrate a solid tumour within it; however, an antegrade pyelogram is indicated in these circumstances to demonstrate the upper tracts (Fig. 5.5b).

Lower Urinary Tract

Useful information on the primary tumour in the bladder may be obtained from the urogram, particularly from the after-micturition film. The shape of the filling defect may indicate whether the tumour is likely to be papillary or solid, and the size and extent of the tumour within the bladder may be revealed. Tumour calcification is rarely seen on the plain film and may be difficult to distinguish from other nearby sources such as the prostate. However, it may be useful when viewed in conjunction with a filling defect and, moreover, it generally indicates that the

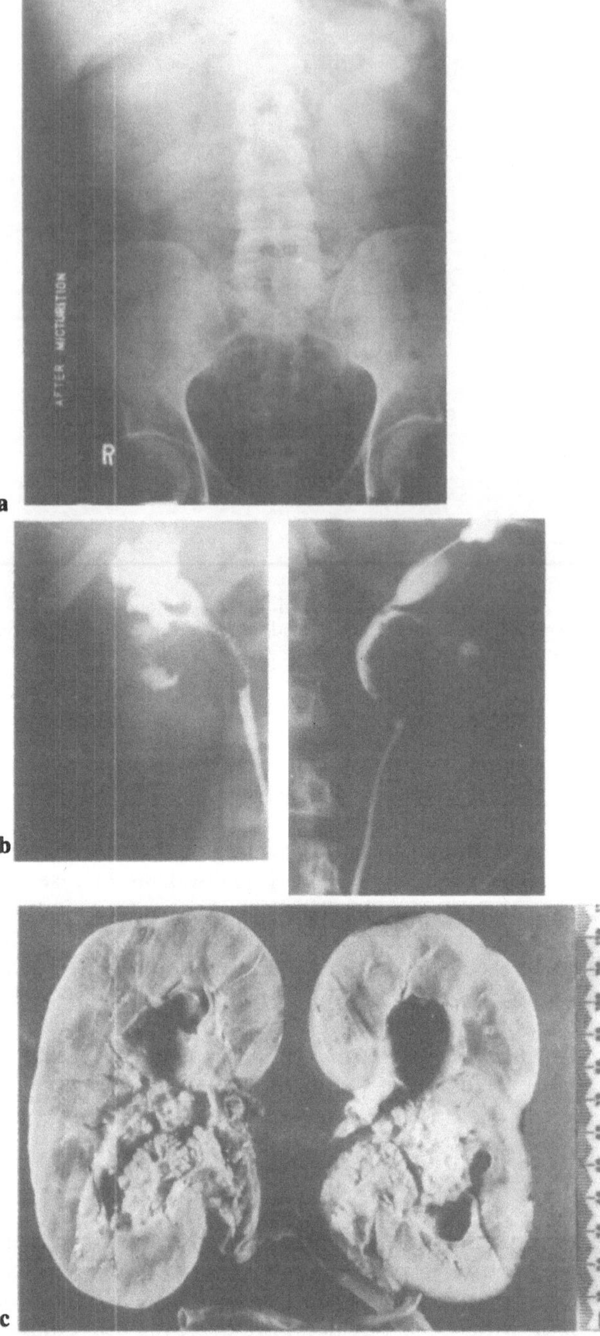

Fig. 5.5a–c. Widespread 'field change' in urothelial carcinoma. Bilateral obstructing renal pelvic carcinomas in a patient with bladder cancer followed for many years. **a** Urography; **b** antegrade pyelograms; **c** operative specimens

tumour is invasive and of a high grade (see Fig. 5.4a). Additional useful information about the state of the patient's lower urinary tract may also be obtained from the IVU film. In particular, the size of the after-micturition residue and the presence of diverticula may have an important bearing on the management.

The importance of the urographic signs of ureteric obstruction in staging bladder cancer has already been emphasised. The corollary is that IVU should always precede cystoscopy. This will forewarn the surgeon that an invasive tumour may exist near to the orifice. The grave disadvantage in delaying urography until after cystoscopy and endoscopic resection of the tumour encountered near to the orifice is that, even if the tumour is superficial, oedema and later fibrosis caused by the operative intervention can obstruct the ureter and thus this valuable index of tumour assessment is lost.

Cystography

A cystogram is only required in the diagnosis and assessment of a bladder tumour when there is suspicion of it arising in a diverticulum which cannot be examined cystoscopically. With care and experience the radiologist can demonstrate a tumour as small as 0.5 cm in diameter. However, CT scanning gives a better image of the diverticulum, the tumour within it and the extent of invasion (see Fig. 5.6c). There are further reasons for performing a cystogram. The first is to assist in planning the radiation fields by demonstrating to the radiotherapist the exact site of the tumour and its relationship to the skin markers. The second is to identify vesicoureteric reflux. This is not uncommon following TUR of bladder tumours in the vicinity of the ureteric orifices. In the context of urothelial cancer reflux might be harmful in two ways: (1) by allowing tumour cells to implant into the upper tracts and (2) by allowing nephrotoxic chemotherapeutic agents instilled into the bladder to reach the kidneys. However, the importance of these two factors is debatable; indeed, reflux may allow a cytotoxic solution instilled into the bladder to come into contact with tumours of the ureter or pelvicaliceal system. Such opportunism has had the desired result on at least one occasion (H. R. England 1978, personal communication).

A persisting urinary tract infection may occasionally be the result of vesicoureteric reflux. Cystography should be considered if symptomatic urinary infections cannot be controlled, as surgical correction of the reflux may be contemplated. Finally, cystography should be done if treatment with intravesical formalin is being considered for the control of intractable haemorrhage. Reflux of formalin into the upper tracts could have fatal consequences (see Chap. 11, p. 265).

Computed Tomography

Primary Tumour

CT scanning of bladder tumours has been considered in several recent publications (Seidelman et al. 1978; Stanley et al. 1978; Kellett et al. 1980; Colleen et al. 1981; Hamlin et al. 1981; Jeffery et al. 1981; Vock et al. 1982).

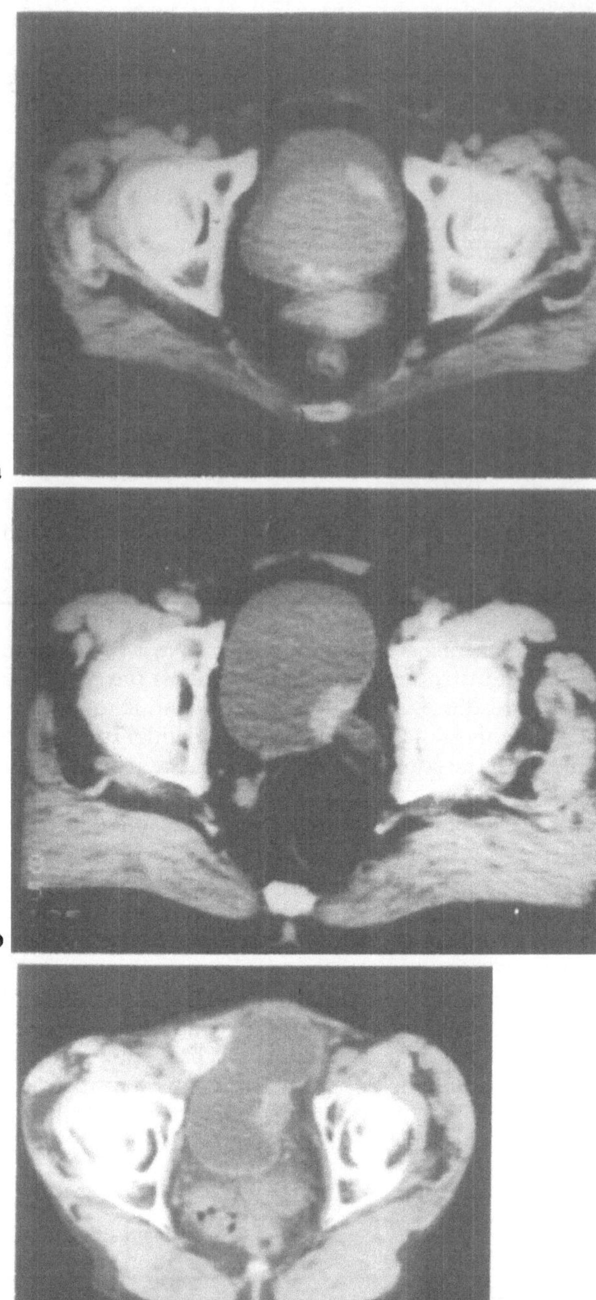

Fig. 5.6a–e. CT scanning in bladder cancer. **a** Multifocal superficial tumours; **b** invasive tumour partially obstructing the ureter; **c** invasive tumour in a bladder diverticulum; **d** tumour invading the seminal vesicles (T4a); **e** lymph node metastases. (Courtesy of Dr. A. Dixon, University of Cambridge Medical School)

Fig. 5.6. *(continued)*

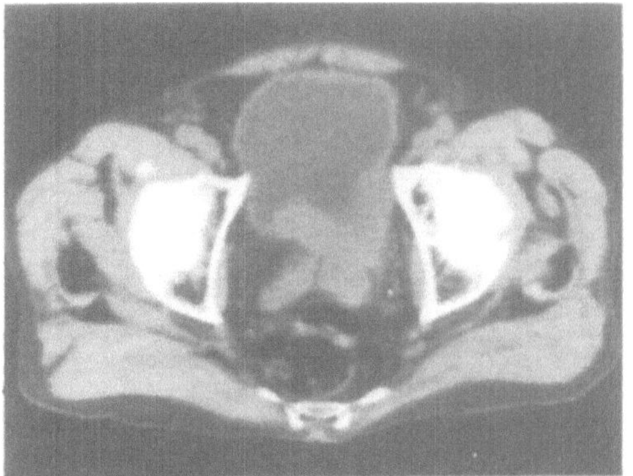

d

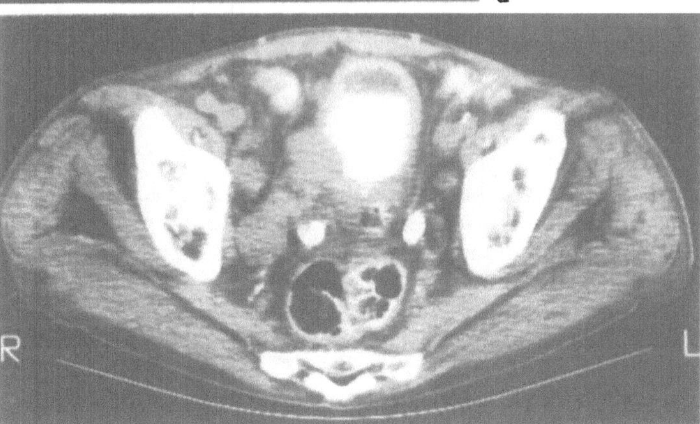

e

Intraluminal tumours of 1.5 cm minimum diameter can usually be identified in the low density urine, though the outline may be sharpened by contrast media or air. This is unnecessary with the newer scanners, though there is still some advantage in outlining the bowel with barium and the vagina with a tampon. Localised thickening or flattening of the bladder wall may be seen and indicates infiltration of the muscle (T2 or T3a). Haziness of the perivesical fat or irregularity of the wall suggest extension beyond the bladder (T3b). A contiguous increase in the tissue density extending to other viscera or the abdominal wall, or obliteration of the angle between the seminal vesicles and the bladder indicates that it is likely to be category T4 (Fig. 5.6a–d). CT can be helpful in the diagnosis and staging of a tumour in a diverticulum (Fig. 5.6c). However, it is not accurate in distinguishing the fact of muscle invasion nor its degree within the bladder wall. It therefore cannot separate a T2 tumour from a T3a tumour. Like other imaging methods it is particularly prone to overstage tumours following even limited operative diagnostic procedures, which can cause inflammation and fibrosis in and around the bladder wall. In advanced disease (T3b and T4), CT imaging becomes more accurate in identifying tumour which has invaded through the bladder wall and beyond (Table 5.1). Here it is definitely superior to the bimanual examination.

Table 5.1. Correlation between the histopathological and CT classification in 77 patients with bladder cancer (Vock et al. 1982)

P	N	CT		
		T<3b	T3b	T4
<3b	52	38	13	1
3b	15	1	14	0
4	10	0	0	10

Concordance: 81%

In the future, improved specificity for lesser degrees of invasion can be expected with the more advanced machines and by ensuring that scanning is done before TUR or biopsy. Its position on the flow chart in Fig. 5.3 is therefore immediately above the point at which a diagnosis of invasive bladder cancer is confirmed.

Metastases

Lymph Node Metastases. The lymphatic drainage of the bladder is shown in Fig. 5.7. The frequency of lymph node metastases corresponds to the progression of the primary tumour, being approximately 25% for tumours within the bladder wall and 60% or more when extension is beyond (see Fig. 5.6e and Chap. 2, pp. 40–41). Accuracy in identification of involved lymph nodes is therefore vital if radical surgery is to be avoided in hopelessly advanced tumours; CT may be more accurate than lymphography (Table 5.2). It may have a particular advantage in that regional nodes in the internal iliac and obturator groups can be identified (Lee et al. 1978; Walsh et al. 1980). It must be realised that the two techniques describe different features of the involved lymph node; CT demonstrates only distortion of the capsule of the node or overall enlargement, whilst lymphography is more sensitive to early changes in the internal architecture caused by metastases.

Distant Metastases (see also section on 'M' staging, p. 104). The CT scan may be extended above the aortic bifurcation to give considerable additional information on the para-aortic nodes and other sites of potential metastatic involvement such as the liver and lungs, but this prolongs the study and increases the cost considerably. It is therefore not justified as a routine unless indicated by other abnormal findings, e.g. elevated liver function tests or ureteric displacement on urography.

Table 5.2. Accuracy of lymphography and CT classification of lymphatic spread in bladder cancer. Both forms of imaging related to histopathological assessment (Vock et al. 1982)

	N	True +	False –	True –	False +	Sensitivity (%)	Specificity (%)	Accuracy (%)
CT	44	16	1	23	4	94	85	89
Lymphography	29	6	7	15	1	46	94	72

Response to Treatment

The rapid and reliable assessment of tumour 'down-staging' by radiotherapy may be of major importance in the early selection of patients for radical cystectomy as opposed to continuing with radiotherapy to a radical dose (van der Werf-Messing 1973). Unfortunately, CT scanning cannot reliably distinguish inflammation and fibrosis around the tumour from the tumour itself. Hence CT can only have a limited role in monitoring the response to radiotherapy.

A second use for CT is in the evaluation of the patient after cystectomy (Lee et al. 1981). This is probably the best technique for distinguishing local recurrent growth from haematoma, urinoma or abscess formation. Although recurrent growth is invariably a poor prognostic sign, its detection may assume greater importance with the development of more effective chemotherapeutic agents. Should local metastases be symptomatic they can be more effectively controlled by radiotherapy if accurately delineated, and here again CT is the best non-invasive imaging technique.

Summary

In the staging of the primary bladder tumour CT becomes more accurate with progression of the tumour beyond category T3a and is certainly more reliable than bimanual examination, particularly in the obese patient. There is little doubt that the accuracy of CT is adversely affected by previous endoscopic surgery and radiotherapy. In the identification of lymphatic metastases, CT can be said to be complementary to lymphography in that the combination gives high specificity and sensitivity.

Lymphography

The increasing popularity of ultrasound and CT scanning may render the investigative technique of lymphography obsolete. Bipedal lymphography can produce excellent visualisation of the external, common iliac and para-aortic lymph nodes. However, the lymphatic drainage of the bladder is first to the perivesical and then to the obturator and internal iliac groups of nodes (Fig. 5.7). It is precisely these nodes which lymphography fails to demonstrate reliably. Published reports show considerable variation in accuracy (Higgs and Macdonald 1968; Lang 1969; Wajsman et al. 1975; Macdonald and Paxton 1976; Turner et al. 1976; Hall 1980; Vinje 1980). One large series reported an accurate correlation with histology in 90% of patients, suggesting that the investigation should always be done in the management of bladder cancer. Subsequent studies may have been subject to more critical appraisal and they emphasise the drawbacks. Discussion of accuracy in correlating clinical with histological variables must be qualified by examining in turn sensitivity and specificity. In the case of lymphography, radiographs and histology of pelvic lymph nodes should be compared node by node. Unfortunately, the criteria for deciding what is abnormal are ill defined, and even experienced radiologists frequently disagree (Hall 1980). To some extent this may derive from the fact that degenerative or lipomatous changes are more common in the older age groups. The specificity of lymphography can be

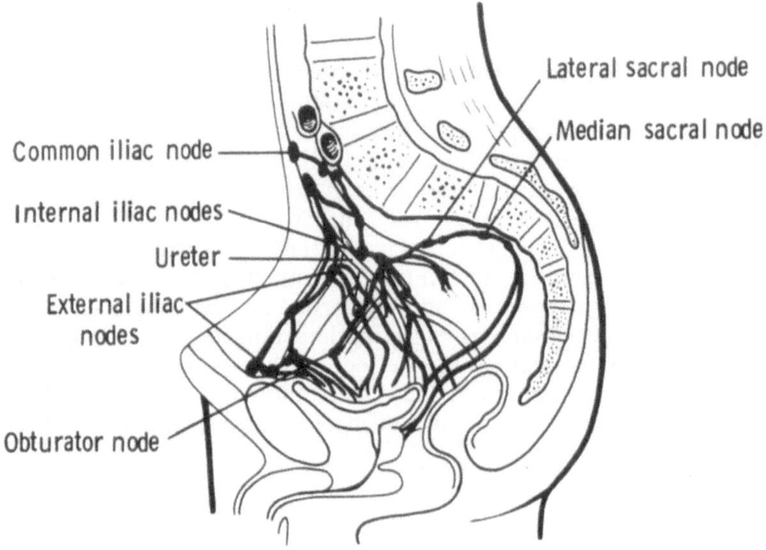

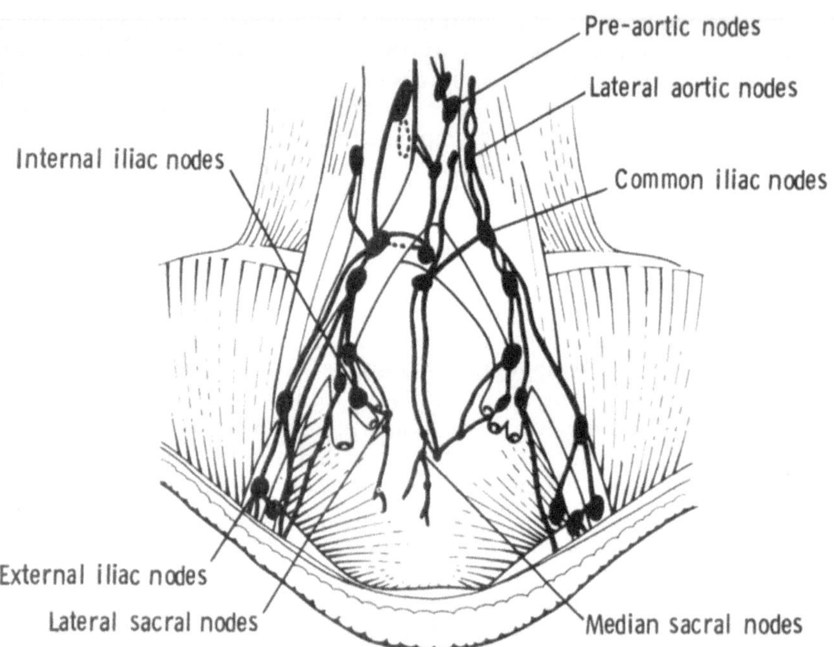

Fig. 5.7a,b. The lymphatic drainage of the bladder. **a** Lateral view; **b** anterior view

improved by treating the lymphangiogram as a dynamic investigation and repeating the films after 4–6 weeks to assess changes in the lymph nodes and perhaps growth of nodal metastases, but such a lengthy delay before a firm diagnosis is established is unacceptable. Lymphangiography is usually compared with the histology of selected lymph nodes rather than with a complete group, which can be obtained only by careful radical lymphadenectomy or by post-mortem dissection. This could certainly lead to apparent false positives. It is now agreed that the false negative rate for lymphangiography is high (poor sensitivity), whereas the false positive rate is lower (reasonable specificity). Thus a positive lymphangiogram may be helpful in combination with other investigations; a negative result contributes rather little.

Fine Needle Aspiration of Pelvic Lymph Nodes

It is likely that the role of both CT scanning and lymphography in the assessment of pelvic lymph nodes will be to demonstrate their position so that fine needle puncture can be performed and the node aspirated for cytological examination. In this respect both investigations may be complementary, but the most important factor may prove to be the accuracy with which these nodes can be punctured (Zornoza et al. 1977; MacIntosh et al. 1979; Zornoza et al. 1981; Wajsman et al. 1982). The major therapeutic decisions regarding surgery, chemotherapy and radiotherapy can only be made if suspicious lymph nodes are shown either histologically or cytologically to contain metastases.

Angiography

For most clinicians pelvic angiography has little to offer in the diagnosis and staging of bladder cancer. However, in some centres it has become established as a second line of investigation. In practice, even the most experienced radiologists find that it is inaccurate in diagnosing early progression and has little advantage over less invasive methods for the more advanced tumours. Moreover, chronic inflammatory disease, tumours of the dome or base of the bladder invading the prostate and the presence of multiple tumours can limit its accuracy (Nilsson 1967; Winterberger et al. 1972; Murphy 1978). In the study by Lang (1980), clinicopathological staging was more accurate for superficial tumours but equal to angiography for those invasive within the bladder wall. The results of this study compare very favourably with the best that can be achieved for tumour staging by CT, but they represent the work of an enthusiast and are unlikely to be emulated.

Hypogastric artery cannulation and angiography may, however, have a role to play in the management of advanced disease for regional perfusion with cytotoxic drugs in high doses or with embolisation of the vesical arteries in cases of intractable haemorrhage (see Chap. 11, p. 274).

Ultrasound

The rapid development of ultrasonographic techniques may, to some extent, have limited the enthusiasm which might otherwise have been due to computed tomography (Barnett and Morley 1976). When both techniques are available to the urologist, there are situations (e.g. the investigation of the renal lump) where a place can be found for each on the flow chart of investigations. The value of external ultrasound in the diagnosis of bladder cancer is equivocal. The situation in which a chance diagnosis of a bladder tumour might be made on ultrasound can only be theoretical, since the initial identification of the growth will always be confirmed by urography, cystoscopy and biopsy. Ultrasound can occasionally make a contribution as an entirely non-invasive technique for staging of bladder cancer (Resnick and Boyce 1979). In a recent survey, Kyle (1982) reported rates of accuracy as high as 85% for early invasive (T2/T3) growths, far surpassing other techniques in this important group of tumours. Nearly comparable results were obtained by Winterberger and Murphy (1974). Unfortunately, more than for any other investigation performed by radiologists the interpretation is highly dependent upon the skill and experience of the investigator, particularly for lesions deep in the pelvis (Morley 1978).

The transrectal probe is less effective in the investigation of bladder tumours than in prostatic carcinoma, where very encouraging results have been obtained. In the study of Harada et al. (1977) extravesical spread was observed in only 67% of proven T4 bladder tumours. Better results have been obtained by transurethral scanning employing a probe incorporated in the cystoscope—a technique developed in Denmark (Holm and Northerved 1974) and in Japan (Nakamura and Niijima 1980, 1981). Whilst a direct comparison has not been made, transurethral ultrasound used by experienced operators is probably comparable with CT in assessing the extent of invasion by a tumour (Schüller et al. 1982). It is equally difficult to distinguish mucosa from muscle, and therefore the fact of invasion is still impossible to establish by a non-invasive technique. Results can also be impaired by gross trabeculation, and the delineation of tumours of the bladder base can be imprecise (Gammelgaard and Holm 1980). Ultrasound cannot differentiate fibrosis caused by treatment from an advancing tumour; however, like CT, ultrasound is effective in identifying tumours in a diverticulum.

'M' Staging

Most clinicians restrict their routine search for metastases to examination of regional and juxtaregional lymph nodes by lymphography, CT scanning and percutaneous node aspiration. A chest radiograph should always be obtained, and the liver function tests, estimation of serum calcium and alkaline phosphatase, together with the isoenzymes if they are elevated, should always be done. A full blood count can provide valuable information, as anaemia is usually a sinister sign of chronic ill-health, though occasionally it can be very specific, e.g. the leucoerythroblastic anaemia of bone marrow infiltration. Similarly a raised erythrocyte sedimentation rate (ESR) in the absence of an obvious acute cause often indicates metastatic disease. The more meticulous the search the more likely are occult metastases to be detected. Murphy (1978) recommended isotopic and radiological bone surveys, bone marrow aspiration for malignant cells and liver scanning, though Lindner and deKernion (1982) found that routine pre-cystectomy radioisotope scans were not cost effective (see also Chap. 6, p. 134). The discovery of metastases should preclude radical treatment, though some surgeons may hope to clear involved regional lymph nodes despite the appalling prognosis. Skeletal involvement occurs terminally and is often symptomatic (Fig. 5.8). Transitional cell carcinoma should probably be added to the list of five primary tumours commonly metastasising to bone, but this assertion may be based on rather misleading evidence. As many as 20% of patients with metastatic disease have skeletal involvement (Murphy 1978; Babaian et al. 1980). The literature is less explicit on the proportion of patients with invasive bladder cancer

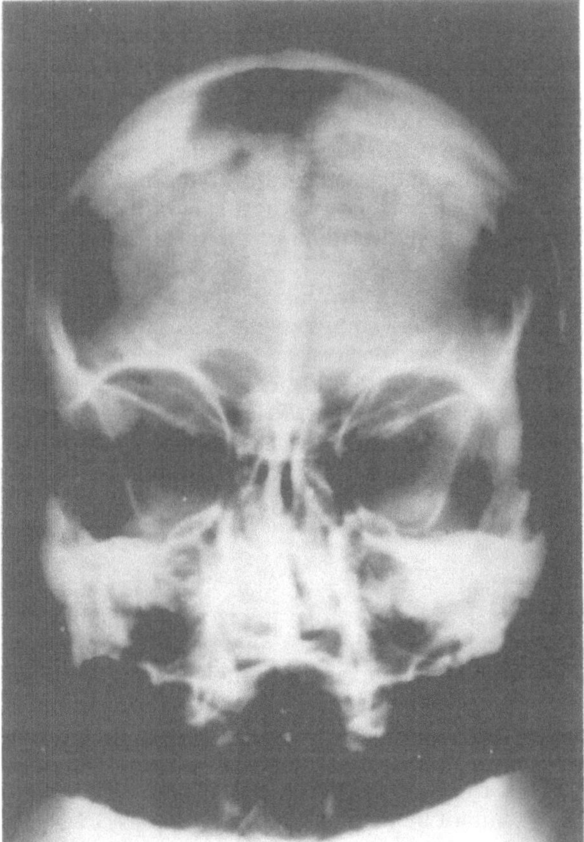

Fig. 5.8. Osteolytic metastasis from carcinoma of the bladder. Patient presented with a discharging lump on the scalp and a frontal lobe disorder

whose asymptomatic bone metastases have precluded treatment. The proportion is likely to be lower than for carcinoma of the breast or prostate, and therefore routine skeletal surveys may not be justified.

Endoscopic Assessment

Technique of Cystourethroscopy

The patient suspected of having a bladder tumour must always be cystoscoped. This procedure should include examination of the urethra and bladder neck. Before the introduction of modern instruments employing fibreoptic illumination and the Hopkins rod lens system, this required use of separate instruments for panendoscopy and cystoscopy. Nowadays most urologists prefer 'to see their way' through the urethra using the direct viewing 0° to 30° telescope and, after entering the bladder, to complete the examination with a 70° telescope. Alternatively a 30° telescope can be used for the whole examination, though special care will then be required to ensure that the anterior wall of the bladder is fully examined. The general availability of a basic kit allows the urologist to examine rapidly the lower urinary tract, biopsy suspicous areas of mucosa and, if necessary, insert ureteric catheters for sampling of upper tract urine and ureterography if there is any doubt that a renal pelvic or ureteric neoplasm coexists. For all these separate procedures the same cystoscope sheath can be used, and trauma to the urethra is thereby minimised.

Availability to the urologist of on-table screening in the operating room provides a facility for more rapid diagnosis and allows ascending ureterography to be done with a bulb-ended catheter. This is in preference to the standard ureteric catheter which must be inserted some way up the ureter, a procedure which is neccessary if the patient has to be moved to the X-ray department. The recent introduction of the ureterorenoscope should now allow visualisation of the ureter and pelvicaliceal system in patients whose ureteric orifices can be suitably dilated.

Anaesthesia

If it seems certain from preoperative investigation that the patient has a bladder tumour, anaesthetic preparation should be such as to allow safe transurethral surgery and adequate relaxation for bimanual examination. This usually entails endotracheal intubation, artificial ventilation and full muscle relaxation. Spinal or extradural anaesthetic can also be used, though it should be remembered that paralysis of lower abdominal musculature entails a block to cord segments as high as T-10. If a large tumour is likely to be encountered, blood should be cross-matched. Clearly these provisions cannot be made on an operating list for every patient who could possibly have a bladder tumour. It is therefore desirable that the urologist should be forewarned. For this reason, and also to facilitate interpretation of non-invasive staging procedures without artefact introduced by treatment, it is preferable that the patient is investigated as fully as possible before surgery.

One exception to this rule may be the patient with recurrent haematuria for which no cause has been apparent. It can be well worth the effort to arrange an emergency cystoscopy during a bleeding episode to identify the source.

In many units diagnostic cystoscopy is done as an outpatient procedure with local urethral anaesthesia. On the continent of Europe these diagnostic procedures are usually done by private urologists, often on an outpatient basis, and this has some advantage in terms of saving anaesthetic and recovery facilities. In general, it is easy to perform in women and possible in men, provided there is no bladder neck obstruction. However, it can be a painful, frightening and embarrassing experience. A patient undergoing this procedure may well be reluctant to return for the long programme of follow-up examinations necessary when bladder cancer is diagnosed. In any case, muscle relaxation cannot be induced, and biopsy and electroresection is impossible. Cystoscopy under local anaesthesia is therefore best avoided if a tumour is suspected, unless the patient's general medical state precludes general anaesthesia or a regional block. In most cases it is unnecessary where day-case theatre facilities are available. The possibility of using small-calibre flexible fibreoptic instruments for cystoscopy has yet to be fully explored, but they could facilitate examination under local anaesthesia and the procedure may once again become popular.

Medium for Cystoscopy

The standard medium for cystoscopy has always been water. However, the small risk of absorption and haemolysis should always be borne in mind. The water should be exchanged for an isotonic, non-ionic solution if an extensive resection is contemplated.

There is some advantage in using carbon dioxide as the medium for cystoscopy in cases in which there is bleeding from a tumour and the bladder is very dirty, when the view through water would always be clouded (Matthews et al. 1983). The insufflation apparatus for laparoscopy can easily be adapted for the standard cystoscope and can be used safely in the bladder.

Describing the Bladder Tumour

At the initial cystoscopy the following points should be recorded:

1. The number of bladder tumours.
2. The site of bladder tumours. These should be mapped out on a chart immediately after cystoscopy. It is important to note their relationship to the ureteric orifices and also to any diverticula which may be present.
3. The size of the tumours. This is often difficult to assess on the inside of the bladder, but the width of the resectoscope loop (7 mm for a 24 French gauge loop) can be used as a measure.
4. The growth pattern—whether the tumour is papillary or solid or both.
5. The base of the tumour—whether it is sessile or pedunculated and its size.
6. The presence of necrosis or calcification.
7. The surrounding mucosa and any changes in the mucosa distant from the tumour. These should be biopsied.

These details were formerly regarded as having considerable prognostic significance in the older tumour registries. They may still be of use in formal research investigations, but in general urological practice the treatment of bladder cancer is determined by stage and grade. Multiplicity is only important in the broadest sense in influencing the choice of cytotoxic drug therapy and occasionally forcing the surgeon to recommend cystectomy when the tumours are so numerous as to defy local control.

The procedure for taking biopsies and resecting bladder tumours is discussed fully in Chapter 8 (see p. 167). If cystoscopy shows no tumour in the bladder cancer follow-up, or if a case of carcinoma in situ is being followed up, the bladder can be 'sampled' by saline barbotage for cytological examination. Using the standard rubber connecting piece and a bladder syringe 50 ml saline can be vigorously injected and withdrawn from the bladder; this procedure should be repeated at least three times and the sample sent for immediate cytological examination.

Bimanual Examination

Pelvic examination should be done before the cystoscopy and resection of the tumour, but this is only useful if it is suspected that the tumour is deeply infiltrating. Occasionally, neoplasms of other pelvic organs, e.g. rectum, cervix and prostate, will be found on this preliminary examination. Such tumours can invade the bladder wall and produce changes which can be difficult to distinguish from a primary urothelial tumor. It is obviously important that the surgeon is forewarned of this before cystoscopy. However, vigorous examination may result in unnecessary bleeding, which will obscure the vision on cystoscopy. It is the bimanual examination after resection of the exophytic portion of the tumour that is essential for the categorisation of the tumour, although the UICC rules require this to be done both before and after the TUR.

Following endoscopic resection and before insertion of the catheter the bladder is carefully palpated bimanually between a finger in the rectum or vagina and the operator's other hand applied firmly over the abdomen. Any residual tumour is carefully palpated to determine its depth of invasion, if it is invading adjacent organs or is fixed to the pelvic wall. Such a clinical assessment depends very much on the experience of the operator for its accuracy. The possible sources of error have been summarised (Wallace 1976); poor abdominal relaxation, particularly in the obese patient commonly invalidates the examination. Unfortunately, bimanual examination is often done as an afterthought when the patient is waking and coughing during extubation. The bladder should be empty and commonly is not. Even when care is taken with these factors tumours may still be missed when situated on the anterior wall behind the symphysis pubis or even in the vault if the abdominal hand palpates too low.

Early authors concluded that the accuracy of clinical staging was disappointing and concurred with the pathological stage in the excised bladder in no more than 50% of cases (Marshall 1952; see Chap. 6 for literature review). Later studies were in general agreement. Kenney et al. (1970) showed concurrence in only 44% of 105 cases with invasive cancer. They demonstrated how thickening in the bladder wall and perivesical tissues resulting from previous treatment, particularly radiotherapy, could be misinterpreted. In their series 40% of cases were understaged before treatment and the same proportion were overstaged after treatment.

Screening

Intuitively it is felt that early investigation of potentially sinister symptoms will lead to the diagnosis of cancer at an early, and therefore curable, stage. However, the results of such a strategy have been generally disappointing. For bladder cancer the provision of 'haematuria clinics' has been thought justified (Wallace and Harris 1965; Turner et al. 1977; Hendry et al. 1981), but the data hardly support this conclusion. Another proposition is that the detection of disease in the preclinical stage by mass screening techniques might be more effective in the control of cancer than 'symptom clinics' with open referral. The benefits of a screening programme can only be assessed by a reduction in mortality. To achieve this, huge numbers of tests may be required. The cost of evaluation will rise with the inevitable presentation of false positives. It has been calculated that in the USA a 50% reduction in mortality from bladder cancer would involve 60 million tests a year, generating 60000 false positives (Morrison 1979). Clearly the cost effectiveness can be improved by examining high-risk groups. The efficacy of such a programme in reducing mortality then depends upon the sensitivities and specificities of risk factors and of the screening methods. It is also influenced by the invasive potential of the tumour or dysplastic epithelial lesions and the efficiency of the follow-up procedure in detecting early progressive disease.

Screening techniques which are at present available and feasible in terms of cost and patient acceptability entail use of impregnated reagent sticks for occult haematuria, urine microscopy and urine cytological examination. Epidemiological high-risk factors used to select groups for screening include exposure to industrial carcinogens, notably the aryl hydrocarbons used in the dye, rubber and cable industries (Hueper 1969; Cole et al. 1972; Davies et al. 1976; Kipling 1976; Lower 1982); employment in industries (e.g. gas, leather) which involve exposure to unidentified carcinogens and have a high risk of bladder cancer; bilharzial infection; analgesic abuse; and heavy cigarette smoking. Other epidemiological factors of potential importance in transitional cell carcinogenesis include artificial sweeteners and chlorination of drinking water. However, the risk is too slight to warrant screening of populations at risk (Doll and Peto 1981).

Cytology

Occupational Bladder Cancer

Urine cytology is the most familiar technique for screening large populations for bladder cancer, although it is neither so effective, nor its use so widespread, as cervical cytology in carcinoma of the cervix. There is now much information available from workers in the chemical industry that has accumulated over many years. Abnormal cytological results leading to full urological evaluation have been reported in 10–70 of 1000 specimens with a false positive rate varying from 10.5% to 15% (Crabbe et al. 1956; El-Bolkainy 1980). The benefits in terms of reduced mortality are still arguable, since a considerable follow-up period is required. From a recent study it was concluded that survival was in fact prolonged in a screened group because more early-stage disease was being diagnosed (Cartwright et al. 1981). Unfortunately, this result was obtained for uncensored data from relatively small numbers of patients. Nevertheless, it is a significant contribution to the literature, which needs to be confirmed.

Bilharzia

The association between bladder cancer and *Schistosoma haematobium* infestation is familiar to most urologists, though the causative factor remains obscure. Bilharzia is common in Egypt (approximately 85% of the population has been infected at some time) and to a lesser extent in other parts of Africa and Arabia. Moreover, carcinoma of the bilharzial bladder is very common (11%–40% of all malignant tumours) where the disease is endemic (Gelfand 1977). A screening programme is therefore likely to be effective. In one such study on the peasant population living in the Nile Delta, 7 patients with carcinoma were identified in 3300 individuals screened (El-Bolkainy et al. 1974).

Phenacetin

Urothelial cancer, with papillary necrosis and interstitial nephropathy, is a complication of excessive use of analgesics containing phenacetin. The association was first established in Sweden and then confirmed in publications from other countries (Bengtsson et al. 1978). It has been estimated that urothelial tumours occur 13 times as frequently in abusers (those taking approximately a 1 kg cumulative dose) than in the normal population. The frequencies for the separate parts of the urinary tract were 77 times for the renal pelvis, 89 times for the ureter and in the bladder 7 times as frequently as in the normal population (Mihatsch et al. 1980). The mechanism of carcinogenesis is likely to be similar to that following exposure to industrial carcinogens (see Chap. 1, p. 7). The induction period in both groups of carcinogens is approximately 20 years. Furthermore, phenacetin is an aromatic amide with an *N*-hydroxylated metabolite related to known industrial carcinogens such as the naphthylamines. In communities prone to analgesic abuse such as are found in Sweden, Switzerland and Australia, the high risk of urothelial cancer would justify a mass screening programme, particularly as such tumours can present many years after administration of the drug has ceased.

Balkan Nephropathy

Transitional cell carcinoma, particularly in the upper urinary tract, is very prevalent in certain parts of Yugoslavia (Petkovic 1975). As in phenacetin abuse, the disease is associated with an interstitial nephropathy. The cause is obscure. Once again, in a population having a large proportion at risk a mass screening programme seems justified.

Random Populations

It is arguable whether screening for a relatively rare disease in the general population is justified on economic grounds (Morrison 1979). The standard techniques of urine cytology are laborious and probably not suitable for screening of large populations (Dimette et al. 1955). The development of automated procedures in cytology, such as flow cytometry, may allow a much wider application of screening urine for malignant cells. Alternatively, the more rapid staining techniques using toluidine blue may increase the number of urine samples that can be examined. In one such survey three cases of bladder cancer were observed from 16062 urine samples selected at random from non-urological patients (Nemoto et al. 1981). Restricting screening facilities to older males also increases the proportion of diagnosed cases of bladder cancer and therefore the cost effectiveness of the programme.

Haematuria

Cytology is established as the only method suitable for screening large populations, yet there is still wide variation in the reported accuracy, due in part to laboratory error in cell preparation but mainly to the differing skills amongst cytologists (Umiker 1964; Theologidis et al. 1971). To some extent this may be rectified by the use of automated techniques of flow cytometry.

On the other hand, haematuria is the presenting symptom in the majority of patients with urothelial cancer, and a logical approach would be to screen populations for the presence of microscopic haematuria. A mass screening programme could be based easily and cheaply on stick testing for haematuria. The sensitivity of every batch of sticks would need to be tested on a standard urine and blood solution. Although the feasibility of such a study has been successfully tested (Freni et al. 1977 a,b), the value of this technique has still to be confirmed in a large-scale prospective study backed up by full urological investigation of all stick-positive cases (Freni and Freni-Titulaer 1977).

Conclusion

It seems unlikely that the morbidity and mortality from bladder cancer will fall significantly as a result of earlier referral or from refinement in existing diagnostic techniques. There have certainly been developments in the assessment of advancing or advanced disease, but their effect is diminished in the face of the generally poor results of the treatment regimens available at present. As soon as an effective systemic therapy becomes available, perhaps in conjunction with improvements in radiotherapeutic techniques, then the diagnosis and staging of established disease will become more critical. Of the available techniques discussed, transurethral ultrasonography and CT scanning are likely to prove the most helpful, provided that they are evaluated by experienced urologists and radiologists and before patients are examined and treated endoscopically. The development of urinary flow cytometry may allow this examination to become routine in diagnosis and follow-up. The development of nuclear magnetic resonance (NMR) scanning is awaited with interest by urologists and uroradiologists.

Early diagnosis before clinical presentation should be the goal, but screening should be limited to manageable numbers by choosing groups of individuals at risk. Unfortunately, such high-risk occupations and habituations account for only a small proportion of patients with bladder cancer. Until a very definite fall in the mortality can be discerned in prospective trials on such patients at risk it is doubtful whether large-scale screening is justified. If so, then screening for haematuria using a standardised sensitive 'stick' test would seem the most appropriate investigation.

References

Allegra SR, Broderick PA, Corvese NL (1972) Cytologic and histologenetic observations in well-differentiated transitional carcinoma of the bladder. J Urol 107: 777–782

Alsabti EA (1979) Prognostic value of urinary fibrinogen degradation products in bladder carcinoma. Eur Surg Res 11: 185–190

Altaffer LF (1982) Paraneoplastic endocrinopathies associated with non-renal genitourinary tumours. J Urol 127: 411–416

Appell RA, Flynn JT, Paris AMI, Blandy JP (1980) Occult bacterial colonisation of bladder tumours. J Urol 124: 345–346

Babaian R, Johnson DF, Llamas L, Ayala AG (1980) Metastases from transitional cell carcinoma of the urinary bladder. Urology 16: 142–144

Barnett E, Morley P (1976) Ultrasound. In: Chisholm GD, Williams DI (eds) Scientific foundations of urology. Heinemann, London, pp 446–458

Bengtsson V, Johansson S, Angervall L (1978) Malignancies of the urinary tract and their relation to analgesic abuse. Kidney Int 13: 107–113

Booth CM, Kellett MJ (1981) Intravenous urography in the follow-up of carcinoma of the bladder. Br J Urol 53: 246–249

Cartwright RA, Cadian T, Garland JB, Bernard SM (1981) The influence of malignant cell cytology screening on the survival of industrial bladder cancer cases. J Epidemiol Community Health 35: 35–38

Chowaniec J, Hicks RM (1977) Ultrastructural changes in experimentally induced bladder tumours. Br J Cancer 35: 254

Cole P, Hoover R, Friedell GN (1972) Occupation and cancer of the lower urinary tract. Cancer 29: 1250–1260

Colleen S, Ek A, Gullberg B, Johansson BG, Lindberg LG, Olsson A (1979) Carcinoembryonic antigen in urine in patients with urothelial carcinomas. Scand J Urol Nephrol 13: 149–153

Colleen S, Ekelund L, Henriksson H, Karp W, Mansson W (1981) Staging of bladder carcinoma with computed tomography. Scand J Urol Nephrol 15: 109–114

Cooper EH, Anderson CK, Steele L, O'Boyle P (1973) Assessment of bladder cancer. Cancer 32: 1263–1266

Crabbe JGS, Cresdee WC, Scott TS, Williams MHC (1956) The cytological diagnosis of bladder tumours amongst dye stuff workers. Br J Industr Med 13: 270–276

Davies JM, Somerville SM, Wallace DM (1976) Occupational bladder tumour cases identified during ten years' interviewing of patients. Br J Urol 48: 561–566

de Voogt HJ, Rathert P, Beyer-Boon ME (eds) (1977) Urinary cytology. Springer, Berlin Heidelberg New York

Dimmette RM, Sproat WF, Klimt CR (1955) Examination of smears of urinary sediment for detection of neoplasms of the bladder. Am J Clin Pathol 25: 1032–1042

Doll R, Peto R (1981) The causes of cancer. Oxford University Press, Oxford

Droller MJ (1981) Prostaglandins and neoplasia. J Urol 125: 757–760

El-Bolkainy MN (1980) Cytology of bladder carcinoma. J Urol 124: 20–22

El-Bolkainy MN, Ghoneim MA, El-Masery BA, Nasr SM (1974) Carcinoma of the bilharzial bladder. Diagnostic value of urine cytology. Urology 3: 319–323

Esposti PL (1981) Urinary cytology for diagnosis, grading and monitoring response to treatment. In: Oliver RTD, Hendry WF, Bloom HJG (eds) Bladder cancer: principles of combination therapy, Butterworths, London, pp 9–17

Esposti PL, Zajicek J (1972) Grading of transitional cell neoplasms of the urinary bladder from smears of bladder washings. A critical review of 326 tumours. Acta Cytol (Baltimore) 16: 529–537

Esposti PL, Moberger G, Zajicek J (1970) The cytologic diagnosis of transitional cell tumours of the urinary bladder and its histologic basis. A study of 567 cases of urinary-tract disorder including 170 untreated and 182 irradiated bladder tumours. Acta Cytol (Baltimore) 14: 145–155

Esposti PL, Tribukait B, Gustafson H (1978) Effects of local treatment with Adriamycin in carcinoma in situ of the urinary bladder: cell morphology and DNA analysis for quantification of malignant cells. In: Edsmyr F (ed) Diagnosis and treatment of superficial urinary bladder tumours. WHO, Montedison, Stockholm

Frable WT, Paxson L, Barksdale JA, Koong WW (1977) Current practice of urinary bladder cytology. Cancer Res 37: 2800–2805

Freni SC, Freni-Titulaer WJ (1977) Microhaematuria found by mass screening of apparently healthy males. Acta Cytol 21: 421–423

Freni SC, Heedrik GJ, Hol C (1977a) Centrifugation techniques and reagent strips in the assessment of microhaematuria. J Clin Pathol 30: 336–340

Freni SC, Dalderup LM, Oudegeest JJ, Wensveen N (1977b) Erythrocyturia, smoking and occupation. J Clin Pathol 30: 341–344

Gammelgaard J, Holm HH (1980) Transurethral and transrectal ultrasound scanning in urology. J Urol 124: 863–868

Gelfand M (1977) Significant advances in the management of bilharzia. Cent Afr J Med 23 (suppl II): 1–2

Hall RR (1980) Lymphangiography in advanced bladder cancer. In: Pavone-Macaluso MP, Smith PW, Edsmyr F (eds) Bladder tumours and other topics in urological oncology, Plenum, New York

Hall RR, Laurence DJR, Neville AM, Wallace DM (1973) Carcinoembryonic antigen and urothelial carcinoma. Br J Urol 45: 88–92

Hamlin DJ, Cockett ATK, Burgener FA (1981) Computed tomography of the pelvis: sagittal and coronal image reconstruction in the evaluation of infiltrative bladder carcinoma. J Comput Ass Tomogr 5: 27–33

Harada K, Ingari D, Tanahashi Y, Watanage H, Saiton M, Mishina T (1977) Staging of bladder tumours by means of transrectal ultrasonography. J Clin Ultrasound 5: 388–392

Harris MJ, Schwinn CP, Morrow IW, Gray RL, Browell BM (1971) Exfoliative cytology of the urinary bladder irrigation specimen. Acta Cytol (Baltimore) 15: 385–399

Hemmingsen L, Rasmussen F, Skaarup P, Wolf H (1981) Urinary protein profiles in patients with urothelial bladder tumours. Br J Urol 53: 324–329

Hendry WF, Manning N, Perry NM, Whitfield HN, Wickham JEA (1981) The effects of a haematuria service in the early diagnosis of bladder cancer. In: Oliver RTD, Hendry WF, Bloom HJG (eds) Bladder cancer: principles of combination therapy. Butterworths, London, pp 19–25

Heney NM, Szyfelbein WM, Daly JJ, Prout GR, Bredin HC (1977) Positive urinary cytology in patients without evident tumour. J Urol 117: 223–224

Hennessey PT, Hurst RE, Hemstreet GP, Cutter G (1981) Urinary glycosoaminoglycans excretion as a biochemical marker in patients with bladder carcinoma. Cancer Res 41: 3868–3873

Higgs B, Macdonald JS (1968) Lymphography in the management of urinary tract tumours. Br J Urol 40: 727–735

Holm HH, Northerved A (1974) Transurethral ultrasonic scanner. J Urol 111: 238–241

Hueper WC (1969) Occupational and environmental cancers of the urinary system. Yale University Press, New Haven, Conn

Jeffrey RB, Palubinskas AJ, Federle MP (1981) CT evaluation of invasive lesions of the bladder. J Comput Ass Tomogr 5: 22–26

Jewett HJ, Strong GH (1946) Infiltrating carcinoma of the bladder. J Urol 55: 366–372

Kellett MJ, Oliver RTD, Husband JE, Kelsey-Fry I (1980) CT scanning as an adjunct to bimanual examination for staging bladder tumours. Br J Urol 52: 101–106

Kenney GM, Hardner GJ, Murphy GP (1970) Clinical staging of bladder tumours. J Urol 104: 720–723

Kipling MD (1976) Occupational considerations in carcinoma of the urogenital tract. Br J Hosp Med 15: 465–472

Klein FA, Herr HW, Whitmore WF, Sogani PC, Melamed MR (1982a) An evaluation of automated flow cytometry (FCM) in detection of carcinoma in situ of the urinary bladder. Cancer 50: 1003–1008

Klein FA, Whitmore WF, Herr HW, Melamed MR (1982b) Flow cytometry follow-up of patients with low stage bladder tumours. J Urol 128: 88–92

Kunit G, Wirl G, Frick J (1980) Collagenase activity in human bladder cancer. In: Pavone-Macaluso M, Smith PW, Edsmyr F (eds) Bladder tumours and other topics in urological oncology, Plenum, New York, pp 107–111

Kyle KF (1982) Ultrasound staging of bladder tumours: a review after six years. Br J Urol 54: 65

Lang EK (1969) The roentgenographic assessment of bladder tumours: a comparison of the diagnostic accuracy of roentgenographic techniques. Cancer 23: 717–724

Lang EK (1980) Angiography in the diagnosis and staging of pelvic neoplasms. Radiology 134: 353–358

Lee JK, Stanley RJ, Sagel SS, McClennan BL (1978) Accuracy of C.T. in detecting intraabdominal and pelvic lymph node metastases from pelvic cancers. Am J Roentgenol Radium Ther Nucl Med 131: 675–679

Lee JK, McClennan BL, Stanley RJ, Levitt RG, Sage SS (1981) Use of CT in evaluation of the post cystectomy patient. AJR 136: 483–488

Leistenschneider W, Nagel R (1980) Lavage cytology of renal pelvis and ureter with special reference to tumours. J Urol 124: 597–600
Lessing JA (1978) Bladder cancer: Early diagnosis and evaluation of biologic potential. A review of newer methods. J Urol 120: 1–5
Lewis RW, Jackson AL, Murphy WM, LeBlanc GA, Meehan WL (1976) Cytology—diagnosis and follow up of transitional cell carcinoma of the urothelium. J Urol 116: 43–46
Lindner A, deKernion JB (1982) Cost-effective analysis of pre-cystectomy radioisotope scans. J Urol 128: 1181–1182
Lower GM (1982) Concepts in causality: chemically induced human urinary bladder cancer. Cancer 49: 1056–1066
McKay HA, Gavrell GJ, Meehan WL, Kaplan RA, LeBlanc GA (1978) Prostaglandin mediated hypercalcaemia in transitional cell carcinoma of the bladder. J Urol 119: 689–692
Macdonald JS, Paxton RM (1976) Lymphography. In: Williams DI, Chisholm GD (eds) Scientific foundations of urology, vol II. Heinemann, London, pp 221–231
MacIntosh PK, Thomson KR, Barbaric ZL (1979) Percutaneous lymph node biopsy to improve lymphographic diagnosis. Radiology 131: 647–649
Marshall VF (1952) The relation of the pre-operative estimate to the pathological demonstration of the extent of vesical neoplasms. J Urol 68: 714–723
Marshall VF (1956) Current clinical problems regarding bladder tumours. Cancer 9: 543–550
Martinez-Piñeiro JA, Muntañola P, Martin MG, Gidalgo L (1977) Fluoroscein urinary cytology in bladder cancer. Eur Urol 3: 142–150
Matthews PN, Skewes DG, Kothari JJ, Woodhouse CRJ, Hendry WF (1983) Carbon dioxide versus water for cystoscopy: a comparative study. Br J Urol 55: 364–366
Mihatsch MJ, Manz T, Knusli HO, Hofer M, Rist M, Guetg R, Rutishauser G, Zollinger HU (1980) Phenacetinabusus III. Maligne Harnwegtumoren bei Phenacetinabusus in Basel (1963–1977). Schweiz Med Wochenschr 110: 255–264
Morley P (1978) Clinical staging of epithelial bladder tumours by echotomography. In: Hull CR, McCready JR, Cosgrove DO (eds) Utrasound on tumour diagnosis. Pitman, London, pp 145–161
Morrison AS (1979) Public health value of using epidemiological information to identify high risk groups for bladder cancer screening. Semin Oncol 6: 184–188
Motomiya Y, Owzono S, Shiomi T, Kondo T, Ijuin M, Okajima E (1979) Studies on lactic dehydrogenase of patients with urinary bladder tumours. Invest Urol 17: 120–124
Murphy GP (1978) Development in pre-operative staging of bladder tumors. Urology 11: 109–115
Nakamura S, Niijima T (1980) Staging of bladder cancer by ultrasonography: a new technique by transurethral intravesical scanning. J Urol 124: 341–344
Nakamura S, Niijima T (1981) Transurethral real time scanner. J Urol 125: 781–783
Nemoto R, Kato T, Shibata K, Kano M (1981) Urinary cytology as a test in mass screening. Tohoku J Exp Med 135: 115–116
Nilsson J (1967) Angiography in tumors of the urinary bladder. Acta Radiol [Diagn] (Stockh) Suppl 263
Petkovic SD (1975) Epidemiology and treatment of renal pelvic and ureteral tumours. J Urol 114: 858–865
Resnick MI, Boyce WH (1979) Ultrasonography of the urinary bladder, seminal vesicles and prostate. In: Resnick MI, Sanders RC (eds) Ultrasound in urology, Williams and Wilkins, Baltimore, pp 220–250
Schmidt JD, Weinstein SH (1976) Pitfalls in clinical staging of bladder tumours. Urol Clin North Am 3: 107–127
Schüller J, Walther E, Schmiedt E, Staehler G, Bauer HW, Schilling A (1982) Intravesical ultrasound tomography in staging bladder carcinoma. J Urol 128: 264–266
Seidelmann FE, Choen WN, Bryan PJ, Temes SP, Kraus D, Schoenrock G (1978) Accuracy of CT staging of bladder neoplasms using the gas filled method: report of 21 patients with surgical confirmation. Am J Roentgenol Radium Ther Nucl Med 130: 735–739
Sherwood T, Davidson AJ, Talner LB (1980) Uroradiology, Blackwell Scientific, Oxford, pp 291–294
Shevchuk MM, Fenoglio CM, Richart RM (1981) Carcinoembryonic antigen in benign and malignant transitional epithelium. Cancer 47: 899–905
Stanley RJ, Sage SS, Fair WR (1978) Computed tomography of the genitourinary tract. J Urol 119: 780–782
Stewart AF (1983) Therapy of malignancy associated hypercalcaemia. Am J Med 74: 475–480
Theologidis AD, Jameson RM, Scott A (1971) The reliability of urinary cytology. Br J Urol 43: 598–602
Tribukait B, Gustafson H, Esposti PL (1979) Ploidy and proliferation in human tumours as measured

by flow-cytofluorimetric DNA analysis and its relation to histopathology and cytology. Cancer 43: 1742–1751
Tribukait B, Gustafson H, Esposti PL (1982) The significance of ploidy and proliferation in the clinical and biological evaluation of bladder tumours. Br J Urol 54: 130–135
Turner AG, Hendry WF, Macdonald JS, Wallace DM (1976) The value of lymphography in the management of bladder cancer. Br J Urol 48: 579–586
Turner AG, Hendry WF, Williams GB, Wallace DM (1977) A haematuria diagnostic service. Br Med J 2: 29–31
Umiker W (1964) Accuracy of cytologic diagnosis of carcinoma of the urinary tract. Acta Cytol 8: 186–191
van der Werf-Messing BHP (1973) Carcinoma of the bladder treated by pre-operative irradiation and cystectomy. Cancer 32: 1084–1088
Vinje B, Skjennald A, Fryjordet A (1980) Lymphography in the evaluation of urinary bladder cancer. Clin Radiol 31: 551–553
Vock P, Haertel M, Fuchs WA, Karrer P, Bishop MC, Zingg EJ (1982) Computed tomography in staging of carcinoma of the urinary bladder. Br J Urol 54: 158–163
Wahren B, Edsmyr F, Zimmerman R (1975) Measurement of urinary C.E.A.-like substances. Cancer 36: 1490–1495
Wahren B, Nilsson B, Zimmerman R (1982) Urinary C.E.A. for prediction of survival time and recurrence of bladder cancer. Cancer 50: 139–145
Wajsman Z, Baumgartner G, Murphy GP, Merrin C (1975) Evaluation of lymphography for clinical staging of bladder tumours. J Urol 114: 712–719
Wajsman Z, Gamarra M, Park JJ (1982) Fine needle aspiration of metastatic lesions and regional lymph nodes in genito-urinary cancer. Urology 19: 356–360
Wakim KG (1971) The pathophysiological basis for the clinical manifestations and complications of transurethral prostatic resection. J Urol 106: 719–728
Wallace DM, Harris DL (1965) Delay in treating bladder tumours. Lancet II: 332–334
Wallace DM (1976) Carcinoma of the urothelium. In: Blandy JP (ed) Urology. Blackwell Scientific, Oxford, pp 774–806
Walsh JW, Amendola MA, Konerding KF, Tiznado J, Hazra TA (1980) Computed tomographic detection of pelvic and inguinal lymph node metastases from primary and recurrent pelvic malignant disease. Radiology 177: 157–166
Walzer Y, Soloway MS (1983) Should the follow-up of patients with bladder cancer include routine excretory urography? J Urol 130: 672–673
Winterberger AR, Murphy GP (1974) Correlation of B-scan ultrasonic laminography with bilateral selective hypogastric arteriography and lymphography in bladder tumours. Vasc Surg 1: 169–176
Winterberger AR, Kenny GM, Choy SW, Murphy GP (1972) Correlation of selective arteriography in the staging of bladder tumours. Cancer 29: 332–337
Zornoza J, Wallace S, Goldstein HM, Lukeman JM, Jing B (1977) Transperitoneal percutaneous retroperitoneal lymph node aspiration biopsy. Radiology 122: 111–115
Zornoza J, Cabanillas FF, Altoff TM, Ordonez N, Cohen MA (1981) Percutaneous needle biopsy in abdominal lymphoma. Am J Roentgenol Radium Ther Nucl Med 136: 97–104

Chapter 6

Classification of Bladder Tumours

G. H. Jacobi, U. Engelmann, R. Hohenfellner

Introduction

Systems for the classification and staging of bladder tumours have slowly been evolving over the past four decades. This process is continuing, for it is abundantly clear that the present systems are not ideal and must be further refined by those using the systems in order to achieve the ideal of a single, internationally accepted and universally applicable system of classification.

Definition of Classification and Staging

The terms 'classification' and 'staging' have never been clearly defined with regard to bladder tumours and they are often used synonymously when they do not in fact have the same meaning. A staging system groups together tumours according to a variety of characteristics of the tumour. When stage groupings are used it may be impossible to separate out from such groupings those factors that are relevant for planning therapy or assessing the prognosis (Wallace 1975). The staging system of Jewett and Strong (Jewett 1952) is applied to bladder tumours at the start of therapy; in each group it incorporates the extent of invasion into the bladder wall together with the presence of nodal or distant metastases.

The classification of a tumour is considerably more precise, as the purpose of classifying a tumour is to describe accurately the tumour according to any number of factors which characterise the biological behaviour of the tumour and are relevant to either the prognosis or planning of treatment. One of the most important points to clarify in any classification or staging system is the difference between the clinical (pre-treatment) and pathological (post-treatment) assessment. Because the same descriptive terms have been used for both they have frequently been confused. A *clinical classification* can be made on all patients with no exclusions, provided that they are fit for IVU and cystoscopy, and can also be performed by all centres. A *pathological classification* can only be made on an operative or post-mortem specimen. While this is obviously more accurate, these cases must inevitably be selected.

A classification of bladder tumours has therefore greater precision and greater flexibility than a staging system. A classification system should fulfil the following requirements:

1. The chosen parameters should have been fully evaluated in clinical studies and be of prognostic significance.
2. The criteria must be standardised and internationally accepted.
3. The examinations necessary for a clinical classification must be as simple as possible to perform in order to assure the widespread use of the system and have an acceptable cost versus benefit relationship (see p. 134). They must be capable of being performed by all clinics that are engaged in the management of bladder cancer, not just the best equipped centres, as they form the basis for all therapeutic methods.
4. The system must be clear, illustrative and concise.

Tumour-Node-Metastases System

The tumour-node-metastases (TNM) system of classification of malignant tumours was developed in France by Pierre Denoix between 1943 and 1952 (UICC 1978). The *Union Internationale Contre le Cancer* (UICC) based their work on his original concepts and presented a TNM system for the classification of bladder tumours in 1963. The first edition of the UICC *TNM Classification of Malignant Tumours*, generally known as the *Livre de Poche*, appeared in 1968. It was well received as being of general interest to clinicians, and the second edition was published in 1974. This classification was unique in that the local tumour stage (T) category corresponded with the histological stages defined in 1974 by the World Health Organisation (WHO) in their pamphlet *Histological Typing of Urinary Bladder Tumours* (Pugh 1981). Wallace et al. (1975) emphasised the value of this classification as being a short, descriptive method for determining the data relevant to the prognosis and therapy. They compared the TNM classification to the *appelation contrôlée* as applied to French wines, i.e. a reliable description of the content (or tumour). At the same time they stressed the fact that the 1974 version of the TNM system was not definitive but rather that it should be further refined and revised by the users.

The third edition of the TNM classification appeared in 1978, and it was planned that this edition 'should remain unchanged for the following ten years unless some major advance in diagnosis or treatment, relevant to a particular site, makes the current classification unrealistic' (UICC 1978). This edition rapidly gained worldwide acceptance and has been recognised for the classification of urological tumours by the WHO and the European Organisation for Research on Treatment of Cancer (EORTC), as well as leading groups outside Europe.

The TNM system classifies tumours by the anatomical extent of the disease, and two classifications are described for each site: (1) the pre-treatment clinical classification, designated TNM, and (2) the post-surgical histopathological

Table 6.1. TNM Pre-treatment clinical classification (UICC 1978)

T —	Primary Tumour
Tis	Pre-invasive carcinoma (carcinoma in situ): 'Flat tumour'
Ta	Papillary non-invasive carcinoma
T0	No evidence of primary tumour
T1	On bimanual examination a freely mobile mass may be felt: this should not be felt after complete transurethral resection of the lesion *and/or* Microscopically, the tumour does not invade beyond the lamina propria
T2	On bimanual examination there is induration of the bladder wall which is mobile. There is no residual induration after complete transurethral resection of the lesion *and/or* There is microscopic invasion of superficial muscle
T3	On bimanual examination induration *or* a nodular mobile mass is palpable in the bladder wall which persists after transurethral resection of the exophytic portion of the lesion *and/or* There is microscopic invasion of deep muscle *or* of extension through the bladder wall. T3a Invasion of deep muscle T3b Invasion through the bladder wall
T4	Tumour fixed or extending to neighbouring structures *and/or* There is microscopic evidence of such involvement T4a Tumour infiltrating the prostate, uterus or vagina T4b Tumour fixed to the pelvic wall and/or abdominal wall
Note: The suffix (m) may be added to the appropriate T category to indicate multiple tumours, e.g. T2 (m)	
TX	The minimum requirements to assess the primary tumour cannot be met
N —	Regional and Juxtaregional Lymph Nodes
N0	No evidence of regional lymph node involvement
N1	Evidence of involvement of a single homolateral regional lymph node
N2	Evidence of involvement of contralateral *or* bilateral *or* multiple regional lymph nodes
N3	Evidence of involvement of fixed regional lymph nodes (there is a fixed mass on the pelvic wall with a free space between this and the tumour)
N4	Evidence of involvement of juxtaregional lymph nodes
NX	The minimum requirements to assess the regional *and/or* juxtaregional lymph nodes cannot be met
M —	Distant Metastases
M0	No evidence of distant metastases
M1	Evidence of distant metastases
MX	The minimum requirements to assess the presence of distant metastases cannot be met

classification, designated pTNM. For the bladder the pre-treatment classification is based on the evidence of a biopsy in addition to clinical examination, and the post-surgical classification includes the evidence from definitive surgery, which may be TUR, as well as a cystectomy specimen.

To carry out a pre-treatment classification it is necessary to standardise the diagnostic procedures that must be applied to all patients. These must be performed to fulfil the minimum requirements of the TNM system and for each category they are as follows:

T Category: Clinical examination, urography, cystoscopy, bimanual palpation under anaesthesia and biopsy or TUR

N Category: Clinical examination and radiography, including lymphography and urography

M Category: Clinical examination, radiography and scintigraphic methods when metastases are suspected

The idea behind the establishment of these minimal requirements is to ensure a comparable quality of staging procedures among different centres so that all centres can participate. The full classification of bladder tumours according to the TNM system is set out in Tables 6.1 and 6.2 and illustrated in Figs. 6.1–6.4.

The version currently in use presents a dual system of classification—a pre-treatment clinical classification and a post-surgical histopathological classification. One of the unique features of the TNM classification of bladder tumours as opposed to tumours at other sites is that the histological findings from a biopsy are used in the pre-treatment clinical classification, whereas for the post-surgical histopathological classification the specimen must be from the definitive surgical treatment.

Table 6.2. pTNM post-surgical histopathological classification (UICC 1978)

pT —	Primary Tumour
pTis	Pre-invasive carcinoma (carcinoma in situ)
pTa	Papillary non-invasive carcinoma
pT0	No evidence of tumour found on histological examination of specimen
pT1	Tumour not extending beyond the lamina propria
pT2	Tumour with invasion of superficial muscle (not more than halfway through muscle coat)
pT3	Tumour with invasion of deep muscle (more than halfway through muscle coat) *or* with invasion of perivesical tissue
pT4	Tumour with invasion of prostate or other extravesical structures
pTX	The extent of invasion cannot be assessed
G —	Histopathological Grading
'G0'	Papilloma, i.e. no evidence of anaplasia
G1	High degree of differentiation
G2	Medium degree of differentiation
G3	Low degree of differentiation *or* undifferentiated
GX	Grade cannot be assessed
L —	Invasion of Lymphatics
L0	No lymphatic invasion
L1	Evidence of invasion of superficial lymphatics
L2	Evidence of invasion of deep lymphatics
LX	Lymphatic invasion cannot be assessed
pN —	Regional and Juxtaregional Lymph Nodes
	The pN categories correspond to the N categories
pM —	Distant Metastases
	The pM categories correspond to the M categories
STAGE GROUPING	
	No stage grouping is at present recommended

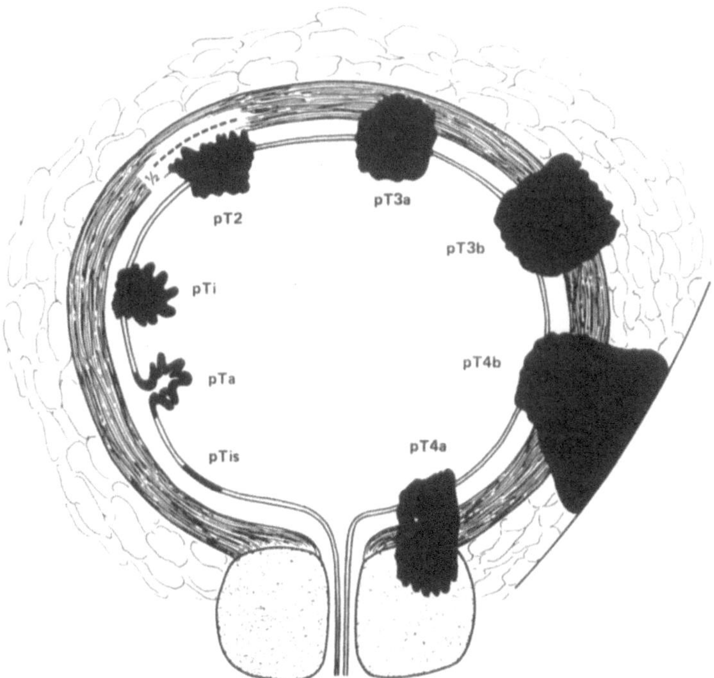

Fig. 6.1. pT-categories in bladder cancer (TNM-system) (UICC 1982)

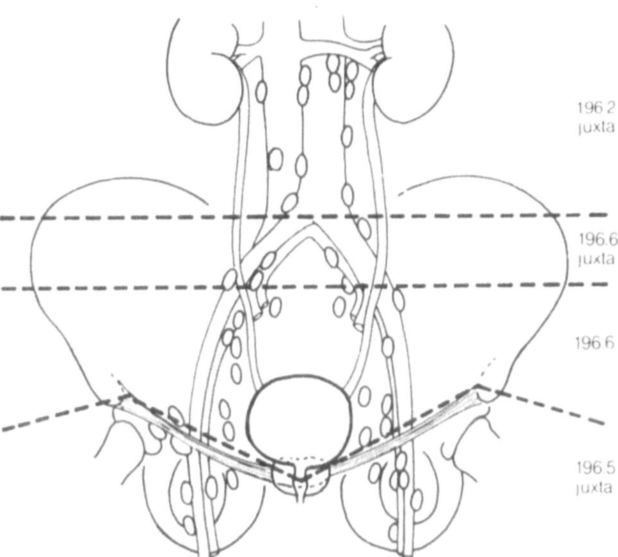

Fig. 6.2. Regional and juxtaregional lymph nodes in bladder cancer. The regional nodes are the nodes below the bifurcation of the common iliac arteries. The juxtaregional nodes are the inguinal, common iliac and para-aortic nodes (UICC 1982)

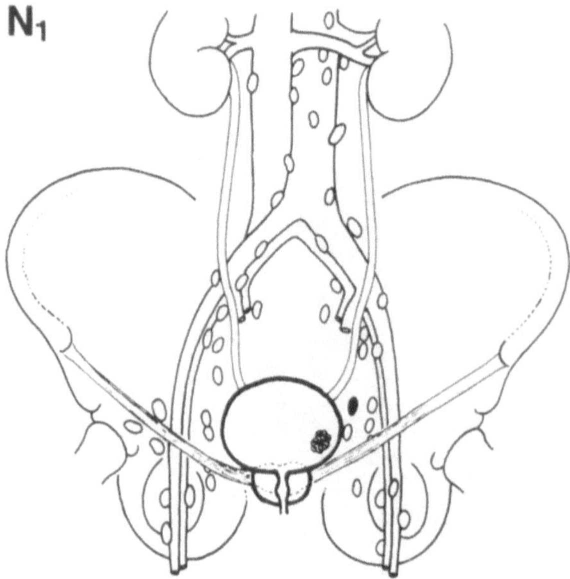

Fig. 6.3. Example of category N1 (UICC 1982)

Once the TNM classification has been given to a tumour it must remain unchanged, as this represents the pre-treatment state of the tumour. However, the use of the TNM system can be further refined and extended by the use of various symbols called 'additional descriptors', which enable this system to be used as a shorthand method of describing the progress of a tumour. The additional descriptors are as follows:

The suffix 'm' means that the tumours are multiple.

The prefix 'y' means that the definitive surgical treatment was preceded by other treatment methods, e.g. instillation therapy.

The prefix 'r' means that the tumour is a recurrence.

The 'r' and 'm' additional descriptors are for use for all tumour sites and their use for bladder tumours has not been strictly defined. The suffix 'm' is usually taken to mean that the tumours are multiple in the bladder at the time of initial assessment and not outside the bladder or multifocal in time as well. The tumour recurrence denoted by 'r' is for a recurrence within the previously treated area and should not be used if the recurrence is in an untreated area elsewhere in the bladder.

The additional symbols C1–C5 represent the 'C-Factor' and denote the degree of certainty with which the TNM categories are allocated (see Table 6.3). The C-factor represents a dynamic category as it can be adapted to new diagnostic findings obtained during the course of the disease and can be periodically re-categorised.

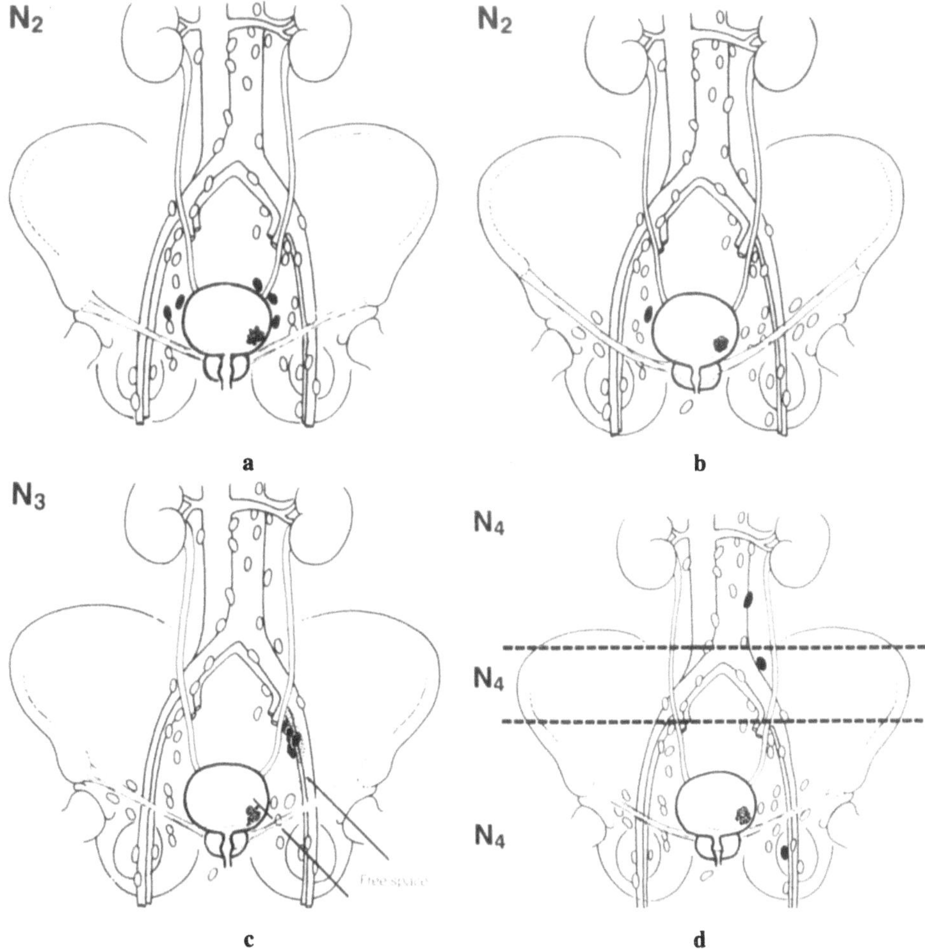

Fig. 6.4. Examples of categories N2 (**a** and **b**), N3 (**c**), N4 (**d**) (UICC 1982)

Table 6.3. C-Factor category (UICC 1978)

C1	Evidence from clinical examination only
C2	Evidence obtained by special diagnostic means
C3	Evidence from surgical exploration only
C4	Evidence of the extent of disease following definitive surgery and including the complete examination of the therapeutically resected specimen
C5	Evidence from autopsy

Example: Degrees of C may be applied to the T, N and M categories. A case might be described as T3C2, N2C1, M0C2

The use of this system is illustrated in the following clinical example: A patient presents with macroscopic haematuria and a filling defect in the bladder is seen on the urogram. On cystoscopy, two papillary tumours are found which are not palpable on bimanual examination under anaesthesia, and the biopsies show that they have not yet infiltrated the lamina propria (Ta(m)C2). Lymphography shows no evidence of lymph node involvement (NOC2). Clinical examination reveals no sign of metastases (MOC1). The definitive surgical treatment is a TUR, which reveals that the lamina propria is invaded (pT1C3 NOC2 MOC1). One year later the patient presents with a recurrence at the original site. Induration is palpable, but the bladder is mobile (rT2C1). After a TUR, the tumour is found to have infiltrated the superficial muscle, but there is no sign of lymph node or distant metastases (rT2C3 NOC1 MOC1). After preoperative systemic chemotherapy the patient undergoes a radical cystectomy. The histopathological examination shows that the tumour invades the deep muscle layers, lymphatic vessels and both obturator node groups (yrpT3 G3 L2 N2 C4).

Bladder tumours can thus be described in detail at the time of diagnosis (TNM), after definitive surgical therapy (pTNM), and also followed in their subsequent development (rTNM). Additional information which is of prognostic importance can also be incorporated, as in the above example. These are the histological grade (G category) and the presence of lymphatic invasion (L category). The UICC system can therefore be made more precise and detailed, but this is at the price of an increase in complexity that is likely to prevent its widespread use and acceptance.

The American System

The results of an autopsy study of 107 bladder cancer patients led Jewett and Strong (1946) to develop a staging system which correlated the probability of the tumour having metastasised with the depth of tumour infiltration and was particularly suitable for the evaluation of cystectomy specimens. Jewett (1952) then reported a series of 80 patients who had had their bladder tumours completely removed by either partial or total cystectomy and demonstrated that the 5-year survival correlated with the depth of infiltration. He concluded that it was of utmost importance to distinguish preoperatively between the superficially and deeply infiltrating tumours and that this could be done by a properly taken biopsy and a pelvic examination under anaesthesia. In the same year, Marshall (1952) reported on a comparison of the preoperative clinical stage and the histopathological findings in 104 patients treated by radical cystectomy. He used a modification of the Jewett and Strong system which has subsequently been known as the Jewett/Strong/Marshall classification, and this has been the system used most frequently for a long time in the USA (Fig. 6.5). The advantage of this system was that it was prognostically relevant as a pathological staging system and easy to apply, but caused confusion because the same terms were used for both the clinical and the pathological staging from the cystectomy specimen. Because a variety of factors are incorporated into one group it is not possible to distinguish cases where neighbouring organs are involved without nodal metastases. The flat carcinoma in situ, as first described by Melicow and Hollowell (1952), cannot be described in this system, nor can the dynamic course of the disease.

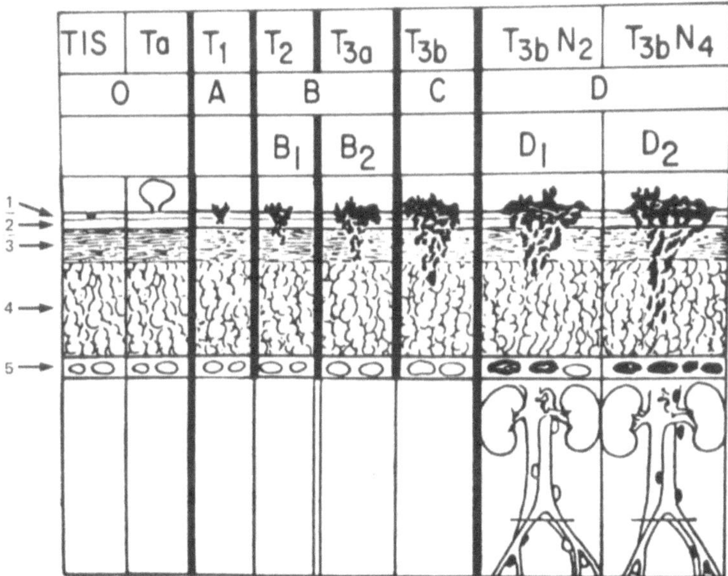

Fig. 6.5. Classification of bladder carcinoma according to Jewett/Strong/Marshall and compared to the AJCC/TNM system. *1*, mucosa; *2*, submucosa: *3*, muscle; *4*, fat; *5*, lymph nodes

The Urological Task Force of the American Joint Committee on Cancer Staging and End Results Reporting (AJCC) published an extended and modified TNM classification in 1967, but this at first met with little enthusiasm. A revised version appeared in 1978, with a second edition being published in 1983 (see Table 6.4). This can be translated without difficulty into the UICC TNM classification, but it should be noted that the 'and/or' clauses of the UICC T-categories have been deleted to give greater emphasis to the histopathology rather than the clinical examination. Thus, one of the goals of any classification has been achieved, namely, that the comparison of treatment and results is possible on an international basis. The substitution of the AJCC classification for the Jewett/Strong/Marshall system is recommended, as the former is now the most precise method for the description of patients with bladder cancer who have been subjected to the various treatment strategies (Prout 1980).

Problems of Bladder Tumour Classification

Carcinoma In Situ

The problems of classification of carcinoma in situ are dealt with in Chapter 7. At present, 'Tis' refers to primary carcinoma in situ, and secondary carcinoma in situ (e.g. T1+Tis) cannot be classified in this system.

Table 6.4. TNM-classification of the American Joint Committee on Cancer (AJCC 1983)

Primary Tumor (T)

The suffix 'm' should be added to the appropriate T category to indicate multiple lesions. Papilloma is classified as 'GO.'

- TX Minimum requirements to assess the primary tumor cannot be met
- T0 No evidence of primary tumor
- Tis Carcinoma *in situ* (If used without subscript. Tis indicates bladder alone)
  - b Bladder
  - u Ureter
  - pr.u Prostatic urethra
  - p.d. Prostatic ducts
- Ta Papillary non-invasive carcinoma
- T1 Carcinoma without microscopic invasion beyond the lamina propria. On bimanual examination a freely mobile mass may be felt; this should not be felt after complete transurethral resection of the lesion
- T2 Microscopic invasion of superficial muscle of the bladder. On bimanual examination there may be induration of the bladder wall, which is mobile. There is usually no residual induration after complete transurethral resection of the lesion
- T3 On bimanual examination there may be induration or a nodular mobile mass palpable in the bladder wall that persists after transurethral resection (T3 may not be used alone)
- T3a Microscopic invasion of deep muscle is defined as histologic evidence of tumor clearly extending through muscle bundles to both edges of a resected specimen
- T3b Invasion into perivesical fat
- T4 Microscopic evidence of muscle invasion: tumour is fixed or invades neighboring structures. The following subclassification should be used when these conditions are met:
- T4a Tumor invading substance of prostate (microscopically proven), uterus, or vagina
- T4b Tumor fixed to the pelvic wall or infiltrating the abdominal wall

STAGE GROUPING

Stage I	T1, N0, M0
Stage II	T2, N0, M0
Stage III	T3a or b; N0, M0
Stage IV	T4, N0, M0
	Any T, N1-N3; M0
	Any T, any N, M1

HISTOPATHOLOGY

The predominant cancer is a transitional cell cancer. Grading of the tumor is as follows:

Tumor Grade (G)

- G1 Well differentiated
- G2 Moderately well differentiated
- G3-G4 Poorly to very poorly differentiated

Use whichever indicator is most appropriate (term or G+ number).

Nodal Involvement (N)

The regional lymph nodes are those within the true pelvis; all others are distant nodes. Histologic examination is required for stages N0 through N3, except for subset 'c.'

- NX Minimum requirements to assess the regional nodes cannot be met
- N0 No involvement of regional lymph nodes
- N1 Involvement of a single homolateral regional lymph node
- N2 Involvement of contralateral, bilateral, or multiple regional lymph nodes
- N3 A fixed mass on the pelvic wall with a free space between it and the tumor

Distant Metastasis (M)

- MX Minimum requirements to assess the presence of distant metastasis cannot be met
- M0 No (known) distant metastasis
- M1 Distant metastasis present
  Specify ____________

Specify sites according to the following notations:

LYM	Distant lymph nodes
PUL	Pulmonary
OSS	Osseous
HEP	Hepatic
BRA	Brain
MAR	Bone marrow
PLE	Pleura
SKI	Skin
EYE	Eye
OTH	Other

POSTSURGICAL TREATMENT
RESIDUAL TUMOR (R)

- R0 No residual tumor
- R1 Microscopic residual tumor
- R2 Macroscopic residual tumors
  Specify ____________

PERFORMANCE STATUS OF HOST (H)

Performance status of the host should be recorded because this information at times is pertinent to the treatment of the patient.

AJCC PERFORMANCE		ECOG SCALE	KARNOVSKY SCALE
H0	Normal activity	0	90–100
H1	Symptomatic but ambulatory; cares for self	1	70–80
H2	Ambulatory more than 50% of the time; occasionally needs assistance	2	50–60
H3	Ambulatory 50% or less of time; nursing care needed	3	30–40
H4	Bedridden; may need hospitalization	4	10–20

Ta and T1 Tumours

It can be virtually impossible to distinguish clinically between a Ta and T1 tumour, and even the biopsy may not be taken from the infiltrating part. Only a complete TUR of the tumour will reveal with any reliability whether the lamina propria is invaded. Computed tomography (CT) and sonography lack the resolution to make this differentiation. Therefore, this differentiation has to be made on a post-surgical basis (i.e. pTa or pT1) and the clinical categories could be merged (Chisholm et al. 1980). The histopathological differentiation may also be difficult and subjective (see Chap. 2, p. 40).

T2 and T3a (B1 and B2) Tumours

The clinical differentiation between infiltration of superficial and deep muscle has been shown to have errors of 20%–40% even with the best clinicians. A transurethral biopsy, even if it could be correctly orientated, cannot distinguish the half-way point in the muscle wall, as this varies with the sex of the patient, the degree of distension and the amount of hypertrophy of the detrusor. Again CT and sonography lack the resolution to do this any better. While the original observations of Jewett and Strong that the presence of deep muscle invasion has a poorer prognosis than when superficial muscle only is invaded remain true, this was based on autopsy and surgical specimens and not on a clinical assessment. Many authors have since reported that there is little difference in survival when the T2 and T3a tumours are assessed clinically (Ritchie et al. 1975; Pearse et al. 1978; Blandy et al. 1980). In most centres both types of tumour are treated radically. In the infiltrating tumours it is the presence of muscle invasion rather than the clinical assessment of its depth that is important to prognosis and therapy.

Further Pathological Classification

Pryor (1973) divided the pT1 tumours into two pathological stages, P1a and P1b, according to whether the stromal core only was infiltrated (P1a) or the true lamina propria (P1b). [The pathological categories (P) were merged into the post-surgical pT categories in 1978.] He reported a significant difference in the 3-year survival between the P1a tumours (77%) and the P1b tumours (64%). Prostatic involvement may either be confined to tumour in the prostatic ducts or consist of direct invasion into the prostatic stroma. The latter has a much worse prognosis, as Schellhamer et al. (1977) have shown, and may be classified separately in a pathological classification (Pugh 1981; see also Chap. 7, p. 150).

Presentation of the Surgical Specimen for Histopathological Staging

The excised bladder is empty and contracted. If it is allowed to fix in this state the tissues will harden, it will be impossible to unfold the bladder and the mucosa will appear as a series of coarse convolutions with deep narrow furrows (Fig. 6.6a). It may be impossible to find small lesions in such a bladder, and the correct assessment of tumour infiltration can be difficult. The specimen may also show a 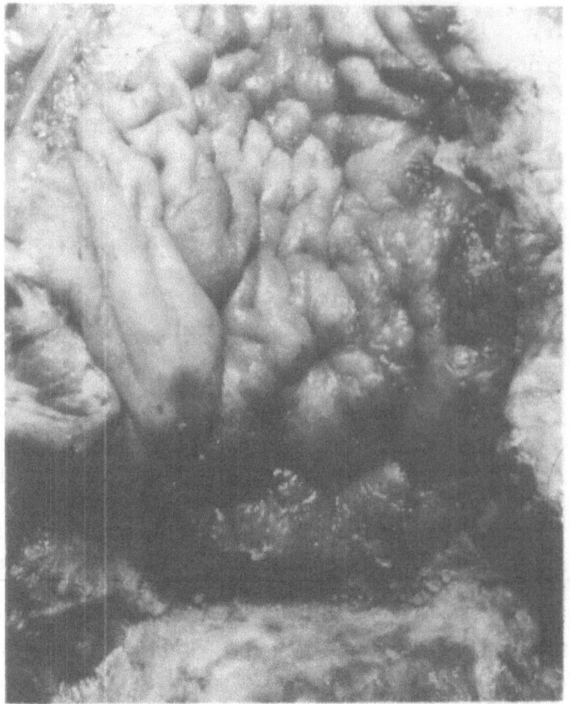

b 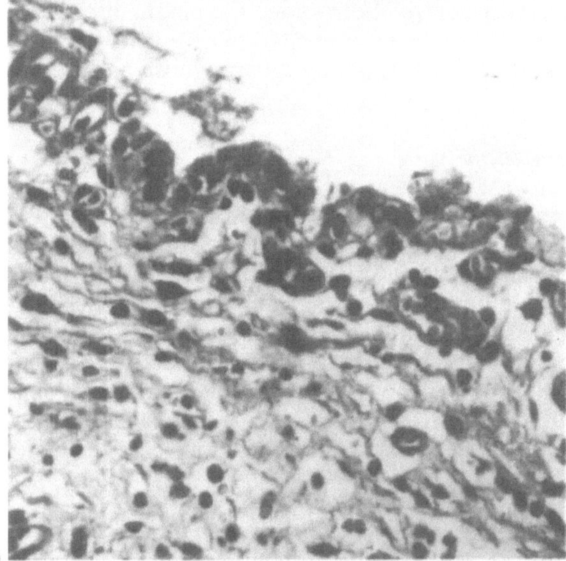

Fig. 6.6. **a** Cystectomy specimen: condition after fixation without filling of the bladder with fixative and ventral incision. The mucosa is hardened by fixation and forms rigid coarse bulges with deep, non-inspectable folds. The result of fixation of the urothelium is especially poor here. **b** Histological section. H & E, × 40. (Courtesy of PD Dr. H. Rumpelt, Institute of Pathology, University of Mainz Medical School)

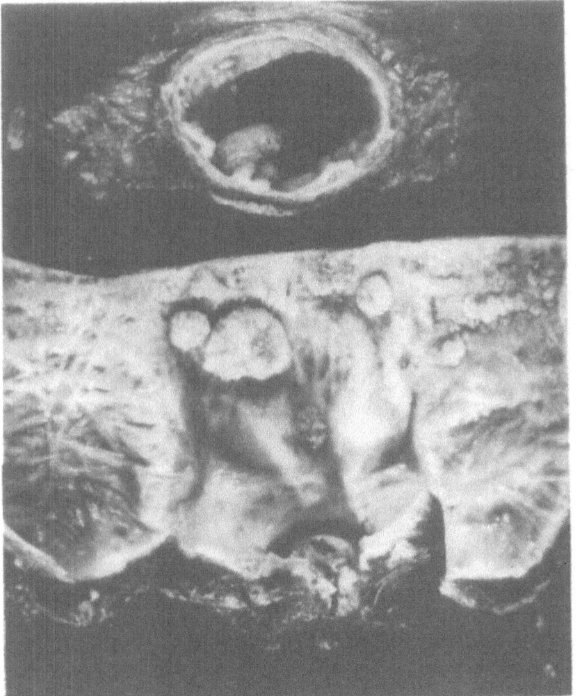

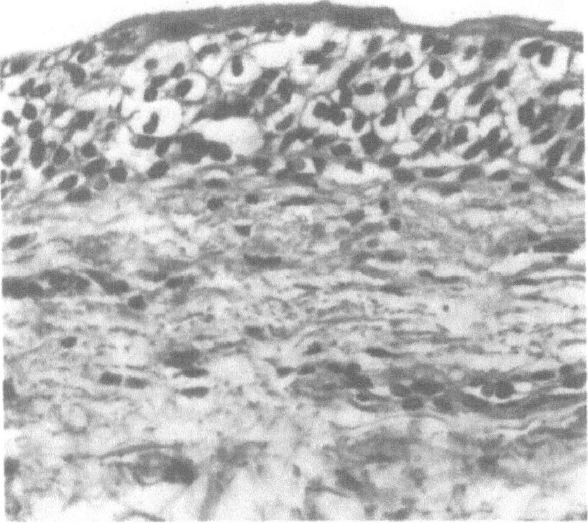

Fig. 6.7. **a** Cystectomy specimen: condition after fixation by filling of the bladder with 200 ml formalin. Half of the bladder has been opened ventrally (*above*), the other half has been cut into 1.5 cm thick slices (*below*). The organ could be easily unfolded. The mucosa can be viewed optimally macroscopically. **b** The histological result of fixation is excellent. H & E, × 240. (Courtesy of PD Dr. H. Rumpelt, Institute of Pathology, University of Mainz Medical School)

severe epithelial desquamation, which may be due either to autolysis resulting from delay in the formalin reaching the centre of such a contracted bladder, or to mucosal damage by the manipulations that the pathologist has to make to examine the interior of the bladder.

If the cystectomy specimen is distended with 100–200 ml of 10% formalin soon after excision and the urethra ligated and the bladder allowed to fix in this state, then it will retain its shape and the detection of any lesion is much easier and more reliable (Austen and Friedell 1965). Giant coronal sections can then be cut (Fig. 6.7a) which give an excellent demonstration of the extent of the infiltration of the tumour, the type of infiltration and the state of the whole urothelium (Soto et al. 1977). The urothelium in such specimens is well preserved (Fig. 6.7b), which permits an accurate evaluation of any accompanying carcinoma in situ and should leave no room for understaging (H. Rumpelt 1983, personal communication.) Correct preservation of the specimen and accurate mapping of the tumour are essentials for the reliable histopathological classification.

Sonography and CT Scanning in Bladder Tumour Classification

Sonography and CT scanning have already been discussed in Chapter 5 with regard to the diagnosis of the bladder tumour. Both procedures may have a contribution to make to the classification of bladder tumours, but must first be critically evaluated. Moreover, both procedures require considerable capital expenditure and neither one is universally available.

Intravesical sonography was at first thought to be useful in the diagnosis of superficial tumours (Prout 1982), but has not yet proved convincing. In experimental investigations on the pig bladder it was impossible to discriminate between the individual layers of the bladder wall using the same techniques. The resolution of intravesical sonography with a 7 mHz transducer was determined to be 0.9 mm lateral discrimination and 1–1.5 mm axial discrimination. As the diameter of sound echos on the monitor also lie within this range, differentiation of tumour tissue from healthy tissue would appear extremely difficult (E. Matouscheck 1984, personal communication). We were unable to determine accurately the extent of tumour infiltration by preoperative sonography in 24 patients who were then treated by a radical cystectomy for infiltrating tumours. The thickness of the bladder wall, a relatively simple parameter to measure, could not be reproducibly determined, as compared to the surgical specimen (Fig. 6.8a–c). Even with ex situ postoperative ultrasound investigation of the cystectomy specimen in a waterbath, the tumour tissue could not always be distinguished from the normal tissue in terms of the echo patterns (Wenderoth et al. 1984).

Before intravesical sonography can be used for the classification of bladder tumours improvements are necessary in the sonographic equipment. The diameter of the probes should be reduced to that of the usual diagnostic cystoscopes, and the resolution and tissue differentiation must be improved, possibly by signal processing, as has been done with prostatic cancer (Walz et al. 1981).

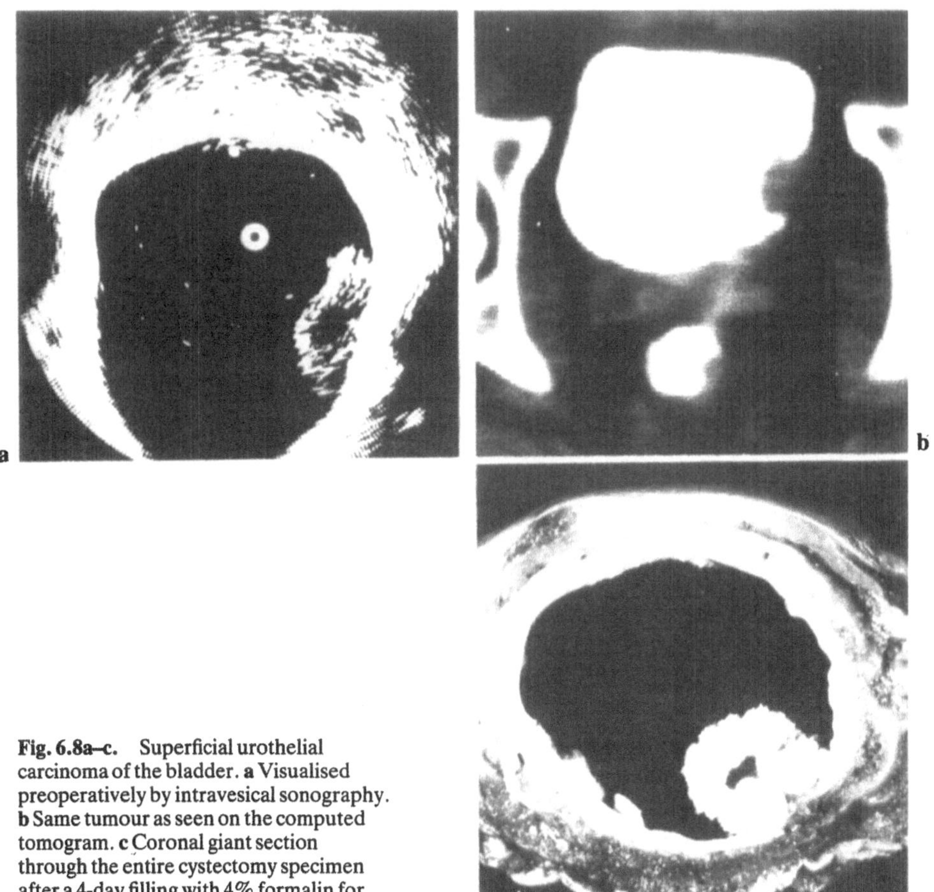

Fig. 6.8a–c. Superficial urothelial carcinoma of the bladder. **a** Visualised preoperatively by intravesical sonography. **b** Same tumour as seen on the computed tomogram. **c** Coronal giant section through the entire cystectomy specimen after a 4-day filling with 4% formalin for fixation; pT1 lesion

CT has possibly greater potential for differentiating the T2 and T3 tumours. The results that have been reported by a number of groups are compiled in Table 6.5. Those investigators who have studied large series of patients who have undergone radical cystectomy—the only reliable method of assessing the value of CT in classifying bladder cancer—have reported accuracy rates of 64%–81% (Koss et al. 1981; Vock et al. 1982; Weinerman et al. 1982; Engelmann et al. 1984). Although the diagnosis of an invasive bladder tumour is possible with CT, it is not yet a reliable means of differentiating the T2 and T3a tumours. In our study of 74 patients in whom CT had been performed prior to radical cystectomy, the number of correctly classified tumours of the 19 patients with pT2 and pT3a tumours depended on the experience of the investigator and varied from 8 to 17 of the 19 patients. In stage T3b tumours there is a tendency to understaging with CT, as the microscopic infiltration in the fat cannot be recognised.

Table 6.5. CT in staging of bladder cancer

Reference	No. of patients	Correlation with clinical finding (Clin.) or histological finding (Histol.)	Operation		Accuracy[a]	
Ahlberg et al. (1982)	46	Clin. 45/46	Cystectomy	5	Correct	8/9
		Histol. 9/46	Partial resection	3	Overstaged	1/9
			Autopsy	1		
Colleen et al. (1981)	24	Clin. 24/24	Cystectomy	17	Correct	15/24
		Histol. 24/24	Laparotomy	7	Overstaged	3/24
					Understaged	6/24
Frödin et al. (1980)	52	Clin. 45/52	Cystectomy	12	Correct	10/12
		Histol. 12/52			Overstaged	2/12
Hodson et al. (1979)	60	Clin. 50/60	Cystectomy	10	No information available on	
		Histol. 10/60			pT-staging	
Jaschke et al. (1981)	20	Histol. 20/20	TUR	17	Correct	16/20
			Cystectomy	1	Overstaged	4/20
			Partial resection	2		
Jeffrey et al. (1981)	22 14/14	Clin. 6/14	Laparotomy	8/14	Correct	6/8
		Histol. 8/14			Understaged	2/8
Kellett et al. (1980)	51	Clin. 51/51	Cystectomy	12/15	Correct	16/20
		Histol. 15/51	Autopsy	1/15	Overstaged	2/15
			Laparotomy	2/15	Understaged	1/15
Koss et al. (1981)	49	Clin. /	Cystectomy	24/25	Correct	16/25
		Histol. 25/49	Laparotomy	1/25	Overstaged	5/25
					Understaged	4/25
Rost et al. (1981)	95	Clin. 95/95	TUR		Correct	13/16
		Histol. 16/95	Cystectomy			
			Autopsy			
Sager et al. (1983)	32	Clin. 32/32	Cystectomy	32	Correct	25/32
		Histol 32/32			Overstaged	7/32
Seidelmann et al. (1978)	21	Histol. 21	Cystectomy	8	Correct	17/21
			Laparotomy	5	Overstaged	4/21
			Biopsy	8		
Schönbauer et al. (1981)	27	Histol. 25/27	TUR	19	Correct	21/25
			Partial resection	2		
			Cystectomy	2		
			Autopsy	1		
			Laparotomy	1		
Vock et al. (1982)	77	Histol. 77	Cystectomy	35	Correct	62/77
			Biopsy	42	Overstaged	14/77
					Understaged	
Weinerman et al. (1982)	54	Histol. 54	Cystectomy	33	Correct	21/33
					Overstaged	7/33
					Understaged	
			TUR/biopsy	21	Correct	20/21

[a] In correlation to histological finding

Lymph node metastases in the true pelvis can be determined by CT with an accuracy of 73%–79% (Table 6.6). The CT cannot detect small metastases that do not enlarge the nodes, and enlarged benign nodes will give false positive results (Morgan et al. 1981; Weinerman et al. 1982). Fine needle biopsies can be taken from any enlarged nodes demonstrated by CT, but a negative result is clinically not useful (Wajsman et al. 1982). Nevertheless, CT is the only non-invasive

Table 6.6. Detection of pelvic lymph node metastases by CT

Reference	No. of patients	Accuracy	Sensitivity	Specificity
Engelmann et al. (1984)	74	99%	100%	98%
Karrer et al. (1980)	44	89%	94%	85%
Koss et al. (1981)	25	92%	60%	100%
Morgan et al. (1981)	34	79%	50%	92%
Walsh et al. (1980)	35	77%	85%	67%
Weinerman et al. (1982)	68	86%	74%	93%

staging procedure for the internal iliac and obturator nodes, as these are not shown by lymphography. CT must therefore be included if any serious attempt is being made to classify the lymph nodes.

The '*Deutschsprachiges TNM Komitee*' Recommendations

In 1981, the clinicians on the National Committee of the UICC on TNM Classification in Germany (*Deutschsprachiges TNM Komitee*; DSK) were asked to assist in the modernisation of the minimal requirements so that in 1988 (the date until which the current TNM version is valid) the updated requirements could be included in the revised TNM classification. The revised requirements as presented and recommended to the DSK (Adolphs and Jacobi 1981) are listed in Table 6.7. It is important to note that in this new version the term minimal is omitted; instead the diagnostic procedures are divided into:

1. Required examinations
2. Special examinations to be performed or recommended in addition
3. Other procedures which can be omitted in certain situations

Table 6.7. Revision of the diagnostic requirements for TNM classification of bladder carcinoma as suggested by the National Committee on TNM Classification [DSK] in Germany (Adolphs and Jacobi 1981)

Category	Required examinations	Special examinations to be performed or recommended in addition	Procedures to be performed in special situations
T	Clinical examination; urography; urethrocystoscopy; biopsy and/or TUR	Bimanual palpation under anaesthesia; sonography; CT-scan	
N	Clinical examination; X-ray diagnosis, including urography	Sonography; CT-scan; biochemical investigations; lymph node biopsy or staging operation	Lymphography
M	Clinical examination; X-ray diagnosis	Sonography; CT-scan; biochemical investigation	

It should be emphasised that these are only recommendations and have not been approved, but they contain proposals that we feel would correct some of the deficiencies of the present classification. The important innovations in the diagnostic procedures are as follows:

1. Bimanual palpation under anaesthesia is no longer a required examination for the T category, but is recommended as a special examination. Thus the bimanual examination is on an equal footing with sonography and CT scanning, as it is no more accurate and probably less objective.
2. Sonography and CT scanning are recommended examinations for all three TNM categories.
3. Lymphography is neither recommended nor required. Instead, lymph node biopsy or a staging operation are especially recommended.
4. The term 'biochemical investigations' has been included to allow for the future development of tumour markers.

Cost Versus Benefit Relationship of the Diagnostic Procedures

As the diagnostic procedures which we order daily depend on recently developed, highly sophisticated, expensive technology we must be aware of what is an acceptable cost versus benefit relationship. The crucial question is how far these should go in the individual case. We must ask ourselves what information on the tumour extent is essential to determine the most rational treatment strategy for the individual patient. The main factor which warrants extensive staging is to determine the possibility of cure; this can justify the use of all diagnostic means to rule out lymphatic and distant spread, regardless of cost, if radical surgery is contemplated.

The goal of innovations or refinements of already established staging procedures is to improve specificity and sensitivity. For 20 years radioisotope methods have been used to supplement conventional radiographic techniques in the assessment of distant metastases. The two most widely used radioisotope techniques in staging urological malignancies are bone and liver scans. As with many other investigations, it sometimes takes years of use until the initial enthusiasm is replaced by a more critical and thus realistic judgement as to their value in routine application for primary staging.

Our experience with bone and liver scans illustrates this point (Hohenfellner and Jacobi 1982). Between 1972 and 1978, 62 bone and 39 liver scans were performed on patients with newly diagnosed bladder tumours who were also considered candidates for radical surgery. The yield of correct positive bone scans was 14.5% and of correct positive liver scans, 7.7%. When we considered the number of patients in whom the scans resulted in a change of treatment policy we found that the predictive staging value of these investigations was extremely low. When this was weighed against the total costs of the work-up we concluded that routine bone and liver scans for all newly diagnosed bladder cancer patients was not justified. It is the responsibility of the larger urological centres to evaluate any newly established staging procedure in this respect.

Laboratory Investigations Contributing to the Classification of Bladder Tumours

Many laboratory investigations have been considered that might add to the classification of bladder tumours. Much time and research have been spent on possible tumour markers; these have been reviewed in Chapter 5. None have proved sufficiently useful to warrant being included in the TNM classification. Other histopathological investigations in addition to grade and invasion may have a significant contribution to make to tumour classification.

Tumour Infiltration Type

Soto et al. (1977) described two types of infiltration in bladder cancers. Tumours can either invade along a broad front with blunt processes or in a more diffuse manner with tentacular processes. The latter type is more often associated with a solid, less well-differentiated tumour and a poorer survival (Jakse et al. 1983).

Blood Group Antigens

Despite the technical problems and problems with interpretation (see Chap. 2, p. 45) this test does give additional prognostic information in superficial bladder tumours. Antigen-positive patients have a better prognosis with a longer tumour-free interval, whereas antigen-negative patients have a poor prognosis and the tumours have a tendency to become invasive and develop metastases (Jakse et al. 1981; Kulkarni et al. 1982).

Immune Status

Many investigations have been performed to try and characterise the immunological status of the patient with a bladder cancer, and these have been reviewed in Chapter 3 (see p. 62). None are of sufficient value to be included in any classification system as yet.

Chromosome Analysis

The analysis of chromosomes in bladder cancer by the 'direct squash technique' was begun by Falor and co-workers in 1968 (Falor 1971; Falor and Ward 1976). The authors drew the following conclusions from the examination of 65 patients with superficial bladder carcinomas who were followed up over 10 years:

Chromosome abnormalities are sensitive tumour markers, and every bladder cancer shows abnormalities. Some tumours have marker chromosomes, and these tumours show a high rate of recurrence and a tendency towards progression in stage and grade (Summers et al. 1981). There is a closer correlation between invasion and chromosome changes than with cellular differentiation (Lamb 1967), and invasive bladder tumours show a high number of marker chromosomes with complex karyotypes (Sandberg 1977). In women with urothelial tumours the concentration of sex chromatin bodies correlates negatively with the mitotic index, de-differentiation and invasion (Atkin and Petkovic 1973; Anichkov and Zus 1980). The cytogenetic analysis of bladder tumours is comparatively simple and inexpensive. It can characterise tumours as to biological behaviour and malignant potential and should now supplement other examinations.

DNA Analysis

The determination of the DNA content of bladder tumours by flow cytometry provides information on the nuclear activity and can be correlated with the tumour grade (Hofstädter et al. 1980; Nelson 1983). Well-differentiated tumours have a diploid DNA stemline, while poorly differentiated tumours are aneuploid (Fosså et al. 1977; Tribukait and Gustafson 1980). The greater the degree of ploidy the greater the risk of tumour recurrence and progression and the poorer the prognosis (Gustafson et al. 1982a,b,c).

Future Perspectives

This chapter has reviewed the various classification and staging systems of bladder tumours with special emphasis on the TNM system. It should be clearly stated that the TNM system is a classification system and that the UICC does not at present recommend a stage grouping for bladder tumours, such as is in use for tumours in many other sites. What we are dealing with at present is the anatomy-related characterisation of the extent of the cancer by the categories T, N and M. From the nine T categories, five N categories and two M categories up to 90 different combinations are possible. We must therefore come to some sort of grouping system in which certain T, N and M categories are combined according to the most clinically relevant prognostic features. Such a combined anatomical and clinical staging could assist with planning treatment strategies. A strictly anatomy-orientated evaluation of a bladder tumour is bound to be incomplete in the living, as our limited staging procedures may well only be describing the 'tip of the iceberg'. The establishment of stage groupings for bladder cancer should be one of the goals for future field studies. Attempts should now be made to develop a treatment-correlated tumour grouping which would enable us to answer the following questions:

1. Which categories of tumour can be cured by a TUR only?
2. Which categories are likely to be cured only by radical surgery?
3. Which categories should be treated with local instillation treatment?
4. Which categories should be considered for adjuvant measures in conjunction with radical surgery, e.g. irradiation or perioperative chemotherapy?
5. In which categories should purely palliative measures only be considered?

We have made many criticisms of the present classification and staging systems. We must now work to bring these together to form some constructive proposals that can be considered for inclusion in the revised version of the TNM classification in 1988. The last, and perhaps the most important, point that we would wish to stress is that all those engaged in the management of bladder cancer throughout the world should strive to 'speak the same language' when reporting on their treatment and results. Unfortunately, nature has not made things so simple that all the staging and classification systems can be made readily interconvertible. Our immediate goal must be to reach a consensus of opinion that will enable us to extract ourselves from this present confused state where some are talking about stages, others about classifications and still others about categories. Only when we are all speaking the same language can we reliably exchange information and enhance our knowledge of bladder cancer on an international basis. Until then we feel that using the TNM system of classification or the AJCC version offers the best solution to these problems.

References

Adolphs HD, Jacobi GH (1981) Recommendations to the DSK (Deutschsprachiges TNM Komittee). In: Spiessl B, Scheibe O, Wagner G (eds) UICC TNM-atlas: illustrated guide to the classification of malignant tumours. Springer, Berlin Heidelberg New York, p 142

Ahlberg NE, Calissendorff B, Wijkström H (1982) Computed tomography in staging of bladder carcinoma. Acta Radiol [Diagn] (Stockh) 23: 47–53

AJCC (1983) American Joint Committee on Cancer. Manual for staging of cancer, 2nd edn. Lippincott, Philadelphia

Anichkov NM, Zus BA (1980) Evaluation of growth rate of human transitional cell tumors according to sex chromatin (barr bodies) content. J Urol 124: 458–460

Atkin NB, Petkovic I (1973) Variable sex chromatin pattern in an early carcinoma of the bladder. J Clin Pathol 26: 126–129

Austen G Jr, Friedell GH (1965) Observations on local growth patterns of bladder cancer. J Urol 93: 224–229

Blandy JP, England HR, Evans JW, Hope-Stone HF, Mair GMM, Mantell BS, Oliver RTD, Paris AMI, Risdon RA (1980) T3 bladder cancer—the case for salvage cystectomy. Br J Urol 52: 506–510

Chisholm GD, Hindmarsh JR, Howatson AG, Webb JN, Busuttil A, Hargreave TB, Newsam JE (1980) TNM (1978) in bladder cancer: use and abuse. Br J Urol 52: 500–505

Colleen S, Ekelund L, Henrikson H, Karp W, Mansson W (1981) Staging of bladder carcinoma with computed tomography. Scan J Urol Nephrol 15: 109–113

Engelmann U, Schild H, Klose K, Schweden F, Jacobi GH (1984) Accuracy of computer tomography in bladder carcinoma—investigation in 74 patients with radical cystectomy. Urologe [A] 23: 161–166

Falor WH (1971) Chromosomes in noninvasive papillary carcinoma of the bladder. JAMA 216: 791

Falor WH, Ward RM (1976) Cytogenetic analysis: a potential index for recurrence of early carcinoma of the bladder. J Urol 115: 49–52

Fosså SD, Kaalhus O, Scott-Knudsen O (1977) The clinical and histopathological significance of Feulgen DNA-values in transitional cell carcinoma of the human urinary bladder. Eur J Cancer 13: 1155–1162

Frödin L, Hemmingsson A, Johansson A, Wicklund H (1980) Computed tomography in staging of bladder carcinoma. Acta Radiol [Diagn] (Stockh) 21: 763–767

Gustafson H, Tribukait B, Esposti PL (1982a) DNA profile and tumour progression in patients with superficial bladder tumours. Urol Res 10: 13–18

Gustafson H, Tribukait B, Esposti PL (1982b) DNA pattern, histological grade and multiplicity related to recurrence rate in superficial bladder tumours. Scand J Urol Nephrol 16: 135–139

Gustafson H, Tribukait B, Esposti PL (1982c) The prognostic value of DNA analysis in primary carcinoma in situ of the urinary bladder. Scand J Urol Nephrol 16: 141–146

Hodson NJ, Husband JE, MacDonald JA (1979) The role of computed tomography in the staging of bladder cancer. Clin Radiol 30: 389–395

Hofstädter F, Jakse G, Lederer B, Mikuz G (1980) Cytophotometric investigations of DNA-content in transitional cell tumors of the bladder. Comparison of results with clinical follow up. Pathol Res Pract 167: 254–264

Hohenfellner R, Jacobi GH (1982) Cost versus benefit relationship of radioisotope scan methods for the primary staging of bladder and testicular cancer. In: Proceedings of the XIXth Congress of the International Society of Urology, San Francisco, Calif, 5–10 September 1982

Jakse G, Hofstädter F, Maerk R (1981) Specific red cell adherence test and unspecific immune response in patients with superficial bladder cancer. Urol Int 36: 171–177

Jakse G, Rauschmeier H, Lentsch P, Hofstädter F (1983) The pattern of tumour invasion—a possibility to classify muscle-infiltrating tumours. Aktuel Urol 14: 179–182

Jaschke W, van Kaick G, Palmtag H (1981) Was leistet die Computertomographie bei der Bestimmung der lokalen Tumorausdehnung vom Blasenkarzinom?—Ergebnisse mit zwei verschiedenen Füllungsmedien. Computertomographie 1: 125–129

Jeffrey RB, Palubinskas AJ, Federle MP (1981) CT evaluation of invasive lesions of the bladder. J Comput Ass Tomogr 5: 22–26

Jewett HJ (1952) Carcinoma of the bladder: influence of depth of infiltration on the 5-year results following complete extirpation of the primary growth. J Urol 67: 672–680

Jewett HJ, Strong GH (1946) Infiltrating carcinoma of the bladder: relation of depth of penetration of the bladder wall to incidence of local extension and metastases. J Urol 55: 366–372

Karrer P, Zingg E, Vock P, Fischedick A, Haertel M, Fuchs WA (1980) Ergebnisse der Computertomographie beim Staging von Blasentumoren. Aktuel Urol 11: 341–344

Kellett MJ, Oliver RTD, Husband JE, Fry IK (1980) Computed tomography as an adjunct to bimanual examination for staging bladder tumours. Br J Urol 52: 101–106

Koss JC, Arger PH, Coleman BG, Muhern CB Jr, Pollack HM, Wein AJ (1981) CT staging of bladder carcinoma. AJR 137: 359–362

Kulkarni JN, Kamat MR, Gangal SG, Talwalkar GV (1982) Cell surface antigen—a study in bladder tumours. J Surg Oncol 19: 14–17

Lamb D (1967) Correlation of chromosome counts with histological appearances and prognosis in transitional-cell carcinoma of bladder. Br Med J I: 273–277

Marshall VF (1952) The relation of the preoperative estimate to the pathologic demonstration of the extent of vesical neoplasms. J Urol 68: 714–723

Melicow MM, Hollowell JW (1952) Intra-urothelial cancer, carcinoma in situ, Bowen's disease of the urinary system: discussion of thirty cases. J Urol 68: 763–771

Morgan CL, Calkins RF, Cavalcanti EJ (1981) Computed tomography in the evaluation, staging and therapy of carcinoma of the bladder and prostate. Radiology 140: 751–761

Nelson RP (1983) New concepts in staging and follow-up of bladder carcinoma. Urology 21: 105–112

Pearse HD, Reed RR, Hodges CV (1978) Radical cystectomy for bladder cancer. J Urol 119: 216–218

Prout GR Jr (1980) Classification and staging of bladder carcinoma. Cancer 45: 1832–1841

Prout GR Jr (1982) Guest editorial: Bladder cancer. J Urol 128: 284

Pryor JP (1973) Factors influencing the survival of patients with transitional cell tumours of the urinary bladder. Br J Urol 45: 586–592

Pugh RCB (1981) Histological staging and grading of bladder tumours. In: Oliver RTD, Hendry WF, Bloom HJG (eds) Bladder cancer: principles of combination therapy. Butterworths, London, pp 3–8

Richie JP, Skinner DG, Kauffman JJ (1975) Radical cystectomy for carcinoma of the bladder: 16 years of experience. J Urol 113: 186–189

Rost A, Wegener OH, Fiedler U (1981) Der Wert der Computer-Tomographie beim Staging von Harnblasen- und Prostatakarzinomen. Z Urol Nephrol 74: 419–425

Sager EM, Talle K, Fosså S, Ous S, Stenwig AE (1983) The role of CT in demonstrating perivesical tumor growth in the preoperative staging of carcinoma of the urinary bladder. Radiology 146: 443–446

Sandberg AA (1977) Chromosome markers and progression in bladder cancer. Cancer Res 37: 2950–2956

Schellhammer PF, Bean MA, Whitmore WP Jr (1977) Prostatic involvement by transitional cell carcinoma: pathogenesis, patterns and prognosis. J Urol 118: 399–403

Schönbauer C, Imhof H, Küster W, Latal D, Kuber W, Reichelt H (1981) Die Computertomographie zur Stadieneinteilung der Blasentumoren. Röntgenblatter 34: 173–175

Seidelmann FE, Cohen WN, Bryan PJ, Temes SP, Kraus D, Schoenrock G (1978) Accuracy of CT staging of bladder neoplasms using the gas-filled method: Report of 21 patients with surgical confirmation. Am J Roentgenol Radium Ther Nucl Med 130: 735–739

Soto EA, Friedell GH, Tiltman AJ (1977) Bladder cancer as seen in giant histologic sections. Cancer 39: 447–455

Summers JL, Falor WH, Ward R (1981) A 10-year analysis of chromosomes in non-invasive papillary carcinoma of the bladder. J Urol 125: 177–178

Tribukait B, Gustafson H (1980) Flow cytofluorometric DNA analyses in bladder carcinoma. Oncology 3: 278–288

UICC (1978) Harmer MH (ed) TNM classification of malignant tumours, 3rd edn. Union Internationale Contre le Cancer, Geneva

UICC (1982) Spiessl B, Scheibe O, Wagner G (eds) TNM-atlas: illustrated guide to the classification of malignant tumours. Springer, Berlin Heidelberg New York

Vock P, Haertel M, Fuchs WA, Karrer P, Bishop MC, Zingg EJ (1982) Computed tomography in staging of carcinoma of the urinary bladder. Br J Urol 54: 158–163

Wajsman Z, Gamarra M, Park JJ, Beckley S, Pontes JE (1982) Transabdominal fine needle aspiration of retroperitoneal lymph nodes in staging of genitourinary tract cancer (correlation with lymphography and lymph node dissection findings). J Urol 128: 1238–1240

Wallace DM (1975) Classification of bladder tumours. Eur Urol 1: 65–67

Wallace DM, Chisholm GD, Hendry WF (1975) TNM classification for urological tumours. Br J Urol 47: 1–12

Walsh JW, Amendola MA, Konerding KF, Tisnado J, Hazra TA (1980) Computed tomography detection of pelvic and inguinal lymph-node metastases from primary and recurrent pelvic malignant disease. Radiology 137: 157–166

Walz PH, Hutschenreiter G, Wessels G, Scheiding U, von Seelen W (1981) Computer evaluation of ultrasound imaging of the prostate for the early detection of cancer. In: Schulmann CC (ed) Advances in diagnostic urology. Springer, Berlin Heidelberg New York, pp 166–170

Weinerman PM, Arger PH, Pollack HM (1982) CT evaluation of bladder and prostate neoplasms. Urol Radiol 4: 105–114

Wenderoth UK, Engelmann U, Walz PH, Jacobi GH (1984) Die intravesikale Sonographie in der Stadieneinteilung des Harnblasenkarzinoms. Verhandlungsbericht der Deutschen Gesellschaft für Urologie. Springer, Berlin Heidelberg New York, pp 215–216

Chapter 7

Carcinoma In Situ

T. B. Hargreave

Definition of Carcinoma In Situ

Anaplasia of the surface epithelium without the formation of papillary structures and without infiltration. (UICC definition)

This lesion has also been called 'flat carcinoma in situ' (Riddle et al. 1976) or 'flat intraepithelial neoplasia' (Barlebo et al. 1972). These are attempts to define the epithelial abnormality where there is an overtly malignant cellular pattern of the epithelial cells but without invasion or papillary growth. Unfortunately, the histological criteria are not clear cut (see Chap. 2, p. 30) and different pathologists will not necessarily agree: One might report severe dysplasia, whereas another may report the same slide to show carcinoma in situ and a third may attempt to grade the in situ change. The problem is compounded by the different clinical patterns of the disease. Some possible criteria for classification of carcinoma in situ are listed in Table 7.1; however, because of the comparative rarity of the lesion, such classification is not usually made and therefore the natural history of the untreated lesion in each category has not been fully documented.

Table 7.1. Some possible classifications of carcinoma in situ

Carcinoma in situ:
With or without exophytic bladder tumour
Near the base or far from exophytic tumour
Localised or generalised
Involving the prostatic ducts or confined to the bladder
Involving the ureters or confined to the bladder
With or without cystoscopically visible alteration in the urothelium
Symptomatic or asymptomatic

Introduction

Flat carcinoma in situ (Tis) was first described by Melicow (1952), who examined sections of mucosa between gross neoplasms in cystectomy specimens. The clinical significance of these lesions has been clarified by later studies. In 1960 Eisenberg et al. reported that patients with mucosal abnormalities peripheral to excised tumours were more prone to develop tumour recurrences. It was subsequently shown by Koss et al. (1969) that men exposed in industry to *para*-aminodiphenyl and who were shedding cancer cells in the urine had flat carcinoma in situ in the absence of cystoscopically visible lesions, and in some cases these lesions progressed to invasive cancer. In 1979, Koss reported further mapping studies and concluded that there are probably two pathways in bladder carcinogenesis: the papillary pathway and the non-papillary pathway. Papillary tumours were considered to be local expressions of the proliferative potential of the urothelium, which, although relatively harmless, may be followed by other manifestations of neoplasia. However, Koss considered the non-papillary flat lesions, notably atypical hyperplasias and carcinoma in situ, to be the principal source of invasive carcinoma. The concept that the papillary tumour is a marker of the malignant potential of the urothelium but that most invasive tumours arise from flat carcinoma in situ is substantiated by a number of studies (Kulatilake et al. 1970; Farrow et al. 1976; Yates-Bell 1979). The time taken for progression from in situ to invasive carcinoma has been reported to be between 26 and 30 months (Melamed et al. 1964) and between 18 and 77 months (Koss et al. 1969), but it may be much longer.

Detecting Early Change

The evidence linking carcinoma in situ to invasive carcinoma has stimulated the search for ways to detect abnormalities at an earlier stage. The hope is that treatment given earlier could alter the neoplastic potential of the urothelium, either by retarding the cascade of changes so that any neoplasia would be manifest only after the person had died of other causes, or by reversing the carcinogenic changes. There is now evidence that cancer is not necessarily an irreversible biological phenomenon; this has been shown by cloning experiments where mice have been grown back from teratoma cells (Mintz and Illmensee 1975).

Newman and Hicks (1978) used the scanning electron microscope (SEM) to examine sections of non-tumour-bearing mucosa from cystectomy specimens which, although normal by light microscopy, had alterations in the luminal membrane. Although these changes can frequently be seen in premalignant urothelium, they can also be found in inflammatory and infective conditions, thus making exact diagnosis difficult.

In an attempt to detect early change D. M. A. Wallace, A. E. Williams and J. Tocher (1980, unpublished data) also used the SEM: 32 biopsies from normal-looking mucosa in patients who had a bladder cancer and 19 biopsies from tumours were processed for SEM. After examination the biopsies were reprocessed for light microscopy. The SEM preparations were scored on a scale of

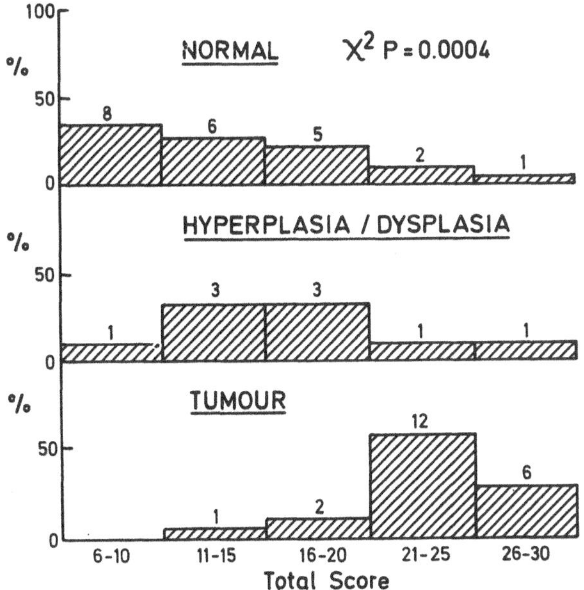

Fig. 7.1. Distribution of SEM. Total score with light microscopy histological type

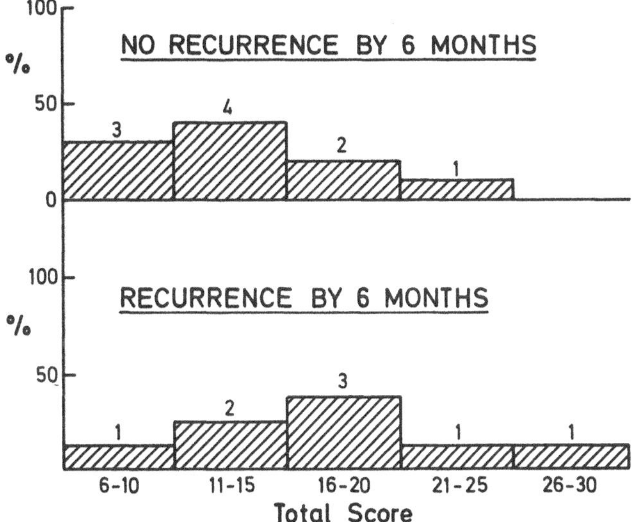

Fig. 7.2. 'Normal' urothelium: variation of SEM ultrastructure score with incidence of tumour recurrence

1–5 according to the following features: cell size, cell shape (whether angular or rounded in outline), intercellular junctions, surface micro-ridges, microvilli and pleomorphism. There were significant differences between the distribution of five out of six of these features (pleomorphism being the exception), between the histologically normal tissue, histologically hyperplastic tissue and tissue taken from the tumours. When the scores were summed an even clearer difference emerged (Fig. 7.1). Only a limited follow-up was available (equivalent to 6 months); when only histologically normal urothelium was considered there was the suggestion that the SEM score might provide an early indication of the patients at risk for tumour recurrence (Fig. 7.2). This preliminary work requires confirmation by a larger series, but this technique may be able to detect neoplastic changes in the luminal surface of the urothelium too subtle to be observed by conventional light microscopy. The advent of newer SEM techniques such as the back-scattered electron mode may allow additional features to be studied, for example the arrangement of the underlying layer of cells and the nuclei.

Another approach has been the use of the red cell adherence test (see Chap. 2), p. 44). This test depends on the fact that malignant urothelial cells may lack the surface blood group antigens. Recent developments, in particular the use of monoclonal antibodies (Finan et al. 1982), have renewed the interest in this test; however, there are still problems with blood group O patients and with the quantification of the test. It remains to be seen whether this test will give better prognostic information than the histological assessment of tumour grade, but it does offer the tantalising possibility that a distinction could be made between apparently similar cases of carcinoma in situ and thereby predict those cases where invasion is imminent.

Fluorescent tumour-localising drugs such as tetracycline have also been tried but have not proved useful, because they are not taken up specifically by malignant or premalignant tissues and because special equipment is required. The attraction of these techniques is that areas of mucosa which appear cystoscopically normal but which are microscopically abnormal could be delineated, thus allowing accurate biopsies and assessment. A technique is being developed which may solve this problem (Kinsey et al. 1978; Kinsey and Cortese 1980; Hisazumi et al. 1984). This system allows normal visual examination through an endoscope with electronic detection of fluorescence induced by haematoporphyrin. Haematoporphyrin is taken up by all tissues, but malignant tissues retain it for longer than normal tissues so that after 48 h the haematoporphyrin left is almost exclusively in malignant tissue, including carcinoma in situ. The haematoporphyrin causes the tissue to fluoresce in ultraviolet light and early reports of the system being used to localise in situ changes are encouraging. In addition to its diagnostic use, haematoporphyrin may have a therapeutic use because in the presence of red light it breaks down to release singlet oxygen, which is very cytotoxic (see Chap. 8, p. 178).

Clinical Presentation of Carcinoma In Situ

The diagnosis of carcinoma in situ is usually made in one of two ways:

1. A patient may have a biopsy taken, usually because of symptoms (symptomatic carcinoma in situ), or because the cytological examination gives a positive result or because there are mucosal changes on cystoscopy.
2. A patient with an overt bladder tumour may have biopsies taken of either normal or abnormal-looking mucosa (carcinoma in situ associated with an exophytic tumour or secondary carcinoma in situ).

These two clinical situations have been called primary Tis and secondary Tis (de Voogt et al. 1977; Jakse et al 1980). It is possible that the categorisations in Table 7.1 will allow further subgroups to be defined, but clinical reports so far usually only distinguish the above two categories.

Patients with symptomatic carcinoma in situ (malignant cystitis) are often young or middle-aged men who present with frequency and dysuria—symptoms that may be mistaken for outflow obstruction—and they usually have haematuria. They may have a constant pain which is either penile, perineal or suprapubic. It is important that this symptom complex is recognised and that a urine sample is sent for cytological examination or that a cystoscopy and biopsies are performed. Carcinoma in situ must be suspected whenever these symptoms occur, particularly in patients who have persisting symptoms after prostatectomy, and also in those cases with abacterial cystitis when there is microscopic haematuria or pyuria.

This group of patients with severe symptoms has a poor prognosis unless radical treatment is undertaken early (Riddle et al. 1976). The clinical course of patients with carcinoma in situ associated with exophytic tumour has not yet been fully documented; there is no doubt that the occasional case may be followed for several years without obvious invasion. However, the close monitoring of symptomatic patients by cytology, endoscopy and biopsies has been compared to watching a time bomb gradually tick off the seconds (Soloway 1981). Confusion between these two patterns of disease as well as between in situ carcinoma and dysplasia has led to variable clinical opinion about the correct management of this condition.

Investigations

Cystoscopic Findings

There is no diagnostic mucosal appearance of carcinoma in situ. In symptomatic cases the mucosa may appear red, inflamed and oedematous; however, biopsies from apparently normal mucosa may also show dysplasia or carcinoma in situ (Table 7.2). The two categories of carcinoma in situ (i.e. symptomatic carcinoma in situ and carcinoma in situ associated with exophytic tumour) are often not distinguished in reported series, and this makes such reports difficult to assess (Schade and Swinney 1968; Cooper et al. 1973; Schade and Swinney, 1973; Heney et al. 1978; Soloway et al. 1978).

It is apparent from the findings listed in Table 7.2 that the presence of a red patch or mossy appearance increases the likelihood that carcinoma in situ will be

Table 7.2. Results of mucosal biopsy in 56 new cases shown according to the worst cystoscopic appearance of the mucosa (adapted from Wallace et al. 1979)

Mucosal appearance	(*n*)	Least favourable mucosal biopsy				
		Normal (%)	Hyperplasia	Mild dysplasia	Severe dysplasia	Carcinoma in situ
Normal	(41)	20 (49)	5	10	1	5
Flat red	(11)	3 (27)	3	0	1	4
Mossy	(4)	1 (25)	0	1	1	1

Table 7.3. Same results as Table 7.2 for 52 patients previously treated by radiotherapy (Wallace et al. 1979)

Mucosal appearance	(*n*)	Least favourable mucosal biopsy				
		Normal	Hyperplasia	Mild dysplasia	Severe dysplasia	Carcinoma
Normal	(10)	3	1	4	1	1
Flat red	(19)	6	5	2	1	5
Mossy	(23)	1	4	4	2	12

found. It is also worth noting that red patches seen at cystoscopy during follow-up after radiotherapy should not be dismissed as radiation reaction (Table 7.3).

Bladder Capacity

The bladder capacity should be measured in all cases of bladder cancer. Reduced capacity in association with red mucosa is one of the features of carcinoma in situ; indeed, the small capacity bladder may be a contraindication to intravesical chemotherapy. If chemotherapy is proposed, serial bladder measurements may give an indication of the response.

Bimanual Examination Under Anaesthesia

In a case of carcinoma in situ there is, by definition, no bimanually palpable lesion. In view of the fact that most invasive cancer is thought to arise from these lesions, bimanual examination is particularly important during the follow-up of treatment, as occasionally invasion may occur without any obvious intravesical projection of the tumour.

Mucosal Biopsy

The advent of small cup biopsy forceps (Fig. 7.3) has meant that it is now possible to sample normal mucosa as well as any suspicious areas in all new cases of

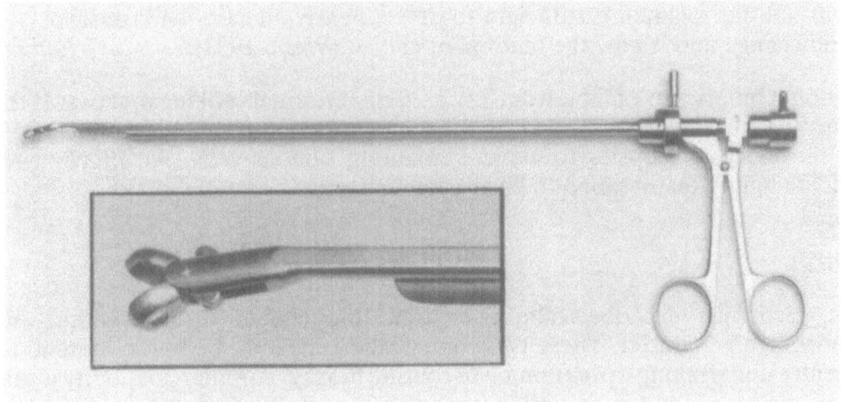

Fig. 7.3. Cup biopsy forceps

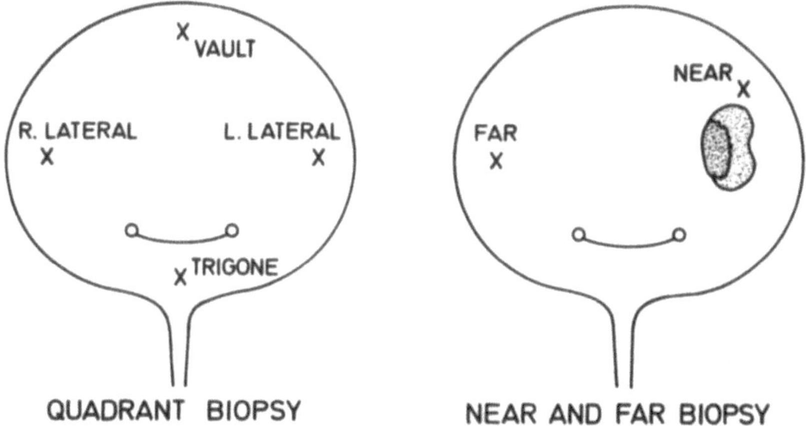

Fig. 7.4. Two systems commonly used for elective biopsy of the apparently normal mucosa

transitional cell cancer of the bladder. The older Lowsley biopsy forceps were too traumatic to allow this sort of routine sampling. The procedure is best undertaken before definitive treatment of any exophytic tumours. Iso-osmotic irrigating fluid should be used, as water causes the surface umbrella cells to desquamate and results in poorer histological preparations. The bladder is filled to approximately two-thirds capacity and the forceps are used to grasp a small portion of mucosa. The purpose of doing the biopsy is to sample the apparently normal mucosa and it is therefore not necessary to dig the forceps in to obtain muscle; indeed, in patients with thin bladders this could be hazardous. There are two commonly used biopsy regimens (Fig. 7.4):

1. Quadrant biopsies—samples are taken from the bladder vault, the right and left lateral walls and from the midline near the trigone.
2. Near and far biopsies—samples are taken from within 2 cm of the base of the primary tumour and from a site on the bladder wall opposite the primary. The

near and far regimen is sufficient to detect nearly all cases with unsuspected field change and is now the method of choice (Webb 1983).

Additional biopsies are taken from any area of abnormal-looking mucosa. If the primary tumour is to be biopsied with the same forceps, this should be undertaken after the mucosal biopsies to avoid implanting tumour cells. All biopsy sites should be lightly diathermied to ensure haemostasis.

Hazards

If the technique described above is used, the chance of perforation and haemorrhage is reduced. These two complications need to be borne in mind by any centre undertaking a programme of routine biopsy. Another possibility is that tumour could be implanted either from another site or from the surface to a deeper layer. There is some experimental and circumstantial evidence that tumour implantation can occur at the time of endoscopic resection and diathermy (Boyd and Burnand 1974; Weldon and Soloway 1975; Page et al. 1978), but only one possible case has been identified at the Western General Hospital, Edinburgh, where a 6-year programme involving several hundred quadrant biopsies has been undertaken.

Another theoretical hazard is that the trauma of the biopsy may accelerate cancerous changes in the mucosa, and it has been said that biopsy should be avoided if at all possible because of this risk (Hicks 1982). The evidence supporting this is experimental only, and there is no clinical evidence that patients who have had multiple mucosal biopsies have more recurrent and invasive tumours. An interesting variation of the biopsy technique is the endoscopic bladder brush technique (Connolly 1979), which can sample cells from wide areas of the bladder for cytological examination; this may be appropriate in cases of carcinoma in situ treated with intravesical chemotherapy where repeated biopsy would otherwise be necessary.

Indications

In the light of the above information some guidelines as to the indications for mucosal biopsy can now be given:

1. Biopsies should be taken of any abnormal-looking areas of urothelium seen in association with exophytic tumour or at cystoscopic follow-up after successful treatment of an exophytic tumour (see Table 7.3).
2. Mucosal biopsies are recommended if urine cytology shows malignant cells in the absence of any exophytic tumour anywhere in the urinary tract.
3. Mucosal biopsies are also recommended if the patient has symptoms of suprapubic or perineal pain which are not explained by urinary infection or obstruction. Such pain may precede the diagnosis of carcinoma in situ by several months, and repeat mucosal biopsies may be indicated after an interval if the results of the first set are normal.
4. At present, routine mucosal biopsy as part of the assessment of a known case of exophytic bladder carcinoma cannot be recommended except as part of a prospective scientific assessment. The natural history of in situ change

associated with exophytic tumour but discovered incidentally is not yet known; a haphazard mucosal biopsy policy with treatment prescribed in an erratic fashion will only confuse an already difficult problem and almost certainly result in overtreatment of patients.

Significance of Results

In the symptomatic group of patients mucosal biopsies are necessary to establish the diagnosis prior to therapy. The question remains whether a programme of routine biopsy of normal mucosa in new bladder tumour cases will yield results which will improve management. Several reports suggest that this will be so. The preliminary results of a prospective surveillance study where mucosal biopsies were obtained from (1) adjacent to the original tumour, (2) lateral to each ureteric orifice and (3) the posterior midline have been reported (Murphy et al. 1979). These results suggest that the presence of hyperplasia, dysplasia and carcinoma in situ may predict subsequent tumour recurrence. The studies by Wolf and Hojgaard (1983) and Schade and Swinney (1983) also support this view. Wolf and Hojgaard (1983) reported on 53 patients with T1 and T2 tumours. In half of the cases concomitant urothelial dysplasia was found and new tumours subsequently occurred in 87% of these cases as compared with 26% who had no mucosal changes. Schade and Swinney (1983) reported the 10-year follow-up of 100 patients who had mucosal biopsies as part of their initial assessment. The outstanding finding was that patients with carcinoma in situ had a significantly worse outcome ($P<0.001$) than those with normal mucosa, regardless of the characteristics of the primary tumour and its grade and stage.

The predictive value of mucosal biopsy is also supported by a prospective study from our own department (Smith et al. 1983): 112 new cases with Ta and T1 exophytic transitional cell cancer had quadrant mucosal biopsies at the initial cystoscopy. Patients with one or more abnormal biopsies (dysplasia or carcinoma in situ) were shown to have a significantly ($P<0.01$) higher probability of recurrence (Fig. 7.5). In all cases the only treatment was endoscopic resection or cystodiathermy of the initial tumour (see also Chap. 8, pp. 164–165).

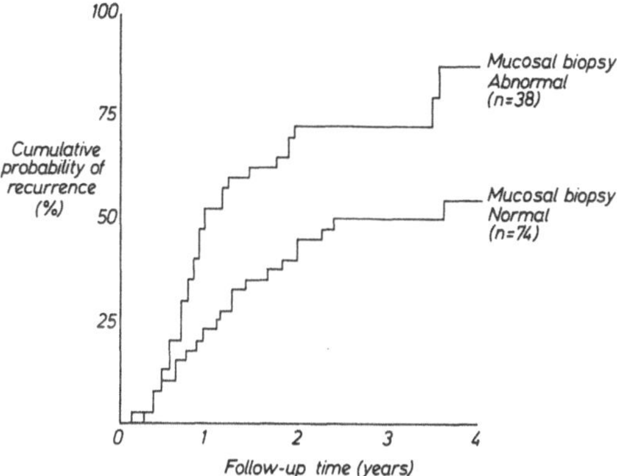

Fig. 7.5. Life table estimate of cumulative probability of transitional cell carcinoma recurrence in 112 patients who initially presented with Ta T1 exophytic tumour. The results are stratified according to the findings from quadrant mucosal biopsy taken at the cystoscopy when the patient first attended as a new untreated case. (Smith et al. 1983)

Further prospective studies were started in the UK by the Medical Research Council in 1981. Until such time as results are clear, and in view of the potential hazards and extra workload for the pathology department, mucosal biopsies are not yet part of the routine preoperative evaluation of all cases, although a strong case can be made out for doing them.

Carcinoma In Situ Involving the Prostate

Farrow et al. (1976) reported mapping studies on 19 total cystectomy specimens from men with symptomatic non-papillary carcinoma in situ and found carcinoma in situ extending into the prostatic ducts in seven cases (37%). In situ and invasive transitional cell carcinoma originating in the prostatic ducts has also been reported by Kirk et al. (1979) and Wolf and Lloyd-Davies (1981). One problem is that the current UICC rules for classification of prostatic involvement are not adequate (see Chap. 6, p. 127). In 27 patients with prostatic involvement by transitional cell carcinoma three subgroups were apparent: (1) prostatic duct in situ carcinoma, (2) non-invasive papillary tumours of the prostatic urethra and (3) direct invasion of the prostate by tumour at the bladder base or bladder neck (Chibber et al. 1981). The last situation is what is meant in the UICC classification as T4a. In situ carcinoma of the prostatic ducts is important because it may occur in conjunction with an in situ change in the bladder and is not apparent unless the prostate is resected. If intravesical chemotherapy is used to treat a male patient with in situ change in the bladder this would seem likely to fail in those cases with prostatic involvement, and consideration needs to be given to transurethral resection of the prostate prior to the chemotherapy. There is not yet enough evidence to recommend routine TUR in all male cases where carcinoma in situ is discovered; therefore, there is a need for prospective clinical studies of the incidence of prostatic involvement in relation to the categories of carcinoma in situ listed in Table 7.1.

Urine Cytology

Urine cytology has theoretical advantages both in the diagnosis and follow-up of in situ cancer. There may be diffuse microscopic lesions which appear normal on cystoscopy and can be missed by mucosal biopsy but which may be detected by cytology. Urine cytology is non-invasive and avoids any risk of stimulating urothelial proliferation by the trauma of a biopsy of an already unstable mucosa (see p. 16). Urine cytology may give false negative results compared with biopsy, but the discrepancy is least in cases of carcinoma in situ and high-grade tumour (Table 7.4). Bladder washing taken by saline barbotage may improve the frequency of positive cytological results (Harris et al. 1971), although the main value of this is in cases of low-grade tumour, as a simple urine cytology usually has a positive result in association with in situ change. Distilled water should not be used as this will produce artefacts and confuse the diagnosis, as has been found in rats (Weinsten et al. 1979).

Table 7.4. Correlation between cytology and biopsy findings at initial and follow-up examinations (adapted from Loening et al. 1978)

Cytology	Biopsy	
	Grade 1	Carcinoma in situ
Negative or normal	17	4
Radiation/drug effect	0	1
TCC or suggestive of TCC	12	20
Carcinoma in situ	0	1
Correlation between biopsy and cytology	41%	80%

TCC, transitional cell cancer

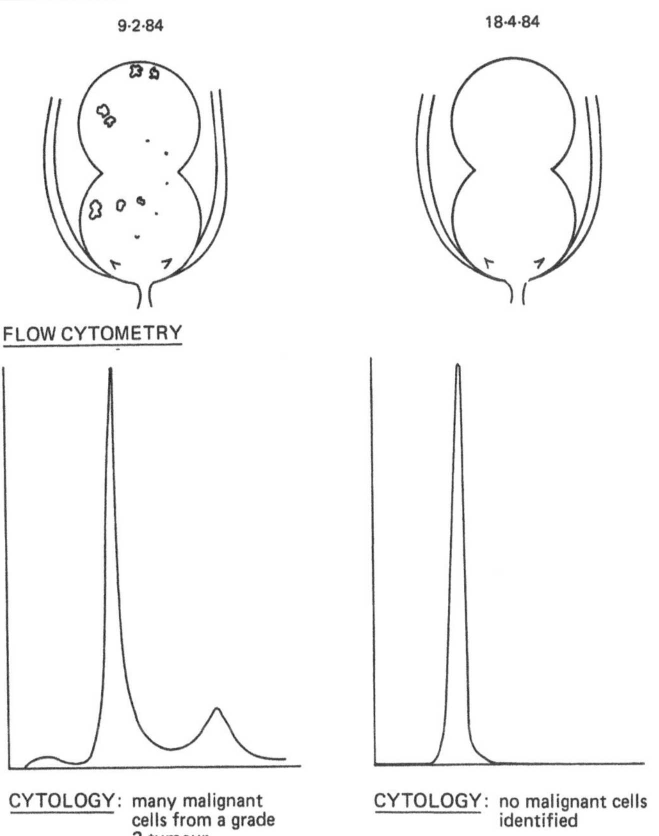

Fig. 7.6. The use of cystoscopy, urine cytology and flow cytometry to monitor the progress of a patient with widespread field change who had intravesical mitomycin C instillations. Note how the bladder has cleared of exophytic lesions, urine cytology has become negative and the peaks of abnormal DNA have disappeared. (Unpublished data from Dr. G. G. Hadjissotiriou, Dr. D. K. Green and Dr. M. A. McIntyre, Dept. of Urology, Western General Hospital, Edinburgh)

An exciting new technique is the application of flow cytometry to cytological specimens taken from bladder washings (Devonec et al. 1981; Farsund et al. 1984). This technique allows objective measurement of DNA and RNA content and may give more exact information when combined with the cytological grade of malignancy (Fig. 7.6). Although the figure illustrates a case with exophytic tumour, the technique is perhaps most appropriate for cytological specimens from patients with carcinoma in situ.

Treatment

There is now recognition that symptomatic carcinoma in situ, as described above, is a highly malignant condition progressing in most cases to invasive and metastasising carcinoma and that early radical treatment is indicated. The choice of radical treatment will depend on the age and general condition of the patient, the severity of symptoms and whether the prostate is involved. Much more controversial is the treatment of in situ change associated with the exophytic tumour; most urologists treat the patient according to the stage and grade of the exophytic lesion, and this treatment is not necessarily altered by the fact that the surrounding mucosa shows carcinoma in situ.

Cystourethrectomy

Riddle et al. (1976) reported the results of treatment of 23 cases of symptomatic carcinoma in situ. Eleven of these patients were treated by cystectomy or cystourethrectomy and one by partial cystectomy. Seven patients were alive at follow-up (mean of 2 years), although two had secondary deposits. Four died of disseminated disease (mean survival of 3 years). The comment was made that although cystectomy was performed for the condition of symptomatic carcinoma in situ, in many cases examination of the cystectomy specimen showed invasion; it is likely that but for the operation all would have developed disseminated disease.

If cystectomy is indicated, the operation should be a radical cystourethrectomy with node dissection because (1) there is frequent involvement of the prostatic urethra, (2) there is frequent unsuspected muscle invasion and (3) nodal metastases may occur rapidly once invasion starts. Utz et al. (1980) also advocate radical cystectomy if the patient is a reasonably good candidate for surgery when the disease is widespread in the bladder and the symptoms are severe. Radical surgery offers the best chance of cure in these patients who have a high risk of developing invasive and metastasising cancers; however, a trial of systemic or intravesical chemotherapy is justified, provided that the response is carefully and critically evaluated.

Radiotherapy

Riddle et al. (1976) reported 11 patients with symptomatic carcinoma in situ who received radiotherapy. The decision to use radiotherapy was often made because of an unwillingness to subject a patient to major surgery for an apparently 'early' disease. One patient remained alive at 8 years, but the histology was unaltered. One patient committed suicide because of continuing perineal pain. One patient died as a result of gastrointestinal complications from the therapy, seven patients died from dissemination bladder cancer (mean survival of 3 years) and one patient died from prostatic malignancy. Riddle's experience suggests that radiotherapy will not prevent metastases from carcinoma in situ, whereas cystectomy may do so. Kulatilake et al. (1970) and Farrow et al. (1977) also report similar poor responses to radiotherapy. Hewitt et al. (1981) does, however, report more favourable responses in 14 patients treated with intracavitary radiation.

Chemotherapy

Systemic Cyclophosphamide

Fifteen patients (14 men and 1 woman) were treated by England and colleagues (1981) with systemic cyclophosphamide. The effect of cyclophosphamide on the bladder was to produce an extensive loss of the mucosa, which later re-epithelialised with a thin but normal mucosa. Six of these patients had severe symptoms of malignant cystitis. The cyclophosphamide was given at first intravenously every 3 weeks for 6 months and then every 6 weeks for 6 months at a dose of 1 g/m^2, but in the light of the results cyclophosphamide therapy is now stopped at 3 months. At 3 months 12 out of 15 patients had a complete response with negative cytological and biopsy results. The remaining three patients showed a marked reduction. There was also a relief of symptoms in five out of six patients with symptoms of malignant cystitis. The therapy caused three patients to have such severe nausea and vomiting that further treatment was refused after 3 months. This complication has led to the search for less toxic cyclophosphamide analogues. 1-Phosphamide, although theoretically less toxic, may in practice have equally severe toxic effects including nausea and diarrhoea (T. B. Hargreave, unpublished data). Systemic cyclophosphamide, in spite of its toxicity, may be an acceptable alternative to radical surgery and does not preclude surgery should it be unsuccessful.

Intracavitary Therapy

The ideal intracavitary agent is effective in penetrating transitional epithelium but will not be absorbed into the circulation and will not have local or systemic effects. Intracavitary therapy has been assessed in cases with extensive or rapidly recurring superficial tumours and as prophylaxis following resection. In these situations the main agents used have been the alkylating agents thiotepa and Epodyl, mitosis blocking agents such as podophyllin or its derivative VM26, and antibiotics such as Adriamycin or mitomycin C. There is much less information about the use of intracavitary therapy with these agents in cases of carcinoma in situ, although promising results have been reported following Adriamycin therapy. If prostatic duct involvement has been found this is a contraindication to intravesical therapy unless a TUR of the prostate is also proposed. Patients should also be assessed for ureteric reflux as this may contraindicate intracavitary therapy if the agent to be used is known to damage the kidney; in fact in some cases it may be advantageous if there is reflux, as in situ lesions extending into the lower ureters will also be treated.

Assessing the Response to Local Chemotherapy

The response to treatment is difficult to assess because symptomatic carcinoma in situ is rare and also because the natural history of carcinoma in situ associated with exophytic tumour is not known. Several methods of assessment may be used.

Timing. Records are kept of time to development of an exophytic tumour, time to development of an invasive recurrence (recurrence showing muscle invasion) and time to death from tumour.

Repeated Mucosal Biopsy. If repeated biopsies are to be carried out then the risk of implantation and possibly the risks of stimulating tumour must be considered (see p. 16). The brush technique described by Connolly (1979) may overcome some of these problems, although the sample obtained is suitable for a cytological diagnosis only and is not a biopsy.

Repeat Urine Cytology. This method has the advantage that it is easy for the patient, non-invasive and is a sample of the whole bladder mucosa.

Symptoms. Successful chemotherapy for symptomatic carcinoma in situ will cause a disappearance of pain. Nevertheless, additional objective measures of response, such as biopsy or cytology, are advisable.

Intravesical Doxorubicin (Adriamycin)

The attractions of doxorubicin when instilled intravesically are (1) that the agent is active against transitional cell carcinoma (Yagoda et al. 1977) and (2) that when instilled it appears to penetrate urothelium up to but not beyond the basement membrane; thus when used by this route it has few systemic effects (Jacobi and Kurth 1980).

Edsmyr (1981) reported treatment with 80 mg Adriamycin dissolved in 100 ml physiological saline instilled into the bladder through a urethral catheter. The catheter was removed and the patient instructed to lie on each side of the body alternately every 15 min. The solution was retained in the bladder for 60 min and then voided. The regimen was repeated each month. This treatment was repeated up to 26 months, according to the cystoscopic findings at follow-up.

Prior to therapy 11 patients had no visible tumour at cystoscopy but the diagnosis had been made by biopsy or cytological examination. A further 19 patients had carcinoma in situ in association with exophytic tumour, which was treated either by resection or radiotherapy. It is not clear how many of Edsmyr's patients fell into the group with symptomatic malignant cystitis and how many were incidentally diagnosed. The results are shown in Table 7.5. The author

Table 7.5. Cytological response to intravesical Adriamycin given for carcinoma in situ (Edsmyr et al. 1979)

Tis		*Tis associated with other tumour*	
No. of patients	11	No. of patients	19
No. of instillations	4–26	No. of instillations	1–20
Cytological remission	Atypia	Cytological remission	Atypia
9/11	1/11	11/19	3/19
82%	9%	58%	16%
91%		74%	

concluded that at least four treatments are necessary in those cases with no other tumour and 11 treatments in those cases associated with exophytic tumour. The most frequent complication of this therapy was a slight reduction in bladder capacity, which occurred in 2 out of 30 patients. Jakse et al. (1980) observed remission in 12 out of 18 patients. Half of the patients were treated with 40 mg Adriamycin in 20 ml saline instilled twice weekly and half received 80 mg Adriamycin in 40 ml saline each month. There was no difference in response rates between the two treatment groups.

Glashan (1982) reported the results of Adriamycin in 21 patients, all of whom had been exposed to industrial carcinogens and in whom urine cytology was diagnostic of carcinoma in situ. Seventeen of these patients also had a red bladder at cystoscopy. A regimen of 50 mg Adriamycin in 50 ml saline retained for 2 h was instituted. This was repeated weekly for 6 weeks. Of the 21 patients 12 showed a complete cytological response and 8 a partial response. All 17 patients with a red bladder showed improved post-therapy cystoscopic appearances.

Other Intravesical Agents

Thiotepa, Epodyl and mitomycin C (Mishina et al. 1982; Prout et al. 1982) have all been used to treat carcinoma in situ with some success. Mitomycin C is worthy of mention as the agent with the most promise. However, a clear evaluation of the role of these agents in carcinoma in situ cannot be made yet for the reasons previously outlined (see also Chap. 10, p. 245).

Intravesical Bacillus Calmette-Guérin

In 1976, Morales et al. reported decreased transitional cell tumour recurrence following repeated instillations of bacillus Calmette Guérin (BCG) into the bladder of nine patients, and subsequently this effect has been confirmed by randomised studies (Brosman 1982; Pinsky et al. 1982). The method of action is unknown, although it is assumed to be an immunotherapeutic effect (see Chap. 3, pp. 68–70). Effectiveness is thought to depend on the ability of the host to react to mycobacterial antigens, a small tumour load and close contact between tumour cells and the BCG (Brosman 1982). Recently Herr et al. (1983) have reported the effect of intravesical and percutaneous BCG on cases with carcinoma in situ.

Forty-one patients with carcinoma in situ in association with stage O, A or B transitional cell cancer were part of a randomised trial of BCG versus endoscopic resection. BCG was administered for 6 weeks both by intravesical instillation (120 mg in 50 ml saline retained for 2 h) and percutaneously (5×10^7 viable units by the multiple tine techniques) beginning 2 weeks after complete endoscopic resection of all visible lesions. Response to therapy was considered complete if the following criteria were met: improved cystoscopic appearance of the bladder mucosa, negative biopsy of any suspicious lesions, negative urine cytological results and improvement in the severity of any voiding symptoms in those patients with symptoms. At 1 year 11 of 17 patients treated by TUR and BCG had no clinical or pathological evidence of carcinoma in situ compared with 2 out of 24 patients treated by TUR alone. These authors also noted two patients who had no residual tumour in the bladder but required cystourethrectomy because of persisting disease in the prostatic ducts (see p. 156). Preliminary results from BCG would appear to rival those reported for Adriamycin, and thus this form of therapy is worthy of further evaluation.

Lasers

There has been limited experience with argon laser treatment for carcinoma in situ (Smith and Dixon 1984). The advantages of the argon laser compared with the neodymium-yttrium aluminium garnet laser are that the burn is superficial and therefore it is possible to treat wide areas of the bladder without causing contracture. Other advantages are that treatment can be performed through a 21 F cystoscope, general anaesthesia is not necessary and bleeding is minimal. The role of laser therapy for carcinoma in situ has yet to be defined, but it may have a place in patients who are unfit for other forms of treatment (see also Chap. 8, p. 177; Chap. 11, p. 273).

Summary

Of the many questions still unanswered about carcinoma in situ one of the most important is how can we predict when it is going to become invasive? Those patients with severe symptoms (malignant cystitis) will require prompt radical treatment, but how long can asymptomatic focal carcinoma in situ be watched? It is a brave patient who allows his doctor simply to observe such lesions. The assessment of response to therapy will remain inadequate until there are better ways to define the disease. The major role for intravesical chemotherapy is likely to be in the treatment of patients with superficial bladder tumours and focal carcinoma in situ. The monitoring of the response to therapy by multiple biopsies and repeated urine cytology should give an indication of the efficacy of the treatment.

The indications for radical cystectomy in this disease will always be relative, as long as there are developments in the field of chemotherapy. While the carcinoma remains in situ it can be cured, and the decision to perform radical surgery must not be left too late.

Extension of in situ carcinoma beyond the bladder into the prostatic urethra and prostatic ducts should be considered before commencing local treatment with intravesical chemotherapy as this is likely to be the cause of treatment failure. The place of TUR of the prostate and prostatic biopsies in patients with carcinoma in situ has yet to be determined.

The encouraging initial results of systemic and intravesical chemotherapy or immunotherapy may save many patients from the prospect of radical surgery. The treatment of in situ bladder cancer with chemotherapeutic agents is perhaps one of the most exciting areas of urological oncology, offering the prospect of a significant alteration in prognosis.

References

Barlebo H, Sorenson BL, Ohlsen AS (1972) Carcinoma in situ of the urinary bladder: flat intraepithelial neoplasia. Scan J Urol Nephrol 6: 213–223

Boyd PRJ, Burnand KG (1974) Site of bladder tumour recurrence. Lancet II: 1290–1292

Brosman SA (1982) Experience with Bacillus Calmette-Guérin in patients with superficial bladder cancer. J Urol 128: 27–30

Chibber PJ, McIntyre MA, Hindmarsh JR, Hargreave TB, Newsam JE, Chisholm GD (1981) Transitional cell carcinoma involving the prostate. Br J Urol 33: 605–609

Connolly JG (1979) Bladder brush. Urology 14: 177–178

Cooper PH, Waisman J, Johnston WH, Skinner DG (1973) Severe atypia of transitional epithelium and carcinoma of the urinary bladder. Cancer 31: 1055–1060

Devonec M, Darzynkiewicz Z, Whitmore WF, Melamed MR (1981) Flow cytometry for follow-up examinations of conservatively treated low stage bladder tumors. J Urol 126: 166–170

de Voogt HJ, Rathert P, Beyer-Boon ME (1977) Carcinoma in situ. In: de Voogt HJ, Rathert P, Beyer-Boon ME (eds) Urinary cytology. Springer, Berlin Heidelberg New York, pp 127–133

Edsmyr F (1981) Intravesical therapy with doxorubicin in patients with superficial bladder tumours. In: Oliver RTD, Hendry WF, Bloom HJG (eds) Bladder cancer: principles of combination therapy. Butterworths, London, pp 107–114

Edsmyr F, Berlin T, Boman J, Esposti PL, Gustagson H, Wikstrom H (1979) Intravesical therapy with Adriamycin in patients with superficial bladder tumours In: Proceedings of the First Conference on Treatment of Urinary Tract Tumors with Adriamycin, Tokyo, 1979, pp 50–57. Obtainable from Montedison Pharmaceuticals

England HR, Molland EA, Oliver RTD, Blandy JP (1981) Systemic cyclophosphamide in flat carcinoma in situ of the bladder. In: Oliver RTD, Hendry WF, Bloom HJG (eds) Bladder cancer: principles of combination therapy. Butterworths, London, pp 97–105

Farrow GM, Utz DC, Rife CC (1976) Morphological and clinical observations of patients with early bladder cancer treated with total cystectomy. Cancer Res 36: 2495–2501

Farrow GM, Utz DC, Rife CC, Greene LF (1977) Clinical observations on sixty-nine cases of in situ carcinoma of the urinary bladder. Cancer Res 37: 2794–2798

Farsund T, Laerum OD, Høstmark J, Jorfald G (1984) Local chemotherapeutic effects in bladder cancer demonstrated by selective sampling and flow cytometry. J Urol 131: 22–32

Finan PJ, Anderson J, Doyle PT, Lennox ES, Bleehen NM (1982) The prediction of invasive potential in superficial transitional cell carcinoma of the bladder. Br J Urol 54: 720–725

Glashan RW (1982) Intravesical therapy with Adriamycin in urothelial dysplasia and early carcinoma in situ. Can J Surg 25: 30–32

Harris MJ, Schwinn CP, Morrow JW, Browell BM (1971) Exfoliative cytology of the urinary irrigation specimen. Acta Cytol 15: 385–399

Heney NM, Daly J, Prout GR Jr, Nieh PT, Heaney JA, Trebeck NF (1978) Biopsy of apparently normal urothelium in patients with bladder carcinoma. J Urol 120: 559–560

Herr HW, Pinsky CM, Whitmore WJ Jr, Oettgen HF, Melamed MR (1983) Effect of intravesical Bacillus Calmette-Guérin (BCG) on carcinoma in situ of the bladder. Cancer 51: 1323–1326

Hewitt CB, Babiszewski JF, Antunez AR (1981) Update on intracavitary radiation in the treatment of bladder tumours. J Urol 126: 323–325

Hicks RM (1982) The development of bladder cancer. In: Williams DI, Chisholm GD (eds) Scientific foundations in urology. Heinemann, London, pp 711–722

Hisazumi H, Misaki T, Mioshi N, Katsusuke N, Misaki T (1984) Whole bladder wall photo radiation therapy for carcinoma in situ: a preliminary report. J Urol 131: 884–887

Jacobi GH, Kurth KH (1980) Studies on the intravesical action of topically administered G3H-doxorubicin hydrochloride in men: plasma uptake and penetration. J Urol 124: 34–37

Jakse G, Hofstadter F, Leither G, Marberger H (1980) Carcinoma in situ of the urinary bladder. A diagnostic and therapeutic challenge. Urologe [A] 19: 93–99

Kinsey JH, Cortese DA (1980) Endoscopic system for simultaneous visual examination and electronic detection of fluorescence. Rev Sci Instrum 51: 1403–1406

Kinsey JH, Cortese DA, Sanderson DR (1978) Detection of hematoporphyrin fluorescence during fibreoptic bronchoscopy to localise early bronchogenic carcinoma. Mayo Clin Proc 53: 594–600

Kirk D, Hinton CE, Shaldon C (1979) Transitional cell carcinoma of the prostate. Br J Urol 51: 575–578

Koss LG (1979) Mapping of the urinary bladder: its impact on the concepts of bladder cancer. Hum Pathol 10: 533–548

Koss LG, Melamed MR, Kelly RE (1969) Further cytologic and histologic studies of bladder lesions in workers exposed to *para*-aminodiphenyl; progress report. J Natl Cancer Inst 43: 233–234

Kulatilake AE, Chisholm GD, Olsen EGJ (1970) In situ carcinoma of the urinary bladder. Proc R Soc Med 63: 95–97

Loening S, Narayana A, Yoder L, Slymen S, Weinstein G, Penick G, Culp D (1978) Longitudinal study of bladder cancer with cytology and biopsy. Br J Urol 50: 496–501

Melamed MR, Voutsa NG, Grabstald H (1964) Natural history and clinical behaviour of in situ carcinoma of the human urinary bladder. Cancer 17: 1533–1545

Melicow MM (1952) Histological study of vesical urothelium intervening between gross neoplasms in total cystectomy. J Urol 68: 261–279

Mintz B, Illmensee K (1975) Normal genetically mosaic mice produced from malignant teratocarcinoma cells. Proc Natl Acad Sci USA 72: 3585–3589

Mishina T, Watanabe H, Fujiwara T, Kobayashi T, Maegawa M, Nakao M, Nakagawa S (1982) Prophylactic use of mitomycin C bladder instillation for preventing the recurrence of bladder tumours. In: Ogana M, Rozencweig M, Staquet MJ (eds) Mitomycin C—current impact on cancer chemotherapy. Exerpta Medica, Amsterdam, pp 153–162

Morales A, Eidinger D, Bruce AW (1976) Intracavitary bacillus Calmette-Guérin in the treatment of superficial bladder tumours. J Urol 116: 180–183

Murphy WM, Nagy GK, Rao MK, Soloway MS, Parija GC, Cox CF, Friedell GH (1979) Normal urothelium in patients with bladder cancer: a preliminary report from the National Bladder Cancer Project Collaborative Group A. Cancer 44: 1050–1058

Newman J, Hicks RM (1978) Detection of neoplastic and preneoplastic urothelia by combined scanning and transmission electron microscopy of urinary surface of human rat bladders. Histopathology 1: 15–135

Page BH, Levinson VB, Curwen MP (1978) The site of recurrence of non-infiltrating bladder tumours. Br J Urol 50: 237–242

Pinsky CM, Camacho FJ, Kerr D, Braun DW, Whitmore WF Jr, Oettgen H (1982) Treatment of superficial bladder cancer with intravesical Bacillus Calmette-Gúerin (BCG). In: Terry W, Rosenberg S (eds) Immunotherapy of human cancer: present state of trials in man, vol 2. Elsevier North Holland, New York, pp 309–312

Prout GR Jr, Griffin PP, Nocks BN, DeFuria D, Daly JJ (1982) Intravesical therapy of low stage bladder carcinoma with mitomycin C: comparison of results in untreated and previously treated patients. J Urol 127: 1096–1098

Riddle PR, Chisholm GD, Trott PA, Pugh RCB (1976) Flat carcinoma in situ of bladder. Br J Urol 47: 829–833

Schade ROK, Swinney J (1968) Precancerous changes in bladder epithelium. Lancet II: 943–946

Schade ROK, Swinney J (1973) The association of urothelial atypism with neoplasia: its importance in treatment and prognosis. J Urol 109: 619–622

Schade ROK, Swinney J (1983) The association of urothelial abnormalities with neoplasia: a 10 year followup. J Urol 129: 1125–1126

Smith JA, Dixon JA (1984) Argon laser phototherapy of superficial transitional cell carcinoma of bladder. J Urol 131: 655–656

Smith G, Elton RA, Beynon LL, Newsam JE, Chisholm GD, Hargreave TB (1983) Prognostic significance of biopsy results of normal looking mucosa in cases of superficial bladder cancer. Br J Urol 55: 665–669

Soloway MS (1981) Editorial comment. J Urol 125: 190

Soloway MS, Murphy W, Rav MK, Cox C (1978) Serial multiple-site biopsies in patients with bladder cancer. J Urol 120: 57–59

Utz DC, Farrow GM, Rife CC, Segura JW, Zincke H (1980) Carcinoma in situ of the bladder. Cancer 45: 1842–1848

Wallace DMA, Hindmarsh JR, Webb JN, Busuttil A, Hargreave TB, Newsam JE, Chisholm GD (1979) The role of multiple mucosal biopsies in the management of patients with bladder cancer. Br J Urol 51: 535–540

Webb JN (1983) The pathology of bladder cancer. In: Smith PH, Prout GR (eds) Urology I. Bladder cancer. Butterworths International Medical Reviews. Butterworths, London, pp 104–124

Weinstein RS, Koo C, Pauli BU, Jacobs JB, Friedell GH (1979) Epithelial injury by cystoscopic fluid. Semin Oncol 6: 257–259

Weldon TE, Soloway MS (1975) Susceptibility of urothelium to neoplastic cellular implantation. Urology 5: 824–827

Wolf H, Hojgaard K (1983) Urothelial dysplasia concomitant with bladder tumours as a determinant factor for future occurrences. Lancet II: 134–136

Wolfe JHN, Lloyd-Davies RW (1981) The management of transitional cell carcinoma of the prostate. Br J Urol 53: 253–257

Yagoda A, Watson RC, Whitmore WF, Grabstald H, Middleman MP, Krakoff IH (1977) Adriamycin in advanced urinary tract cancer: experience in 42 patients. Cancer 39: 279–285

Yates-Bell AJ (1979) Carcinoma in situ of the bladder. Br J Surg 58: 359–364

Chapter 8

The Treatment of Superficial Bladder Tumours

E. J. Zingg and D. M. A. Wallace

Introduction

Treating a patient with a superficial bladder tumour has responsibilities far beyond performing a good TUR of the tumour. Choosing the optimum treatment policy for the patient depends on the urologist having a wide understanding of the disease, a sound knowledge of bladder tumour pathology and a critical appraisal of all the therapeutic modalities available. Treatment is likely to be prolonged over many years, and the follow-up is an essential part of this treatment. The urologist must set out prepared to use all the available forms of treatment, including intravesical chemotherapy and total cystectomy. If he is not, the patient should be referred on at an early stage, rather than persist with ineffective treatment for this may deny the patient the opportunity of cure.

The terms 'superficial' and 'infiltrating' are used loosely to describe tumours of the bladder and need to be defined clearly. They are in fact the crudest of stage groupings and the term 'superficial tumour' has encompassed tumours of widely differing prognoses. Over the last three decades the use of the term 'superficial tumour' has changed as studies have been made of the deteriorating prognoses of tumours with increasing depths of infiltration. The limitations of conservative therapies for muscle-infiltrating tumours have also been established.

Jewett and Strong (1946) were the first to point out the relationship between the depth of infiltration and the prognosis on the basis of post-mortem studies. They originally had just three stages—A, B and C. These were modified and then extended by Marshall (1952) and later the UICC introduced the TNM system (see Chap. 6, p. 118). In both these systems the tumours that were infiltrating muscle were divided according to whether they had infiltrated further than half the depth of the muscle or not. Those tumours that had infiltrated up to this halfway point were grouped together as superficial tumours on the basis that the prognosis was similar and that they could be treated by less radical means.

Today the term 'superficial bladder tumour' has become more restricted in its use. Muscle infiltration of any degree is associated with a reduced life expectancy. The depth of muscle infiltration is particularly hard to determine clinically without the full thickness of the bladder wall being available for pathological assessment. Therefore, all tumours infiltrating muscle will be dealt with in the chapter on invasive tumours (Chap. 9) and this chapter will deal only with the management of those tumours of categories Ta and T1 (stage O and A). When interpreting and comparing the results of the treatment of superficial tumours in the literature it is important to establish if the data include tumours that are invading superficial muscle.

Superficial bladder tumours exhibit a wide spectrum of neoplastic activity, and rational management depends on a careful assessment of all the factors likely to influence the subsequent behaviour of the urothelium. The initial resection of the primary tumour is usually not a major procedure, but the subsequent surveillance of the patient and the management of the neoplastic diathesis form a sizeable proportion of the urologist's workload and may tax all of his therapeutic skills and judgement. It is therefore essential to have a clear understanding of the natural history of this disease and its risk factors and it is important for the urologist to understand and to work with the close cooperation of a pathologist.

Natural History and Pathology

The natural history of superficial bladder cancer is dominated by two properties: the tendency for tumours to be multifocal in time and place, and the tendency for these tumour recurrences to undergo progression. At presentation 28%–35% of cases have more than one tumour in the bladder (O'Flynn et al. 1975; Lutzeyer et al. 1982). The incidence of recurrent tumour in the bladder after endoscopic treatment of the primary tumour has been reported to be between 40% and 87%, with the majority of reports giving an incidence of around 70% (Varkarakis et al. 1974; Lutzeyer et al. 1982). Whether these are strictly 'recurrences' or 'new occurrences' is a matter of debate while their aetiology remains uncertain (see p. 165). Recurrent tumours may occur at the original site in the bladder (perhaps the only true recurrences, see p. 166), elsewhere within the bladder or elsewhere within the urinary tract. Recurrent tumours are more likely to be multifocal (45%) and also more likely to develop further recurrences (84%) than the primary tumours (Lutzeyer et al. 1982).

Progression may be defined as any change in the characteristics of a recurrent tumour that increases its threat to the patient and is principally a change in grade, depth of invasion or the development of metastases. The risk of tumour progression for Ta and T1 tumours is 7%–22% (Barnes et al. 1977; Mackenzie et al. 1981; Lutzeyer et al. 1982; Dalesio et al. 1983; Heney et al. 1983). The cancer death rate is clearly one of the end points by which tumour progression can be assessed. This is between 4% and 12% for Ta and T1 tumours of all grades (Pryor 1973; Williams et al. 1977; Anderström et al. 1980; England et al. 1981; Pocock et al. 1982).

Superficial bladder cancer is a heterogeneous group of tumours, with some following a benign course while others are clearly lethal. A number of characteristics of these tumours have been studied in order to define those patients who are at greatest risk of developing tumour recurrences and tumour progression so that more effective additional therapy might be instituted at an earlier stage. These have included the presence and depth of invasion, tumour grade, size, multiplicity, abnormalities on selected mucosal biopsies, deletion of blood group antigens (see Chap. 2, p. 44), and results of flow cytometry, cytological examination and chromosome studies (see Chap. 6, p. 135).

Risk of Developing Tumour Recurrences

The grade, lamina propria invasion, multiplicity and size of the tumour and abnormal mucosal biopsies have all been found to correlate with the tumour recurrences in various studies. Heney et al. (1982) have used these five factors together with urine cytology to divide patients into low- and high-risk groups. Those with negative predictors had recurrence rates below 70%, while those with positive predictors had recurrence rates above 70% (see Fig. 8.1). Other authors have reported that stage and grade did not affect the recurrence rate (England et al. 1981; Smith et al. 1983) and Dalesio et al. (1983) reported that the most important factor that influenced the recurrence rate was the number of tumours present at diagnosis.

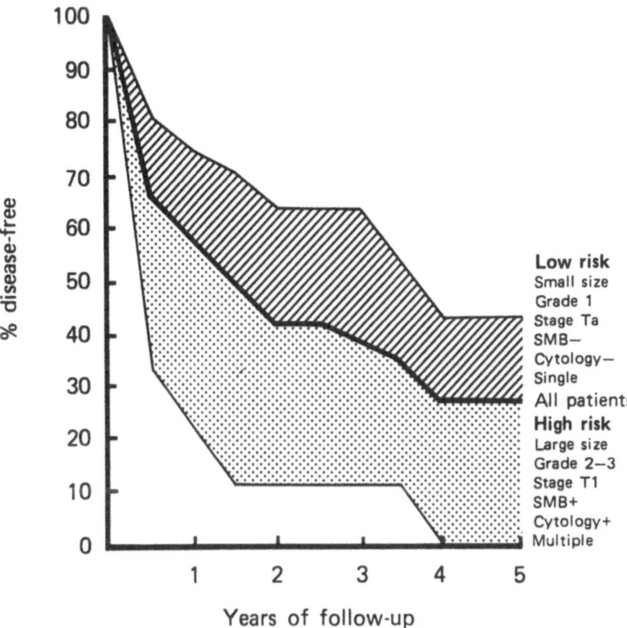

Fig. 8.1. The percentage of patients free of bladder tumour over 5 years' follow-up. The disease-free curves for patients with 'positive' predictors all fell below the common line (*dotted area*), whereas the disease-free curves for patients with 'negative' predictors fell above the line (*shaded area*) (Heney et al. 1982)

There are many factors that influence the results of selected mucosal biopsies. The number of biopsies taken, the sites chosen for biopsy, how close to the tumour base they are taken and the cystoscopic appearance of the mucosa (Wallace et al. 1979) will all influence the proportion of abnormal biopsies as well as the pathological interpretation and grading of the changes. Heney et al. (1983) found a significant difference in recurrence rate between those patients who had normal or only mild dysplasia and those who had moderate to severe dysplasia in their mucosal biopsies. Wolf and Hojgaard (1983) reported a recurrence rate of 87% when dysplasia was present, as compared with 26% when it was absent, but this series included some T2 cases.

Risk of Tumour Progression

Tumour progression is of greater importance than the recurrence rate as this is clearly more life-threatening and may require more radical treatment. The factors that correlate with tumour progression are essentially the same as those for tumour recurrence: invasion of the lamina propria, grade, multiplicity, size of the primary tumour and urothelial abnormalities on mucosal biopsies (Lutzeyer et al. 1982; Heney et al. 1983; Narayana et al. 1983). Table 8.1 shows the number of tumours undergoing progression, which is defined as muscle invasion or metastases, according to grade for pTa and pT1 tumours (Heney et al. 1983). In this study there were no significant differences in the incidence of progression between Grade 1 and Grade 2 tumours. The difference in progression rate was only significant when the tumours were more than 4 cm and when there were more than three tumours present.

Table 8.1. Progression by grade for categories pTa and pT1 (Heney et al. 1983)

	G1	G2	G3
pTa	2/85 (2%)	3/50 (6%)	1/4 (25%)
pT1	0/7	6/29 (21%)	13/27 (48%)

Lutzeyer et al. (1982) reported that the risk of progression of primary pTa and pT1 tumours was 20% and 24% respectively. The risk of progression of a solitary pTa or pT1 tumour (both primary and recurrent) was 18% and 33%, whereas if they were multiple it was 43% and 46% respectively.

Abnormalities of the non-tumour-bearing mucosa, especially carcinoma in situ, indicate a poor prognosis. Schade and Swinney (1983) carried out a 10-year follow-up of 92 cases of bladder cancer in which mucosal biopsies had been taken and found that cases with evidence of carcinoma in situ on biopsy had a significantly worse outcome than those with normal or non-malignant changes, regardless of the characteristics of the primary tumour and its grade or stage. Ten of the 37 patients with carcinoma in situ and 5 of 54 with dysplasia died of bladder cancer. Similar findings were reported when carcinoma in situ was found in the incidentally resected mucosa adjacent to a bladder tumour (Althausen et al. 1976).

The use of blood group antigen deletion to predict which patients with superficial tumours will develop invasion has become a topic of considerable interest. This test has already been reviewed in Chapter 2 (see p. 45), and many questions raised about the validity of the test. Can this test be used to make decisions about the management of patients with bladder tumours? The report of Catalona (1981) and the results of Gunter et al. (1983), who reported a false negative rate of 10% (i.e. tumours that were predicted to invade and did not), suggest that this test cannot be relied on for making decisions of such therapeutic importance, though it is a highly significant test for identifying those patients with potentially invasive lesions.

Tumour Recurrence—Field Change or Implantation?

Superficial bladder tumours have been initiated by urine-borne carcinogens (see Chap. 1, p. 7). The whole urothelium has been exposed to these carcinogens, and the bladder, being the storage organ, has been exposed for the longest time. Urothelial carcinogenesis is a process that takes from 10 to 30 years, and it is therefore to be expected that following exposure to a carcinogen bladder tumours will be multifocal and will appear over a period of many years. The careful histological examination of the non-tumour-bearing urothelium in patients with bladder cancer shows neoplastic and preneoplastic changes in a high proportion of cases. Soto et al. (1977) studied cystectomy specimens from 45 patients with bladder cancer, examined the bladders by taking giant histological sections through the whole bladder and built up a map of the whole surface of the bladder by using step sections. In 33 of the 43 cases of invasive cancer, carcinoma in situ was found adjacent to the tumour and over two-thirds of these cases had two or more non-contiguous areas of carcinoma in situ. In 10 cases there was no adjacent carcinoma in situ and the tumours appeared to be histologically unifocal. This figure is comparable to the 30% of superficial tumours that do not have any recurrence.

Selected mucosal biopsies in patients with superficial bladder tumours have shown that neoplastic or preneoplastic changes may be found in 30%–70% of cases (Eisenberg et al. 1960; Schade and Swinney 1968; Cooper et al. 1973; Heney et al. 1978; Soloway et al. 1978). As discussed above, these changes correlate closely with the subsequent development of recurrent tumours. Whilst a proportion of cases (less than 30%) may have a unifocal lesion, the majority of cases with bladder cancer have histologically detectable premalignant urothelial changes present at the time of diagnosis of the first tumour. The time taken for these changes to progress to overt tumour formation and the factors that bring about the final propagation of tumour growth are not yet determined.

While it is likely that the principal cause of tumour recurrence is through a 'field change' in the urothelium, there is some evidence that implantation of tumour cells may play a part. This evidence is derived from a number of sources:

1. *Experimental studies*. Using a murine model Weldon and Soloway (1975) showed that when a cell suspension from a transplantable syngeneic bladder tumour was instilled into the normal mouse bladder very few tumours could be implanted. When the mucosa had been previously damaged by prior instillation of the cytotoxic agent MNU or by electrocautery of the bladder (Solway and Masters 1980) then the incidence of tumour implantation was very much higher. The tumour cell suspension that was used came from a poorly

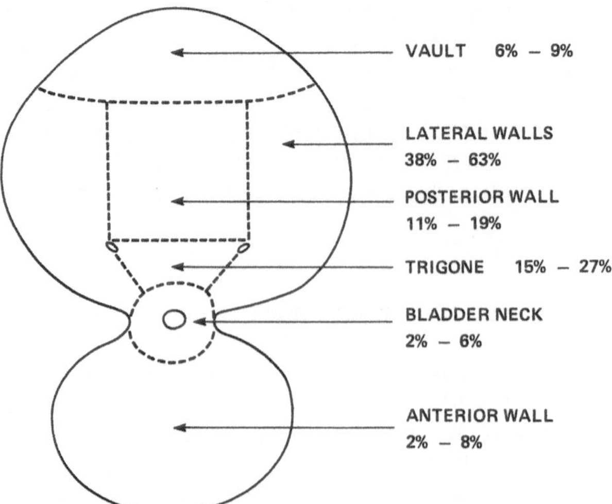

Fig. 8.2. The sites of initial bladder tumours

differentiated invasive bladder tumour that had been induced by the prolonged feeding of FANFT and which had already been serially transplanted. While this evidence shows that tumour cell implantation can occur, there is no evidence as yet that well-differentiated tumours can be implanted and grow to form papillary tumours.

2. *Location of the primary and recurrent tumours*. The typical site for a primary tumour is on the lateral wall adjacent to the ureteric orifice (Fig. 8.2). Primary tumours rarely occur in the vault, or on the anterior wall or around the bladder neck. The distribution of recurrent tumours within the bladder is very different. The region of the vault of the bladder, especially around the air bubble, is a common site for tumour recurrences, as is the region of the anterior wall and bladder neck. Boyd and Burnand (1974) reported on 32 patients with well-differentiated non-invasive transitional cell carcinomas of the bladder, of whom 31 developed recurrences. Only two of the primary tumours occurred in the vault of the bladder, whereas 29 of the 31 cases with recurrent tumours had a recurrence in the vault. Page et al. (1978) reported that in 43 of 56 cases of non-infiltrating primary tumours the tumour was adjacent and lateral to the ureteric orifice and that none of the primary tumours were in the vault in the region of the air bubble. The recurrent tumours were much less restricted in their sites and occurred on the posterior-superior walls in 41% and adjacent to the air bubble in 8% of a total of 578 tumour recurrences. It was postulated that this different distribution of recurrences was caused by tumour implantation. An alternative explanation is that the endoscopic treatment provided a stimulus to cell proliferation in these areas. The location of so many tumours in the region of the air bubble is of interest. The gas in this bubble after endoscopic resection or diathermy will contain hydrogen and carbon monoxide rather than air (Davis 1983). It is possible that this gas has a damaging effect on the mucosa that allows tumour cells to implant or provides a stimulus to cell proliferation in this area.

3. *Marker chromosomes*. Chromosome analyses of bladder tumours have shown that these tumours have abnormal chromosomes which include marker chromosomes (Falor and Ward 1977). These marker chromosomes are abnormal chromosomes that reappear in the metaphases and that do not conform to any of the morphological patterns of the normal karyotype. When a marker chromosome is present it may reappear in some of the recurrent tumours. Tumour implantation is the most likely explanation for this observation but intraepithelial spread of neoplastic cells during the long latent period or a multifocal origin of the same marker chromosomes are other possible explanations.
4. *Results of single-dose chemotherapy*. Several studies have now shown that a single dose or a short course of intravesical chemotherapy given immediately after TUR of bladder tumours reduces the recurrence rate (Burnand et al. 1976; Gavrell et al. 1978; Abrams et al. 1981; England et al. 1981). Whether this treatment is effective by preventing tumour cell implantation or by acting on the early stages on tumour formation in the urothelium that has just received a proliferative stimulus is not known.

There is therefore no good evidence as yet that the high recurrence rate of the well-differentiated papillary tumours is caused by tumour implantation, though it should be borne in mind as a possible mechanism of spread, especially when dealing with a poorly differentiated tumour. At the follow-up cystoscopy great care must be taken to visualise the areas where recurrent tumours are likely to develop, such as the anterior wall. Even when the result of cystosocopy is negative, bladder washings may detect unsuspected in situ changes and influence the follow-up. Recurrent tumours may change their character and therefore it is a sound policy to resect them for histological examination rather than destroy them with diathermy.

Transurethral Resection

The therapeutic objectives in the initial treatment of superficial tumours are to remove completely the tumour or tumours, to assess the need for further therapy and to plan the follow-up. The standard initial method of management is a TUR. This should achieve the complete removal of the tumour and also enables the urologist to submit the whole tumour for histological examination. A decision to perform only a biopsy may be taken if the tumour appears to be deeply infiltrating or if a complete TUR is not possible, either because the tumour is too large or because it arises in a diverticulum.

Anaesthesia

Bladder tumours can be resected using regional or general anaesthesia, but a thorough bimanual examination requires good relaxation (see Chap. 5, p. 108). One particular problem encountered in resection of bladder tumours is stimulation of the obturator nerve, which lies close to the lateral wall of the

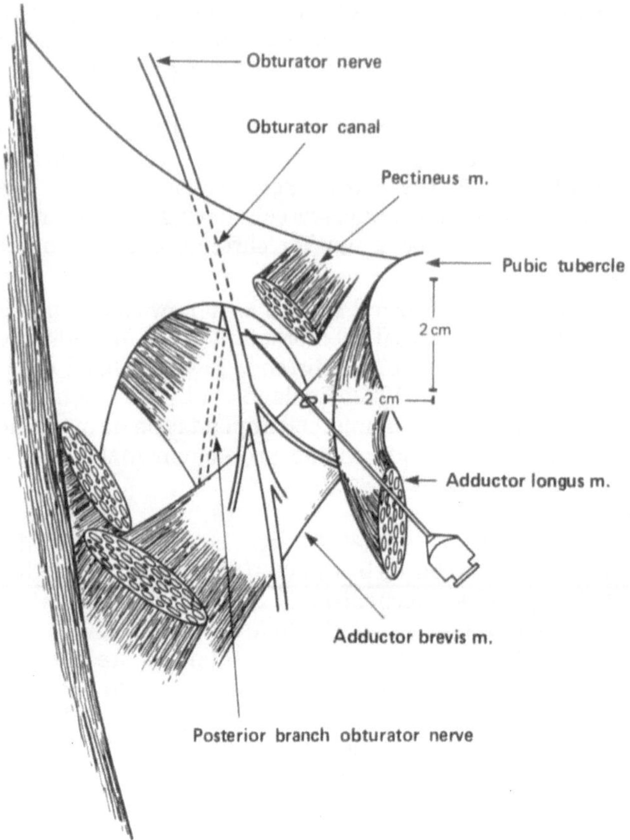

Fig. 8.3. The anatomy of the obturator nerve and the landmarks for obturator block

bladder in the obturator fossa. It may be stimulated when the high-frequency cutting current is partially rectified by arcing between the resectoscope loop and the bladder wall (Fastenmeier and Flachenecker 1981). The resulting direct current stimulates the nerve and the mass contraction of the adductor muscles causes a sudden and violent movement of the patient. When this happens there is a risk that the loop will perforate the bladder wall. Fortunately, this perforation is extraperitoneal and can be managed conservatively, but this repeated 'obturator kick' is dangerous and can prevent the complete resection of the tumour.

One way of preventing this is for the anaesthetist to paralyse the patient with a short-acting depolarising agent such as suxamethonium. This will give up to 5 min of relaxation, which will usually suffice, but can only be used with general anaesthesia. When regional anaesthesia is used or when it is known that a large tumour must be resected close to the obturator nerve then an obturator nerve block can be employed (Augspurger and Donohue 1980). Local anaesthesia is injected through a long needle inserted 2 cm lateral and caudal to the pubic tubercle and the needle is walked off the inferior border of the superior pubic ramus in order to meet the obturator nerve where it lies in the obturator canal. Injection here will block the main trunk before it divides (Fig. 8.3).

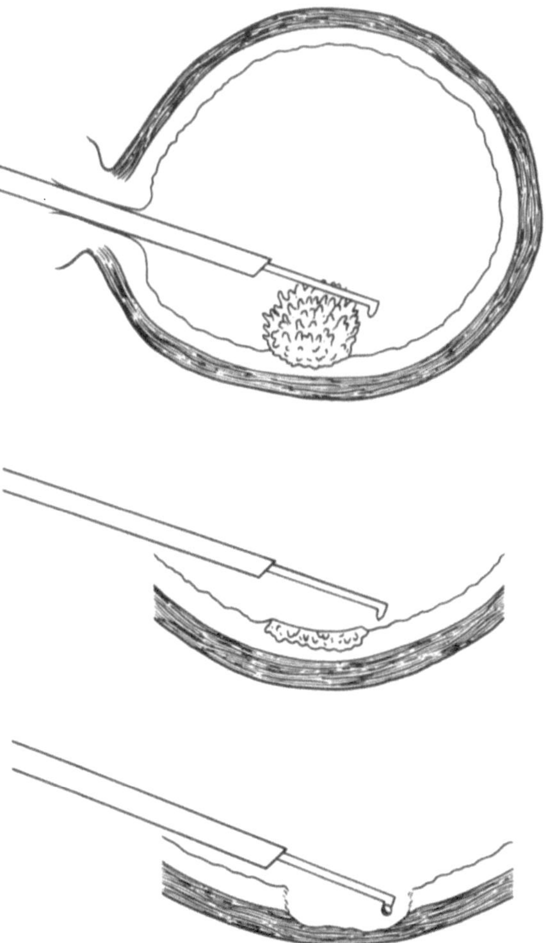

Fig. 8.4. Technique of resecting a bladder tumour: First resect the exophytic portion, then resect the base down into muscle and send specimens separately. Finally, resect the surrounding mucosa and secure haemostasis

Technique

The detailed description of the techniques of transurethral surgery is beyond the scope of this book. However, there are certain points of technique that are important when resecting bladder tumours. The standard resectoscope is adequate for resecting nearly all bladder tumours, but there are certain advantages in using a continuous irrigation resectoscope. The use of this instrument allows the operator to resect in a bladder that has a relatively fixed volume, which means that the tumour that is being resected is not always moving away as the bladder distends. The risk of perforation is reduced by not resecting when the bladder is either collapsed or overdistended.

The irrigating fluid used can be either water or glycine. While water has the theoretical advantage that it will cause the rapid lysis of malignant cells, it has the disadvantage that morbidity will be greater if significant amounts are absorbed (Dick et al. 1980).

As outlined in Chapter 5 (see p. 107) the procedure begins with a careful inspection of the whole bladder and urethra by passing the cystoscope under vision. The location of all tumours and their appearance should be noted. Resection of multiple tumours should be carried out in a systematic fashion and a careful check made at the end to ensure that all tumours have been dealt with. If there are tumours on the base of the bladder it is best to begin resecting there as that is where the blood and tumour fragments collect and these will obscure the tumours if that area is done last. When resecting a large tumour or an area of tumour it is best to start at the side furthest from the urethral meatus and to work towards it. Resection should be carried down to the muscle and then into the muscle. It is safe to resect deep into the muscle in the extraperitoneal areas of the bladder down to where the perivesical fat begins to be seen. However, in the peritoneal areas of the vault the resection into muscle should be carried out cautiously, especially in elderly women in whom the bladder wall may be very thin.

When resecting the larger tumours the bulk of the tumour should be resected and washed out. The base of the tumour should be resected down into the muscle and sent as a separate specimen (Fig. 8.4). The pathologist can then turn most of his attention to examining this specimen to determine whether or not muscle is invaded. The tumour margins can also be sent as separate specimens as this is the area that might show secondary carcinoma in situ or even submucosal spread. The cold cup biopsy forceps can be used to take biopsies from the base of a tumour. This may be safer in the vault of the bladder and may avoid diathermy artefacts.

Initial treatment of what is thought to be a superficial tumour by diathermy coagulation alone is inappropriate treatment as it destroys the tumour without obtaining any material for histological examination, and therefore the subsequent management of the patient cannot be planned on a rational basis. Treatment by biopsy and coagulation is also not to be recommended as the histological assessment is inadequate and the extent of coagulation is poorly controlled. Moreover, it can be dangerous and may be a completely inadequate form of therapy.

Special Problems

Tumour at the Ureteric Orifice

The typical site for a primary bladder tumour is adjacent and lateral to the ureteric orifice. Large tumours in this region may obscure the orifice and in this situation it is important to check that there is no delay on the IVU to suggest that there is infiltration or that tumour may be growing in the intramural ureter. There need be no hesitation in resecting the ureteric orifice or intramural ureter if this is required to remove the tumour adequately. If reflux occurs it seldom causes problems (Amar and Das 1983), and the ureter is not liable to develop stricturing unless diathermy is used (Booth and Kellett 1981). Three out of 34 patients who had tumours in the vicinity of the ureteric orifice treated by TUR only developed mild upper tract obstruction, while 8 of 17 patients treated by cystodiathermy became obstructed, 4 severely; interstitial or external radiotherapy also increased the risk of stricturing (Booth and Kellett 1981).

Tumour in a Diverticulum

Resection of tumours in bladder diverticula may be prevented because (1) access to the diverticulum may be impossible and (2) there is no real thickness of muscle to resect into. If the tumour is infiltrating there is very little tissue for it to penetrate before it reaches perivesical fat (category T3b). Tumours arising in small diverticula may be treated by biopsy and diathermy, but any large diverticulum containing tumour is best treated by a partial cystectomy. Recurrent tumours in a bladder with multiple diverticula are an indication for the early adoption of intravesical chemotherapy.

The Huge Tumour

Occasionally a patient will present with tumour filling or covering most of the bladder. Resecting these tumours can be extremely taxing for both the patient and the urologist, and some of these tumours must be considered too big to be safely or adequately resected endoscopically except by a very experienced resectionist. In this situation intravesical chemotherapy is ineffective; radiotherapy should not be used merely because of the bulk of tumour present, which may well still be superficial. The large superficial papillary tumour is very suitable for treatment with Helmstein's hydrostatic distension (Helmstein 1972). The blood supply to these long-fronded tumours is easily occluded by this treatment and they readily necrose and slough off afterwards (see p. 264 for details of treatment.).

Concomitant Prostatic Hyperplasia and Outflow Obstruction

Bladder tumours and prostatic hyperplasia with obstruction are common conditions and frequently occur together. When it is necessary to resect both a bladder tumour and the prostate then the bladder tumour should be resected first. Complete haemostasis must be achieved, and all the tumour chips must be evacuated and the base of the tumour carefully inspected before continuing with resecting the prostate. If haemostasis is not good or the bladder wall has been perforated then the prostatic resection should be deferred. Occasionally the mere bulk of the prostate prevents access to tumours near the bladder neck and the prostate will have to be resected in order to get to the bladder tumours (Fig. 8.5). In general, if a TUR needs to be performed it should be a complete resection rather than one which leaves the prostate half resected.

The potential hazards of combining these two procedures are that tumour will be implanted into the prostatic urethra and that the additional trauma will result in an increased recurrence rate (Hinman 1956). Two large studies by Laor et al. (1981) and Greene and Yalowitz (1972) have shown that combining the two procedures did not result in either an increased recurrence rate or an increase of

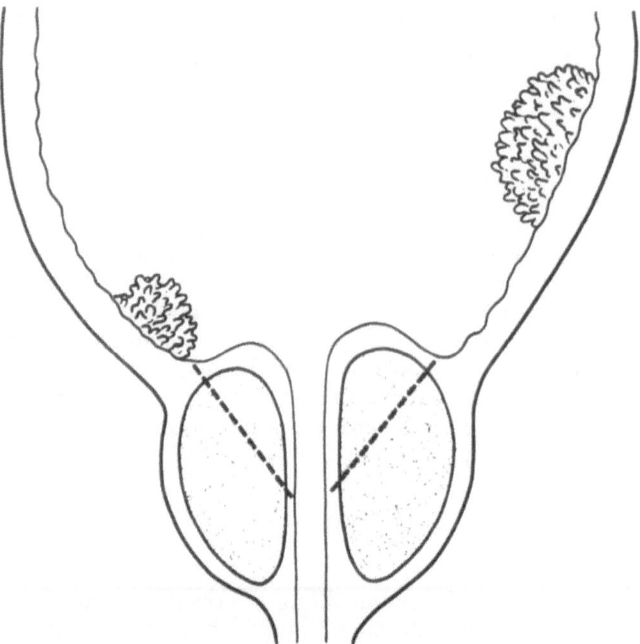

Fig. 8.5. The enlarged prostate may prevent tumours near the bladder neck from being adequately resected. The prostate must be resected first

tumour recurrences in the prostatic urethra. The two procedures can therefore be combined, but great vigilance will be needed in the early postoperative period as the risk of haemorrhage is greater.

Complications

The main complications of TURs of bladder tumours are haemorrhage, infection, perforation, TUR reactions and vesicoureteric reflux. Dick et al. (1980) reviewed the complications of TUR of bladder tumours in 373 patients. Haemorrhage requiring transfusion occurred in 13%, infection in 24% and there were five intraperitoneal and 38 extraperitoneal perforations, giving an overall rate of 5% for perforations. The postoperative mortality for the 373 patients was 1.3%, or 0.6% for the 834 procedures. The same mortality of 0.6% was quoted by Cifuentes Delatte et al. (1982) for 2143 endoscopic resections of bladder tumours.

The management of the haemorrhage is by careful coagulation at the time of the resection and care of the catheter following resection. If all the clot is evacuated and the bladder allowed to stay collapsed and empty then the bleeding from a resected bladder tumour will nearly always stop. Bladder tumours are frequently infected (see Chap. 4, p. 80) and these should be treated with the appropriate antibiotics preoperatively. Prophylactic, short-course antibiotics need not be given routinely except for the high-risk cases such as those with diabetes, valvular heart disease and prostheses.

Perforations of the bladder may occur into the peritoneum (Fig. 8.6) or into the extraperitoneal tissues. Extraperitoneal perforations are not uncommon and may

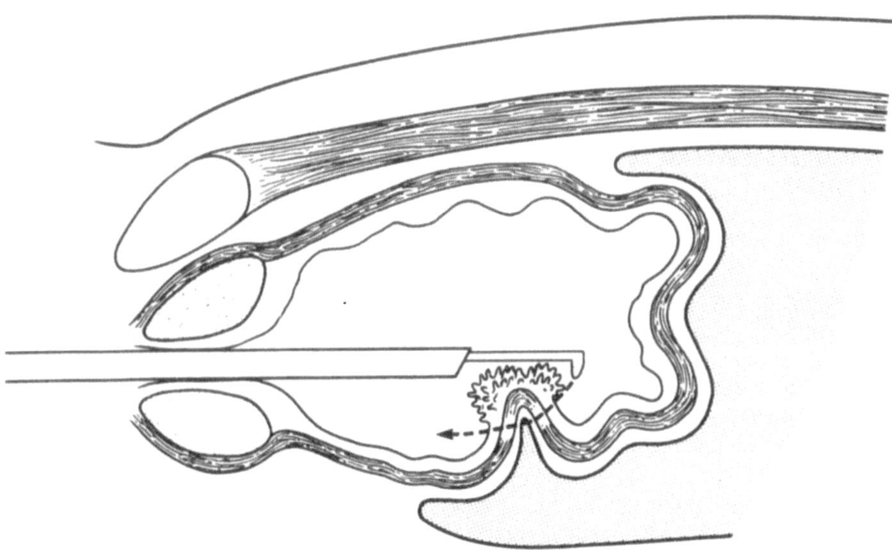

Fig. 8.6. An intraperitoneal perforation may occur either when resecting a partially collapsed bladder or when resecting a fully distended thin-walled bladder

be more frequent than is realised when resections are made deep into the muscle of the lateral wall. Serious complications are few following an extraperitoneal perforation and the only treatment is to leave a catheter for 24–48 h. An intraperitoneal perforation should be suspected if there is a disparity in the amount of fluid going in and coming out of the bladder or if the patient becomes hypotensive and peripherally vasoconstricted during the resection. Afterwards the patients may have abdominal distension, tenderness and guarding. The diagnosis is usually made from the clinical signs but occasionally a cystogram may be necessary. An intraperitoneal perforation should be treated by an immediate laparotomy and oversewing of the perforation and peritoneal lavage. Even though numerous tumour chips have gone into the peritoneal cavity the risk of tumour implantation is negligible, as only one case has been reported (Marberger 1977).

In contrast to the prostate there is very little absorption of the irrigating fluid during the resection of a bladder tumour, and absorption is only likely to be a problem when the bladder wall has been resected. Usually the resection stops at this stage but may go on if the prostate is also to be resected or if there are multiple bladder tumours to be resected.

Vesicoureteric reflux can occur following resections of the ureteric orifice and of tumours in the vicinity of the orifice. The overall incidence of reflux following resections of bladder tumours is 5% (Toggenburg and Brand 1979); however, when the ureteric orifice is resected, 70% develop reflux, and 47% when the resection is in the vicinity of the orifice (Hartung and Hegemann 1981). Renal damage is extremely unlikely to occur just as a result of the reflux, and symptomatic urinary infections are also rare. There is, however, the risk that the reflux will allow tumour cells to implant into the upper tracts. Hartung and Hegemann (1981) reported seven cases of renal pelvic transitional cell carcinomas occurring following TUR of bladder tumours and of these seven patients six had reflux.

Other Modes of Therapy

Helmstein's Bladder Distension

This technique was first used by Helmstein in 1966 for the treatment of bladder carcinomas. It was originally thought that this would be effective treatment for invasive cancers (Helmstein 1972), but further experience with this technique has shown that it gives poor results with invasive cancers, although it can be good palliative treatment and is very effective at controlling haemorrhage (see Chap. 11, p. 265). In the series reported by Helmstein (1972) and by England et al. (1973) the patients with multiple papillary superficial tumours responded well, with the bladder nearly always being cleared of tumour. The bulky, long-fronded, non-invasive papillary tumour is most vulnerable to being made ischaemic by the hydrostatic pressure within the bladder, and it is only in this type of tumour that Helmstein's bladder distension is recommended as the initial therapy.

The Helmstein's bladder distension must last for a period of 6 h to destroy the tumour, and therefore an epidural anaesthetic is required. A specially designed balloon catheter is inserted into the bladder and distended with a hydrostatic pressure of 125 cm of water: 25 cm of water pressure is needed to overcome the elastic resistance of the balloon and the 100 cm of water is equivalent to 75 mmHg, which will occlude the blood supply to the inside of the bladder. This pressure should not be exceeded as there is a risk that the bladder will rupture. If the patient's diastolic blood pressure is lower than 75 mmHg, then the pressure should be reduced accordingly. The patient must be closely monitored during treatment to ensure that this pressure is not exceeded. Patients who have had previous surgery to the bladder or radiotherapy should be treated with great caution because of the increased risk of rupture.

This treatment is therefore only for carefully selected patients in whom the bladder is filled with superficial papillary tumours which are too extensive to resect transurethrally. Although the number of cases reported is small it is unlikely that this procedure reduces the recurrence rate.

Partial Cystectomy

A partial cystectomy would seem to be a logical form of treatment for a localised bladder tumour but it has several major disadvantages: Bladder tumours are usually not localised, tumour recurrences after partial cystectomy may be difficult to treat and partial cystectomy cannot be repeated. Esch and Rummelhardt (1973) reported that in 30% of partial cystectomy specimens they found tumour at the resection edges, and therefore many of these operations did not achieve an adequate clearance. In these cases multiple mucosal biopsies were not performed preoperatively. There is also a risk that tumour will be implanted into the wound, which is very distressing for the patient and difficult to treat. The development of the resectoscope and the increase in experience of urologists in resecting bladder tumours has provided an effective alternative therapy which avoids most of the complications of open resections and has a much lower morbidity and mortality.

From the published results it can be seen that the 5-year survival following partial cystectomy for pTa and pT1 tumours is 50%–70%, the operative mortality is 1%–7% and the risk of tumour implantation is 1%–3%. However, very little can be concluded from these reports as the numbers are small, the cases are selected and the criteria for selection are not clearly defined (Zingg and Zeltner 1980).

There are two well-established indications for partial cystectomy: (1) the tumour arising in a diverticulum and (2) the adenocarcinoma of urachal origin arising in the vault of the bladder. Very occasionally a patient presents with such bad coxarthrosis that endoscopic access to the bladder is impossible and a partial cystectomy may be considered. There are certain other situations where a partial cystectomy may be considered but the following criteria must be met:

1. The tumour is solitary.
2. Multiple mucosal biopsies show no evidence of premalignant change.
3. The tumour is in the mobile part of the bladder and an adequate clearance (3 cm) can be obtained.
4. There has been no previous radiotherapy.
5. The tumour does not infiltrate into deep muscle.

When a partial cystectomy is to be performed, preoperative flash radiotherapy should be given to reduce the risk of wound implantation (van der Werf-Messing 1978).

Open cystodiathermy excision of bladder tumours should be condemned as an operation as it achieves no more than a TUR but has an unacceptable morbidity and mortality.

Radiotherapy

External Beam Megavoltage Therapy

Radiotherapy has been used in the treatment of selected cases of superficial bladder cancer, usually those with a bad prognosis, and the results have been poor. Whitmore and Prout (1982) reported eight cases of stage O and A bladder cancer treated with radiotherapy which all later required cystectomy for either tumour recurrence or severe radiation cystitis. In their review of the literature they concluded that complete responses could be obtained in 78% of superficial tumours with radical radiotherapy, but more than 50% developed recurrences within 5 years of follow-up. The treatment of recurrent superficial tumours after radiotherapy is hazardous because of the increased risks of perforation, haemorrhage and severe bladder contracture. Also, assessment of the depth of invasion is more difficult because of the radiation fibrosis around the bladder. For this reason salvage cystectomy may be delayed too long and the tumour found to be incurable.

A low dose of prophylactic radiotherapy was also found to be ineffective in preventing tumour recurrences (Page et al. 1979): 750 cGy were given a few days after transurethral resection of non-infiltrating bladder tumours in 29 patients; 12 of these and 11 of the 27 control patients developed recurrences after less than 4 years of follow-up.

External beam radiotherapy, therefore, has no role in the management of superficial bladder tumours and should only be considered for the treatment of elderly patients with T1 Grade 3 tumours.

Interstitial Irradiation

Nearly all the patients who have been treated with interstitial irradiation have been selected because of poor risk factors, and usually the tumours have been small, localised and frequently invading muscle. As with partial cystectomy, there are no controlled trials and the selection criteria of the reported series are not always apparent.

Four different sources have been used for interstitial irradiation of bladder cancer: gold grains, iridium wires, tantalum wires and radium needles. All these sources must be inserted at open operation as there is as yet no satisfactory endoscopic method for inserting the source. This has to be done with great care in order to get the correct dosimetry. Intracavitary irradiation is practised in very few centres and the reported results of Hewitt et al. (1981) are comparable to those of interstitial irradiation.

The largest experience with the treatment of superficial bladder tumours with interstitial irradiation is reported by van der Werf-Messing and Hop (1981): 197 patients with category T1NXM0 tumours were treated by interstitial radium and were compared with 148 patients with the same category of tumour who were treated by TUR alone. This was not a controlled or prospective trial but the two groups were reported to be comparable. They concluded that patients with T1NXM0 bladder tumours treated by TUR alone had a significantly higher chance of dying of carcinoma of the bladder than if they had been treated by radium implant. There was also a striking difference in the recurrence rate: 20% of the TUR group and 80% of the radium group were recurrence free at 5 years. More patients in the TUR group needed to undergo cystectomy or radical external beam radiotherapy. Complications were relatively few in the radium group, and bladder contracture was not a major problem, despite the fact that the bladder received a relatively high radiation dose.

Williams et al. (1981) reviewed 180 patients treated by either gold grain or tantalum wire implants. The tumours that had been selected for treatment were either T1 or T2 tumours which were solitary and less than 4 cm in diameter. The tumours were categorised retrospectively and the 5-year survival for pTa tumours was 73% and for pT1 tumours 57%. The overall mortality was 1.4%. Scar implants occurred in 2% of the cases, and 16 of the 47 T1 patients developed recurrent tumours in the bladder. One finding of note was that the presence of carcinoma in situ in the bladder did not adversely affect the result.

Interstitial irradiation can therefore be carried out with relatively low morbidity and mortality and can reduce the incidence of both bladder recurrences and progression of Ta and T1 tumours. It is, however, a very expensive form of treatment and few centres are equipped and have the necessary expertise to carry out interstitial irradiation, especially with radium. The results of interstitial irradiation must now be compared with adjuvant intravesical chemotherapy in prospective controlled trials.

Lasers

The clinical use of laser technology has scarcely passed its infancy and treatment of tumours is at a very early stage of development. The features of the light emitted by a laser (*L*ight *A*mplification by the *S*timulated *E*mission of *R*adiation) are that it is of a fixed frequency with a parallel beam that is coherent (ordered and predictable in time and space). Laser light is almost monochromatic. There are many different devices for producing lasers and they are named according to the medium which is used to produce the laser beam. Those that are being used clinically are the carbon dioxide, neodymium-yttrium aluminium garnet (Nd-YAG) and the argon lasers (see also the section on transurethral laser irradiation in Chap. 11, p. 273).

The laser can be finely controlled by adjusting the total power input and the size of the beam at the target. The energy of a laser is absorbed by the target tissue as heat. The biological effects depend principally on the energy density, the wavelength, the duration and the tissue treated. These effects range from biostimulation at the very lowest energy levels, through biosuppression to photocoagulation and eventually tissue vapourisation at the highest energy levels.

The volume of tissue that is heated before the superficial cells are destroyed varies with the wavelength of the laser used. For the carbon dioxide laser (wavelength 10.6 μm) the energy is absorbed by water and there is therefore rapid vapourisation of tissue at the point of impact with very little surrounding tissue damage. This makes it a precise cutting tool and it can be used as a knife. The other two lasers have shorter wavelengths and the energy is not absorbed by water. They produce tissue damage to a depth of approximately 1 mm for the argon laser and 5–8 mm for the Nd-YAG laser. This makes them particularly suitable for treating bleeding vessels and for destroying tumour tissue up to a maximum depth of 8 mm.

The above three types of lasers have been used in the treatment of superficial bladder tumours and have been reviewed by Hall (1982). The carbon dioxide laser cannot be used in water and the bladder must be filled with carbon dioxide, nor can it be used with a flexible fibre and this presents great technical difficulties when used within the bladder. The argon and Nd-YAG lasers can both be used through water in the bladder and can be transmitted along a flexible single-quartz fibre.

The advantages in using a laser for the treatment of superficial bladder tumours are that the depth of tissue damage can be controlled much more precisely than with electrocautery; there may be selective early sealing of lymphatics, which may prevent tumour spread; and the vapourisation of the tumour may prevent tumour implantation. The Nd-YAG laser completely destroys a block of tissue with sharply defined margins. Electrocautery only partially destroys the deeper tissues, leaving islands of cells that can regenerate. Scarring is therefore more extensive with the laser but tumour destruction more likely to be complete. The use of the argon laser in the bladder causes no pain and can be used without anaesthesia, but some sensation is felt with the Nd-YAG laser. Haemorrhage is also better controlled than with cystodiathermy.

The disadvantages with the laser are that it produces complete destruction of the tumour without obtaining any tissue for histological examination. It therefore cannot replace the resectoscope but must be used in conjunction when histological specimens are required. It is unlikely that there would be any time saved by using the laser for larger tumours and the equipment at present is large and expensive.

Several centres are now using lasers for the treatment of superficial bladder tumours and the results are comparable to those achieved by conventional endoscopic treatment. Hofstetter et al. (1982) have treated 152 patients with bladder tumours and found that the Nd-YAG laser may be superior to TUR for multiple small tumours, but they state that prospective controlled trials are required before any conclusions can be drawn. So far there is no clear advantage for using a laser and it is unlikely that lasers will be widely adopted for clinical use in treating bladder cancer. However, the most important place of lasers may be in the recently developed use of photodynamic therapy for bladder cancer.

Photodynamic Therapy

The porphyrins are a group of compounds that can sensitise tissues to light. A derivative of the haematoporphyrin group (Hpd) has been shown to be selectively taken up by malignant tissue, and this has enabled Hpd to be used both diagnostically and therapeutically in a number of different types of tumour. One of the first tumours to be studied for photodynamic therapy was bladder cancer (Kelly et al. 1975).

When Hpd is injected into the blood stream it is absorbed by most tissues but is selectively retained by malignant tissues. This is partly because it is more rapidly eliminated from the normal tissues, so that by 72 h the differential between the normal and the malignant tissues is maximal. When illuminated with violet light of wavelength 405 nm the Hpd fluoresces. This has been used in the location of carcinoma in situ and early tumours, especially in the bronchus (Kinsey et al. 1978). The fluorescence is usually of a low level and needs amplification to detect reliably the malignant tumour tissue. When exposed to red light of wavelength 630 nm the Hpd releases the highly reactive singlet oxygen, which causes cell death. This property has been used to treat tumours that are accessible to light such as tumours of the skin, bronchus and bladder. Light of this wavelength is delivered by specially designed lasers.

In the bladder there is a wide therapeutic ratio as the normal bladder is relatively resistant to photodynamic therapy (Benson et al. 1983). The preliminary trials have shown that it can be effective treatment for carcinoma in situ and superficial bladder tumours (Benson et al. 1983; Hisazumi et al. 1983; Tsuchiya et al. 1983). It is unlikely to be effective therapy for large tumours or deeply invasive tumours because the uptake is uneven and the depth of penetration of red light into the tissues is only about 1 cm.

The future development of this technique will depend firstly on isolating the most active constituent of Hpd or producing new photosensitisers that are taken up more selectively by malignant tissue. Secondly, the technical problems of delivering the correct amount of light of the specific wavelengths to the whole surface of the bladder must be overcome, and finally more sensitive methods must be developed for detecting the low levels of fluorescence produced by carcinoma in situ and dysplastic lesions.

Follow-up

Early Repeat TUR

In order to reduce the errors in assessing tumours of categories Ta and T1 (which may be of the order of 20%–30%) an early repeat TUR (*nach Resektion*) may be carried out. The cystoscopic appearances and bimanual findings after a TUR will be unreliable for assessing residual tumour as the inflammatory reaction and oedema take approximately 6 weeks to resolve. The purpose of the early repeat TUR is therefore to resect the original tumour site down to muscle for further histological examination. This is best carried out between 3 and 6 weeks.

The cases in which this is indicated are those where the findings will substantially alter the treatment policy. These are cases of pT1 tumours in which muscle invasion might have been missed in the first TUR and cases of T2 tumours in which management by TUR alone is being considered and in which the finding of muscle invasion in the second TUR specimen would indicate more radical therapy.

Cystoscopy

Regular follow-up cystoscopic examinations of the bladder are mandatory in patients with superficial bladder tumours because of the high recurrence rates. Symptoms, such as haematuria, cannot be relied upon for the detection of recurrences at an early stage (Miller et al. 1969). The risk of developing a recurrence falls in a roughly exponential fashion after TUR, and therefore the intervals between cystoscopies can be lengthened accordingly. The first cystoscopy should be done at 3 months and, if there is no recurrence, the intervals thereafter should be determined by the presence of the risk factors described earlier. When the risks of developing recurrence and progression are low then the patient can be examined by cystoscopy at 6-monthly intervals for the next year and then at yearly intervals. If high-risk factors are present then the patient should stay on a regimen of cystoscopies 3-monthly for a year and then 6-monthly for 2 years before moving to yearly examinations, provided that he or she remains recurrence free. The development of a recurrence should reduce the next interval to 3 months.

Cytology

When a patient is recurrence free after 5 years of annual cystoscopies then the chances of developing a recurrence are very small and are probably less than 5%. Annual cystoscopies after 5 years are therefore not likely to be cost effective and the annual cystoscopy can be replaced with a urine cytology examination. This at least should ensure an annual medical consultation during which the patient can be directly questioned about haematuria and other symptoms. It is unwise to dismiss these patients from follow-up completely. There are, however, no good data on the prolonged follow-up of such patients based on urine cytology.

When the bladder is seen to be free of recurrence, bladder washings can be taken for cytological examination. A positive finding indicates the need for close follow-up, whereas if it is negative the patient may be left for up to 1 year.

Intravenous Urography

Urothelial cancer is a multifocal disease and patients with bladder cancer are also at risk of developing tumours in their upper tracts. When superficial tumours of the bladder are considered, the risk of developing an upper tract tumour is 0.26%–1.5% (England et al. 1981; Walzer and Soloway 1983). This is in contrast to an incidence of 3.3-4% for patients undergoing cystectomy for bladder cancer (Schellhammer and Whitmore 1976; Zincke et al. 1984) and an incidence of 44%–55% of patients with upper tract tumours developing a bladder tumour. Routine IVU is not likely to be cost effective in the early detection of upper tract tumours as these are rare and may occur over a prolonged period after the initial resection. Upper tract tumours occurred up to 14 years after the initial resection in the series reported by England et al. (1981).

Booth and Kellett (1981) assessed the results of IVUs in 250 patients being followed-up for carcinoma of the bladder. Three ureteric tumours were found and these all occurred in 40 patients with active recurrent disease. Upper tract obstruction was found in 18 cases who had previously had tumours treated in the vicinity of the ureteric orifice. These authors suggest that after treatment of a tumour at the ureteric orifice the function of the upper tracts should be followed by renography.

IVU should be carried out on patients being followed for superficial bladder tumours in any of the following circumstances:

1. When results of cytological examination are positive and no tumour is found in the bladder.
2. When there has been haematuria and no tumour is found in the bladder.
3. When recurrent tumours occur in and around the ureteric orifice, as their treatment by cystodiathermy or radiation may cause obstruction, or there may be tumour in the lower ureter or in the kidneys.
4. In patients with uncontrolled tumours in whom there is an appreciable risk of upper tract tumours and in whom a change of therapy is indicated such as cystectomy.
5. When the patient has upper tract symptoms such as loin pain.

Intravesical Chemotherapy

Intravesical chemotherapy has become one of the most important topics in the treatment of bladder cancer. This form of therapy is now widely adopted and several different agents are being used. There are many pertinent questions on the use of intravesical chemotherapy for superficial bladder cancer and the available data should be critically examined. This subject will therefore be covered in detail in Chapter 10 (see p. 235).

Systemic Therapy for Superficial Tumours

Retinoids

Vitamin A belongs to a group of compounds known as the retinoids, which influence the differentiation and proliferation of epithelial tissues. The potential for vitamin A to reduce proliferation and improve differentiation of the urothelium and thereby reduce the recurrence rate of superficial bladder tumours was first recognised by Evard and Bollag (1972). Experimental studies with animal models have shown that a number of different retinoids are capable of reducing the incidence of tumours in animals fed on the carcinogens FANFT and BBN. The toxic side effects of vitamin A and most of the analogues have precluded their clinical use in the management of recurrent bladder tumours until the development of the aromatic analogues, such as etretinate, which may be much less toxic and more effective.

Two clinical studies have now been reported on the use of etretinate in the management of superficial bladder tumours (Alfthan et al. 1983; Studer et al. 1984). Both studies indicate that the toxicity is acceptable and that it is effective in reducing the recurrence rate. An oral compound that is both effective and of acceptable toxicity will be of great value in the management of superficial tumours, and the results of more extensive and comparative trials must be awaited with interest before this form of therapy can be widely adopted.

Vitamin B_6 (Pyridoxine)

The excretion of abnormal tryptophan metabolites in the urine may be associated with an increased risk of developing bladder cancer (see Chap. 1, p. 12). The excretion of these abnormal metabolites can be corrected by giving vitamin B_6. In a study by Byar and Blackard (1977) patients with pTa and pT1 tumours were given either placebo, pyridoxine or intravesical thiotepa after TUR. There was no significant reduction in the recurrence rate with either thiotepa or pyridoxine therapy; however, the subjects were not stratified according to the excretion of abnormal tryptophan metabolites before starting treatment, and pyridoxine therapy may only be effective in those patients excreting abnormal amounts of tryptophan metabolites. Further trials of pyridoxine therapy, where the patients are stratified according to the excretion of abnormal metabolites after a tryptophan load, have been carried out and the results are awaited.

Oral Methotrexate

Methotrexate is active against transitional cell carcinomas as judged by its effect on metastatic disease (see Chap. 10, p. 248). It is absorbed from the stomach and is excreted mostly unchanged in the urine. Hall et al. (1981) reported that a dose of 50 mg orally gave cytotoxic levels in the urine for at least 8 h and was free of serious toxicity. In a phase 2 study 16 patients with rapidly recurring multiple Ta and T1 bladder tumours were treated with 50 mg weekly for 18 months. Eleven patients had a reduction in the size, number and frequency of tumours and the other five did not respond, with two of them requiring a cystectomy. This report is encouraging and further controlled trials are required.

Total Cystectomy

Total cystectomy is the treatment of choice when conservative therapies for superficial bladder cancer have failed. The essential aspects of the management of those patients who have not responded to treatment is the selection of cases and the timing of cystectomy. When performed too readily cystectomy inflicts unnecessary morbidity and mortality, whereas if left too late it will be a therapeutic failure and the opportunity for cure will be lost.

There are few indications for cystectomy as the primary treatment for bladder cancer that does not invade muscle. When multifocal disease presents with extension beyond the bladder into the prostatic urethra or prostatic ducts then failure of conservative therapy is likely and the treatment is cystectomy. Patients with multifocal poorly differentiated T1 tumours have a poor prognosis but may be controlled by intravesical chemotherapy. Many urologists would, however, consider these patients for primary cystectomy.

The definition of failure of control is crucial for the selection of cases for cystectomy. How many different conservative therapies should be tried? How long can they be pursued before the risk of losing the chance of cure outweighs the possibility of control of the disease with preservation of bladder and sexual function? Uncontrolled pTa tumours that start to invade the lamina propria and recurrent T1 tumours that begin to invade muscle are clearly failing on conservative therapy, whereas those pTa tumours that remain non-invasive can continue to be treated conservatively. The development of tumours outside the bladder in the prostate, anterior urethra and lower ureters is an indication for cystectomy. When recurrent tumours are confined to the bladder the question is how long can conservative therapy by TUR or intravesical chemotherapy be continued before abandoning it for a cystectomy. Fitzpatrick et al. (1979) reported on the treatment with intravesical Epodyl of patients with multiple recurrent tumours not controlled by endoscopic surgery: 24 patients did not respond to Epodyl and were treated for an average of 2.8 years; 13 required cystectomy and 6 radiotherapy; the 5-year survival was 43%, and 13 patients died of bladder cancer. The authors concluded that failure to clear the bladder after 12 months of treatment is an indication for radical treatment and considered that the high bladder cancer mortality in this group was due to conservative treatment being continued for too long.

Bracken et al. (1981) reported a series of 109 patients with superficial bladder cancer treated by cystectomy in which the policy was to carry out cystectomy at a much earlier stage than in the series above. The median number of TURs before cystectomy was two; 27.5% of the patients had had more than five and 10% more than ten TURs. The indication for cystectomy was tumour in the prostatic urethra in 26 patients; 2 patients had carcinoma in situ in the prostatic ducts. The rest had endoscopically uncontrolled bladder tumours or had carcinoma in situ (5 cases primary and 17 cases secondary). There were 3 postoperative deaths in this series (2.75%); 14 cases developed local recurrence or distant metastases, and the 5-year survival was 76%. Urethral cancer was found in 9% of the male patients. Urethrectomy was performed in 72 males and was omitted in 23 males. One of these later developed an invasive urethral recurrence which was not controlled by further surgery and chemotherapy.

When cystectomy is carried out in time for superficial bladder cancer the results are good. When it is left too late the results are as poor as for deeply invasive disease. The morbidity and mortality of cystectomy must be weighed not only against the potential of cure of this disease but also the avoidance of multiple hospital admissions for TURs and intravesical chemotherapy.

Evaluation of Results

Recurrent superficial bladder cancer is a disease that is difficult to measure precisely. The number of tumours present cannot always be assessed as they may be confluent and involve wide areas of the bladder. The proportion of the surface of the bladder involved can only be guessed at on cystoscopy. The rate at which tumours are recurring is also difficult to measure and depends on examination of the bladder at fixed intervals. This is not always possible in clinical practice. There are, however, several aspects of this disease that can be used to assess the therapeutic or prophylactic effect of different forms of therapy.

1. *Percentage free of recurrent tumours* over the period of follow-up.
2. *Time to the first recurrence.* This may be relevant for prophylactic therapy, but cystoscopies must be carried out at fixed intervals.
3. *Recurrence rate.* This has been determined by dividing the total number of visits at which recurrences were present by the total patient-months of follow-up and is expressed as the recurrence rate/100 patient months (Schulman et al. 1982). Again, cystoscopies must be carried out at the same intervals for all patients.
4. *Development of invasion and metastases.* Assessment of this has all the errors that have been described in Chapters 5 and 6, but they will be reduced by observing the patient for longer.
5. *Survival.* This may be quoted as the overall survival or may be adjusted for the expected survival of the population being studied.
6. *Deaths from bladder cancer.* This may be the ultimate measure of therapeutic failure; however, the death rate from bladder cancer is low in superficial disease and may not be sensitive enough to detect therapeutic effects.

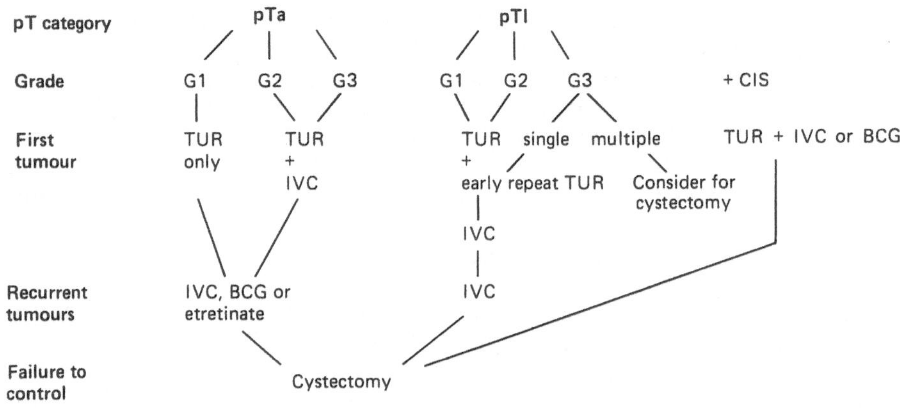

Fig. 8.7. An outline of the management of superficial bladder tumours at the Department of Urology at the University of Berne. *IVC*, intravesical chemotherapy; *CIS*, carcinoma in situ

Adopting a Treatment Policy

A wide range of therapeutic modalities for superficial bladder tumours have been presented in this chapter (see also Chap. 10). It is essential for the urologist to have clearly defined policies for the management of these tumours, and the various treatments should not be selected on a casual basis. The urologist may prefer to participate in controlled clinical trials and this is to be commended. A brief outline of the management policies at the University of Berne is presented in Fig. 8.7 to serve as an illustration, and similar policy outlines should be available for all urological clinics. There are several important questions which must be answered when formulating a treatment policy for superficial bladder tumours:

1. Which tumours can be treated by endoscopic resection alone and for which tumours is intravesical chemotherapy indicated after the initial TUR?
2. Which recurrent tumours need intravesical chemotherapy and what is the drug of choice?
3. When intravesical chemotherapy fails to eradicate the tumours should a second-line drug be tried?
4. When and for which patients is cystectomy indicated?
5. Is there a role for radiotherapy, either interstitial or external beam?
6. What should be the follow-up policy for the different categories of patient?

References

Abrams PH, Choa RG, Gaches CGC, Ashken MH, Green NA (1981) A controlled trial of single dose Adriamycin in superficial bladder tumours. Br J Urol 53: 585–587

Alfthan O, Tarkkanen J, Gröhn P, Heinonen E, Pyrhönen S, Säilä K (1983) Tigason (etretinate) in prevention of recurrence of superficial bladder tumours. A double-blind clinical trial. Eur Urol 9: 6–9
Althausen AF, Prout GR, Daly JJ (1976) Non-invasive papillary carcinoma of bladder associated with carcinoma in situ. J Urol 116: 576–579
Amar AD, Das S (1983) Vesicoureteric reflux in patients with bladder tumours. Br J Urol 55: 483–487
Anderström C, Johansson S, Nilsson S (1980) The significance of lamina propria invasion on the prognosis of patients with bladder tumours. J Urol 124: 23–26
Augspurger RR, Donohue RE (1980) Prevention of obturator nerve stimulation during transurethral surgery. J Urol 123: 170–172
Barnes R, Hadley H, Dick A, Johnston O, Dexter J (1977) Changes in grade and stage of recurrent bladder tumours. J Urol 118: 177–179
Benson RC, Kinsey JH, Cortese DA, Farrow GM, Utz DC (1983) Treatment of transitional cell carcinoma of bladder with haematoporphyrin derivative phototherapy. J Urol 130: 1090–1095
Booth CM, Kellett MJ (1981) Intravenous urography in the follow-up of carcinoma of the bladder. Br J Urol 53: 246–249
Boyd PJP, Burnand KG (1974) Site of bladder tumour recurrences. Lancet II: 1290–1292
Bracken B, McDonald MW, Johnson DE (1981) Cystectomy for superficial bladder cancer. Urology 18: 459–463
Burnand KG, Boyd PJR, Mayo ME, Shuttleworth KED, Lloyd-Davies RW (1976) Single dose intravesical thiotepa as an adjuvant to cystodiathermy in the treatment of transitional cell bladder carcinoma. Br J Urol 48: 55–59
Byar D, Blackard C (1977) Comparisons of placebo, pyridoxine and topical thiotepa in preventing recurrence of stage 1 bladder cancer. Urology 10(6): 556–561
Catalona WJ (1981) Practical utility of specific red cell adherence test in bladder cancer. Urology 18: 113–117
Cifuentes Delatte L, Garcia de la Pena E, Vela Navarrette R (1982) Survival rates of patients with bladder tumours. An experience of 1744 cases (1950–1978). Br J Urol 54: 267–274
Cooper PH, Waisman J, Johnston WH, Skinner DG (1973) Severe atypia of transitional epithelium and carcinoma of the urinary bladder. Cancer 31: 1055–1060
Dalesio O, Schulman CC, Sylvester R, De Pauw M, Robinson M, Denis L, Smith P, Viggiano G (1983) Prognostic factors in superficial bladder tumours. A study of the European Organisation for Research on Treatment for Cancer: genitourinary tract cancer cooperative group. J Urol 129: 730–733
Davis TRC (1983) The composition and origin of the gas produced during urological endoscopic resections. Br J Urol 55: 294–297
Dick A, Barnes R, Hadley H, Bergman RT, Ninan C (1980) Complications of transurethral resection of bladder tumours: prevention, recognition and treatment. J Urol 124: 810–811
Eisenberg RB, Roth RB, Schweinsberg MH (1960) Bladder tumours and associated proliferative mucosal lesions. J Urol 84: 544–550
England HR, Rigby C, Shepheard BGF, Tresidder GC, Blandy JP (1973) Evaluation of Helmstein's distension method for carcinoma of the bladder. Br J Urol 45: 593–599
England HR, Paris AMI, Blandy JP (1981) The correlation of T1 bladder tumour history with prognosis and follow-up requirements. Br J Urol 53: 593–597
Esch W, Rummelhardt S (1973) Blasenteilresektion beim fortgeschrittenen Blasenkarzinom. Helv Chir Acta 40: 459–461
Evard JP, Bollag W (1972) Konservative Behandlung der rezidivierenden Harnblasenpapillomatose mit Vitamin-A-Säure. Schweiz Med Wochenschr 102: 1880
Falor WH, Ward RM (1977) Prognosis in well-differentiated noninvasive carcinoma of the bladder based on chromosomal analysis. Surg Gynecol Obstet 144: 515–518
Fastenmeier K, Flackenecker G (1981) High frequency technology: applications and hazards. In: Mauermayer W (ed) Transurethral surgery. Springer, Berlin Heidelberg New York, pp 47–60
Fitzpatrick JM, Khan O, Oliver RTD, Riddle PR (1979) Long term follow-up in patients with superficial bladder tumours treated with intravesical Epodyl. Br J Urol 51: 545–548
Gavrell GJ, Lewis RW, Meehan WL, Leblanc GA (1978) Intravesical thiotepa in the immediate postoperative period in patients with recurrent transitional cell carcinoma of the bladder. J Urol 120: 410–411
Greene LF, Yalowitz PA (1972) The advisability of concomitant transurethral excision of vesical neoplasia and prostatic hyperplasia. J Urol 107: 445–447
Gunter PA, de Abela-Borg J, Pugh RCB (1983) Urothelium and the specific red cell adherence test. Br J Urol 55: 10–16

Hall RR (1982) Report to the standing committee on urological instruments: Lasers in urology. Br J Urol 54: 421–426

Hall RR, Herring DW, Gibb I, Heath AB (1981) Prophylactic oral methotrexate therapy for multiple superficial bladder carcinoma. Br J Urol 53: 582–584

Hartung R, Hegemann M (1981) Implantationsmetastasen in den oberen Harnwegen durch resektionsbedingten vesikoureteralen Reflux. Aktuel Urol 12: 202–205

Helmstein K (1972) Treatment of bladder carcinoma by a hydrostatic technique. Report on 43 cases. Br J Urol 44; 434–450

Heney NM, Daly J, Prout GR, Nieh PT, Heaney JA, Trebeck NE (1978) Biopsy of apparently normal urothelium in patients with bladder carcinoma. J Urol 120: 559–560

Heney NM, Nocks BN, Daly JJ, Prout GR, Newall JB, Griffin PB, Perrone TL, Szyfelbein WA (1982) Ta and T1 bladder cancer: Location recurrence and progression. Br J Urol 54: 152–157

Heney NM, Ahmed S, Flanagan MJ, Frable W, Corder MP, Hafermann MD, Hawkins IR (1983) Superficial bladder cancer: progression and recurrence. J Urol 130: 1083–1086

Hewitt CB, Babiszewski JF, Antunez AR (1981) Update on intracavitary radiation in the treatment of bladder tumours. J Urol 126: 323–325.

Hinman F (1956) Recurrence of bladder tumors by surgical implantation. J Urol 75: 695–696

Hisazumi H, Misaki T, Miyoshi N (1983) Photoradiation therapy of bladder tumours. J Urol 130: 685–687

Hofstetter A, Schmiedt E, Staehler G (1982) Endovesikale Zerstoerung von Blasentumoren mit dem Neodym-YAG-Laser. Urologe [A] 21: 9–11

Jewett HJ, Strong GH (1946) Infiltrating carcinoma of the bladder: relation of depth of penetration of the bladder wall to incidence of local extension and metastases. J Urol 55: 366–372

Kelly JF, Snell ME, Berenbaum MC (1975) Photodynamic destruction of human bladder carcinoma. Br J Cancer 31: 237–244

Kinsey JH, Cortese DA, Sanderson DR (1978) Detection of haematoporphyrin fluorescence during fibreoptic bronchoscopy to localise early bronchogenic carcinoma. Mayo Clin Proc 53: 594–600

Laor E, Grabstald H, Whitmore WF (1981) The influence of simultaneous resection of bladder tumours and prostate on the occurrence of prostatic urethral tumours. J Urol 126: 171–172

Lutzeyer W, Rubben H, Dahm H (1982) Prognostic parameters in superficial bladder cancer: an analysis of 315 cases. J Urol 127: 250–252

Mackenzie N, Torti FM, Faysal M (1981) The natural history of superficial bladder tumours. Proc Am Assoc Cancer Res 22: 198

Marberger H (1977) Die Transurethrale Resektion als Palliativbehandlung beim Blasenkarzinom. In: Verhandlungsbericht der Deutschen Gesellschaft für Urologie, vol 29. Springer, Berlin Heidelberg New York, p 19

Marshall VF (1952) The relation of the preoperative estimate to the pathologic demonstration of the extent of vesical neoplasms. J Urol 68: 714–723

Miller A, Mitchell JP, Brown NJ (1969) The British Bladder Tumour Registry. Br J Urol (Suppl), pp 1–64 (Chap 3 The natural history of bladder tumours, pp 17–25)

Narayana AS, Loening SA, Slymen DJ, Culp DA (1983) Bladder cancer: Factors affecting survival. J Urol 130: 56–60

O'Flynn JD, Smith JM, Hanson JS (1975) Transurethral resection for the assessment and treatment of vesical neoplasms. Eur Urol 1: 38–40

Page BH, Levison VB, Curwen MP (1978) The site recurrence of non-infiltrating bladder tumours. Br J Urol 50: 237–242

Page BH, Levison V, Curwen MP (1979) A trial of prophylactic radiotherapy for non-infiltrating bladder tumours. Br J Urol 51: 197–199

Pocock RD, Ponder BAJ, O'Sullivan JP, Ibrahim SK, Easton DF, Shearer RJ (1982) Prognostic factors in non-infiltrating carcinoma of the bladder: a preliminary report. Br J Urol 54: 711–715

Pryor JP (1973) Factors influencing the survival of patients with transitional cell tumours of the urinary bladder. Br J Urol 45: 586–592

Schade RO, Swinney J (1968) Precancerous changes in bladder epithelium. Lancet II: 943–946

Schade ROK, Swinney J (1983) The association of urothelial abnormalities with neoplasia: a 10-year follow-up. J Urol 129: 1125–1126

Schellhammer PF, Whitmore WF (1976) Transitional cell carcinoma of the urethra in men having cystectomy for bladder cancer. J Urol 115: 56–60

Schulman CC, Robinson M, Denis L, Smith P, Viggiano G, de Pauw M, Dalesio O, Sylvester R (1982) Prophylactic chemotherapy of superficial transitional cell bladder carcinoma: An EORTC randomised trial comparing thiotepa, an epipodophylotoxin (VM26) and TUR alone. Eur Urol 8: 207–212

Smith G, Elton RA, Beynon LL, Newsam JE, Chisholm GD, Hargreave TB (1983) Prognostic significance of biopsy results of normal looking mucosa in cases of superficial bladder cancer. Br J Urol 55: 665–669
Soloway MS, Masters S (1980) Urothelial susceptibility to tumour cell implantation. Influence of cauterisation. Cancer 46: 1158–1163
Soloway MS, Murphy W, Rav MK, Cox C (1978) Serial multiple-site biopsies in patients with bladder cancer. J Urol 120: 57–59
Soto EA, Friedell GH, Tiltman AJ (1977) Bladder cancer as seen in giant histologic sections. Cancer 39: 447–455
Studer UE, Biedermann C, Chollet D, Karrer P, Kraft R, Toggenburg H, Vonbank F (1984) Prevention of recurrent superficial bladder tumours by oral etretinate: preliminary results of a randomised, double blind multicenter trial in Switzerland. J Urol 131: 47–49
Toggenburg H, Brand H (1979) Die klinische Bedeutung der Vesikorenalen Reflux nach Elektroresektion von Blasentumoren. Helv Chir Acta 46: 405–408
Tsuchiya A, Obara N, Miwa M, Ohi T, Kato H, Hayata Y (1983) Haematoporphyrin derivative and laser photoradiation in the diagnosis and treatment of bladder cancer. J Urol 130: 79–82
van der Werf-Messing BHP (1978) Cancer of the urinary bladder treated by interstitial radium implant. Int J Radiat Oncol Biol Phys 4: 373–378
van der Werf-Messing BHP, Hop WCJ (1981) Carcinoma of the urinary bladder (category T1NXM0) treated either by radium implant or by transurethral resection only. Int J Radiat Oncol Biol Phys 7: 299–303
Varkarakis MJ, Gaeta J, Moore RH, Murphy GP (1974) Superficial bladder tumour. Aspects of clinical progression. Urology 4: 414–420
Wallace DMA, Hindmarsh JR, Webb JN, Busuttil A, Hargreave TB, Newsam JE, Chisholm GD (1979) The role of multiple mucosal biopsies in the management of patients with bladder cancer. Br J Urol 51: 535–540
Walzer Y, Soloway MS (1983) Should the follow-up of patients with bladder cancer include routine excretory urography? J Urol 130: 672–673
Weldon TE, Soloway MS (1975) Susceptibility of urothelium to neoplastic cellular implantation. Urology 5: 824–827
Whitmore WF, Prout GR (1982) Discouraging results for high dose external beam radiation therapy in low stage (O and A) bladder cancer. J Urol 127: 902–905
Williams GB, Trott PA, Bloom HJG (1981) Carcinoma of the bladder treated by interstitial irradiation. Br J Urol 53: 221–224
Williams JL, Hammonds JC, Saunders N (1977) T1 bladder tumours. Br J Urol 49: 663–668
Wolf H, Hojgaard K (1983) Prognostic factors in local surgical treatment of invasive bladder cancer, with special reference to the presence of urothelial dysplasia. Cancer 51: 1710–1715
Zincke H, Garbeff PJ, Beahrs JR (1984) Upper tract transitional cell cancer after radical cystectomy for bladder cancer. J Urol 131: 50–52
Zingg EJ, Zeltner T (1980) Partial cystectomy. In: Pavone-Macaluso M, Smith PH, Edsmyr F (eds) Bladder tumours and other topics in urological oncology. Plenum, New York, pp 201–205

Chapter 9

The Treatment of Muscle Invasive Bladder Cancer

E. J. Zingg, P. N. Plowman, D. M. A. Wallace, P. C. Peters and J. P. Blandy

Introduction

When a bladder tumour invades into the muscle it is an ominous prognostic sign: The patient has at best little more than a 50% chance of surviving the disease. The probability of there being nodal or distant metastases at presentation is high and there is limited scope for curative therapy. Of patients presenting with bladder cancer 25%–35% have tumours that are already invading muscle. Most of these will not have clinically apparent metastases, and therefore curative treatment will be attempted. If this is to be achieved then treatment must be radical. However, in many cases there will already be microscopic metastases, and radical treatment of the primary tumour all too often turns out to be but a palliative measure. A thorough assessment of the tumour and full investigation of the patient to search for metastases (see Chap. 5) are essential before radical local therapy. At the present time only those cases that are without clinically detectable distant metastases should be considered for curative therapy.

There are three main approaches to the primary management of invasive bladder cancer: radical surgery, radical radiotherapy and a combination of preoperative radiotherapy and surgery. None of these has a clear advantage over the others and all seem to be reaching towards a barrier of about 50% 5-year survival which is determined more by the nature of the disease than by the efficacy of local therapy. The debate at present is about how best to achieve local control. The challenge for the future is to find effective systemic therapy for the microscopic metastases that can be integrated into the present treatment regimens. When such treatment is available then we may substantially alter our present management of the primary tumour. The choice of treatment at present depends on a great many factors. In the first two parts of this chapter all three methods of treatment are reviewed. In the final two parts the contrasting policies adopted by two different centres are described; both are personal views on the management of invasive bladder cancer.

The wide diversity of opinion over the primary management of invasive bladder cancer has existed for many years, yet few controlled clinical trials have been conducted that might resolve which is the best treatment for each category of patient. Why is there such a paucity of randomised controlled clinical trials such as the four reported by Prout et al. (1971), Wallace and Bloom (1976), Miller (1977) and Anderström et al. (1983)? These trials require large numbers of comparable patients. When the selection criteria for such trials are defined it becomes apparent that these cases are not very common in a single centre; therefore, recruitment will be slow and the trial must become a multicentre study if it is to achieve a statistically meaningful result. Such trials are difficult to run, and maintaining agreement and consistency among the different centres requires a great amount of effort on the part of all the contributors. In the collaborative study of the Urological Cancer Research Group reported by Prout et al. (1971) 185 of the 427 patients entered were found to be ineligible. The multicentre study undertaken by the Institute of Urology and Royal Marsden Hospital took ten years to accrue 199 patients from eight different centres (Wallace and Bloom 1976).

In contrast to such studies there is an abundance of reports on the results of non-randomised and uncontrolled treatment of patients who are usually highly selected. This data is of limited value as such reports cannot readily be compared one with another to draw conclusions about methods of treatment. There are three main reasons for this: selection of patients, staging errors and changes over periods of time.

Selection may operate in several ways from the total number of patients with bladder cancer in a population to the actual inclusion of an individual case into a series which is being reported. Few centres have a 'captive' population for treatment, and thus the first way selection may operate is that certain cases may never be referred to a particular hospital. There may be many reasons for this, including social, economic, geographical and personal, but general practitioners are also free to refer patients according to the treatment policies adopted by the various hospitals. At the centres conducting the studies patients may be selected in and selected out of the study according to a number of stated and unstated criteria. Individual clinicians must retain the right to treat each individual patient as they feel appropriate. All series will have patients that should have been included according to the selection criteria but who have been excluded for a variety of reasons, most of which will not be reported. Many such patients will be excluded because of factors that place them in a higher risk group; their inclusion would therefore adversely affect the overall results.

The importance of selection would not be so great if there were a staging and classification system that was perfect and we knew that the cases were exactly comparable in each series. However, staging systems are far from perfect (see Chap. 6), and many of the differences in the results of non-randomised series between different centres could be accounted for by differences in their staging techniques. Randomised trials are the only way of overcoming this problem and they require large numbers of patients from multiple centres.

Finally, there have been many new developments over the last three decades, not just in surgery, but also in radiotherapy and general medical care. Both diagnostic and therapeutic skills have changed, and there is limited value in using historical series as controls or comparing results of series from different periods of time.

There are many more factors that the clinician must consider, in addition to studying the literature, before deciding on a treatment strategy for invasive bladder cancer. It is up to the urologist to judge how best to treat the patient according to the means available. Populations differ in their cultural, social and economic background and these differences must be taken into account. Despite the need for controlled trials and the benefit of having clearly laid-down treatment policies for bladder cancer in each institution, every patient must always be treated as an individual.

Part 1. Surgery

E. J. Zingg and D. M. A. Wallace

Conservative Surgery

The original purpose of dividing the muscle invasive tumours clinically into those that penetrate only into superficial muscle from those that penetrate into deep muscle was to distinguish the tumours which could be treated with conservation of the bladder from those which required radical therapy. The results of conservative surgery for T2 tumours are poor whether treated by TUR or by partial cystectomy. Barnes et al. (1977) reported a 5-year survival of only 31% for 75 patients with stage B tumours. This result is comparable to the results of more aggressive therapy, but it should be remembered that these patients were selected as being suitable for treatment by TUR and therefore were likely to have smaller tumours.

When treated equally radically there is little difference in the results of the T2 and T3 tumours (Skinner 1977). In one series they even had a poorer survival (Blandy et al. 1980). The poor prognosis for the T2 tumour therefore justifies the decision to treat it as aggressively as the more deeply invasive tumours, particularly when poorly differentiated.

Certain carefully selected cases may, however, be considered for treatment by TUR alone. These patients should have tumours that are small, papillary T2 tumours and are well or moderately differentiated. When such a tumour is managed by TUR alone then it is essential that an early repeat TUR of the tumour site is carried out at 3–6 weeks; if there is any tumour remaining which is invading muscle then that tumour must be treated as a T3 tumour.

A segmental resection may also be carried out for invasive tumours, according to the criteria already discussed in Chapter 8 (see p. 175). Such patients will always be highly selected and little can be derived from the published data except that the results—47%–75% survival for T2 or B1 cases—are comparable to those for patients treated by more radical therapy. A short course of preoperative radiation should be given to prevent possible wound implantation.

Total Cystectomy

Definitions

The term 'simple cystectomy' is used to describe the removal of just the bladder in cases of diseases confined to the bladder. When the bladder is removed in cases of malignant disease then the procedure is a radical cystectomy. It is understood that this means the removal of the bladder together with the prostate and seminal vesicles in the male and the whole urethra, anterior vaginal wall, uterus and adnexae in the female. The procedure can be extended to include bilateral removal of the regional lymph nodes (obturator, external, internal and common iliac groups of nodes). The principle of radical cancer surgery is to remove the tumour-bearing organ together with its surrounding tissues and the regional lymph nodes.

Radical cystectomy has played a central role in the management of invasive bladder cancer for many years. This is a major operation which results in the loss of normal bladder and sexual function and requires the construction of a definitive form of urinary diversion. Selection of patients for this operation must be one of the most carefully considered decisions that the urologist must make.

Indications

The indications for primary management of invasive bladder tumours by cystectomy will vary according to the opinions of the individual urologist. Each urologist must decide what is the best treatment in his hands, in his hospital and for each individual patient. Radical cystectomy should be discussed in those cases that are beyond the scope of conservative treatments. The indications for cystectomy can be considered in terms of curative or palliative treatments and are listed in Table 9.1.

Table 9.1. Indications for cystectomy

Curative intent:

1. Infiltrating bladder cancer (T3 and T4a), especially:
   a) >3 cm diameter
   b) multifocal
   c) obstructed ureter
   d) prostatic infiltration
   e) at base of bladder
2. Multifocal papillary tumours (T1 and T2)
   a) failed intravesical chemotherapy
   b) widespread carcinoma in situ
   c) rapidly recurring and progressing
3. Recurrent or residual tumour after radiotherapy

Palliative

1. Contracted bladder with severe symptoms
2. Massive bleeding not controlled by conservative measures

Selection

Age alone is not a contraindication to cystectomy and diversion. Patients over 80 years old may successfully undergo this operation, though the operative morbidity and mortality will be higher. Social rehabilitation of such elderly patients is possible, provided that they are carefully selected (Zingg et al. 1980; Zincke 1982). The patient's general health is of prime importance, and the cardiovascular and respiratory systems should be fully assessed as for any patient coming to major surgery. Impaired renal function is not infrequently encountered in such patients and may result from previous surgery or pyelonephritis, as well as obstruction. Moderate impairment of function with plasma creatinines up to 250 mmol/litre is not a contraindication.

The intellect and psychological make-up of patients is of considerable importance. They must not only be very well motivated to go through with the operation, postoperative recovery and rehabilitation, but must fully understand the necessity for the operation and its consequences. The full social and physical rehabilitation of patients is only possible if they are able to care for the diversion by themselves and return to an active life.

Preoperative Preparation

It should be axiomatic that before such major surgery the patient must be made fully aware of the nature of the operation, including the possible complications, the loss of the normal bladder function, the diversion, the loss of sexual potency in the male and the loss of the vagina in the female. The possibility of later reconstructive surgery to restore potency can be mentioned to the male patient. The prospect of a urinary diversion and the need to wear an external appliance may be very difficult for the patient to accept. Ample time must be taken to discuss this both by the medical staff and the stoma therapist, who should see the patient preoperatively. Patients may be more ready to accept the stoma and external appliance when they have had a chance to wear such an appliance preoperatively and also to meet a patient of the same sex who already has a diversion in order to discuss potential problems and to talk about their anxieties. It is also useful to involve spouses of patients in the discussion at this stage.

Stoma Site

The position for the stoma must be chosen with great care by the surgeon and marked preoperatively. It is important to look at the abdomen with the patient lying, sitting and standing in order to choose the optimal site for the stoma. The stoma must never be placed in a skin crease or else it will inevitably leak, and it should be away from the iliac crest. The flange should not be pushed up in the sitting position or else the appliance will tend to shear off. If the surgeon is unsure about a proposed site the patient can wear a partly filled bag for a day to test its positioning.

Physiotherapy

The patient should receive pulmonary physiotherapy and be fully familiar with the breathing exercises that will be essential postoperatively. Intensive physiotherapy preoperatively is the most effective measure to prevent postoperative pulmonary complications (Schoenenberger 1984).

Bowel Preparation

The human gastrointestinal tract is a huge reservoir of bacteria, where the concentration of bacteria steadily increases from the stomach, which is nearly free of bacteria when empty, to concentrations of 10^5–10^8 in the distal small bowel and up to 10^{11} in the colon. Thorough mechanical cleansing of the bowel is the most effective way to reduce the risk of contaminating the operative field and also facilitates the surgery and postoperative recovery. Bowel cleansing is predominantly carried out by orthograde lavage (Hewitt et al. 1973), which can be accomplished in 2–4 h and is the procedure of choice when thorough preparation is required. However, this procedure must be performed with caution in patients with cardiac or renal failure. When physiological saline or Ringer's lactated solution is used, then fluid and acid-base disturbances are minimal. Alternatively, oral mannitol with fluids or simply oral magnesium sulphate may achieve satisfactory clearing of the bowel without the need for passing a nasogastric tube, but take a little longer.

Surgical Technique

For full details of the operative techniques of removing the bladder the reader is referred to the definitive texts on operative surgery. However, there are many important points of technique which should be discussed here. The patient should be supine or in a modified lithotomy position if a synchronous urethrectomy is to be carried out. The bladder is catheterised, and a rectal tube may be inserted to facilitate the separation of the prostate from the rectum. The stoma site is marked with a scratch and the abdomen is then opened with a midline incision skirting the umbilicus on the opposite side to the stoma. If there are obvious metastases the procedure should be abandoned after frozen section confirmation unless a palliative cystectomy is indicated. The procedure begins with the pelvic lymph node dissection. The lateral margin of this dissection is the genitofemoral nerve lying on the psoas muscle, although many surgeons only go as far lateral as the femoral artery in order to avoid the risk of lymphoedema of the leg. The upper and lower limits of the dissection are 2–4 cm above the bifurcation of the common iliac artery down to the origin of the inferior epigastric vessels. The nodal tissue is then swept medially off the iliac vessels taking the anterior branches of the hypogastric artery. It is not necessary to ligate the main trunk of the hypogastric artery; indeed it may be dangerous to do so. The nodes are dissected out of the obturator fossa, care being taken not to injure the nerve. They are labelled according to their origin and sent for frozen section (see p. 196).

If the nodes are found to be free of metastases on microscopic examination then the bladder is removed. The ureters should be divided at least 10 cm above the bladder as the probability of finding carcinoma in situ in the distal ureter is 10%–12% (Sharma et al. 1970; Wallace 1973). The cut ends of the ureters will be further trimmed when the diversion is carried out, and these pieces should be sent for histological examination. The vesical branches of the internal iliac artery are clipped or ligated and divided. The peritoneum is incised right down into the pouch of Douglas and the plane between the rectum and prostate found by blunt dissection. This may be difficult if there has been previous transurethral surgery to the prostate or radiotherapy and may be done more safely through a separate perineal incision. The pelvic fascia lateral to the prostate is incised and the deep pedicles are clamped and divided. This dissection can either be carried out from above downwards or else the membranous urethra can be divided and the prostate turned upwards and the pedicles divided in the opposite direction. Bleeding should be controlled by transfixation sutures, with the pelvic floor closed and the cavity packed while the diversion is performed.

Lymph Node Dissection

Between 20% and 25% of patients coming to cystectomy for bladder cancer have metastases in the pelvic lymph nodes and the prognosis is extremely poor. If these nodes are metastatic is radical surgery justified or can a meticulous node dissection be of therapeutic benefit? Do the pelvic nodes need to be examined by frozen section before the bladder is removed? Does this procedure add to the morbidity of the whole operation?

Opinions are divided on the therapeutic value of the pelvic lymphadenectomy. Daughtry et al. (1977) reported that no patients survived more than 20 months after cystectomy if the nodes had metastases and concluded that there was no justification in performing a pelvic lymphadenectomy. In contrast, Skinner (1982a) reports a 36% actuarial survival of 36 patients with metastatic nodes who had undergone a meticulous pelvic node dissection at the time of radical cystectomy, and concluded that this procedure can cure some patients with nodal metastases. Smith and Whitmore (1982) have reported a large series of 134 patients with nodal metastases in whom the overall survival was only 7% but was 17% for the 30 patients with only N1 disease. Many other centres have reported similar results (Table 9.2), but the numbers are small and there is rarely sufficient detail reported with regard to the site, size and number of positive nodes.

Table 9.2. Reported survival of patients with nodal metastases

Reference	No. of patients	Percentage survival (5-year)
Whitmore and Marshall (1962)	13	16
Dretter et al. (1973)	35	13
Laplante and Brice (1973)	39	13
Reid et al. (1976)	24	21
Clark (1978)	12	25
Smith and Whitmore (1981)	134	7
Bloom et al. (1982)	15	16
Skinner (1982a)	36	36

When pelvic lymph node metastases are palpable there is little doubt that the disease is disseminated and beyond the scope of local surgery. When the disease is microscopic and confined to one or two nodes then it is controversial as to whether to abandon the cystectomy; it is clearly possible to achieve a few long-term survivors in this group by meticulous surgery, but the majority will still die of bladder cancer within 2 years (Studer et al. 1983). One factor that influences the reported results is how meticulous is the examination of the nodes: The more sections that are cut from each node the more chance the pathologist has of detecting microscopic metastases (see Chap. 2, p. 44). This variation in pathological technique may account for some of the variation in results as the technique of the pathologist and the size and site of the metastases are seldom reported. There is insufficient time to examine tissue sent for frozen section in as great detail as tissue that is fixed, so if metastases are found on frozen section it is likely that they are widespread and the prognosis is correspondingly poor.

When the lymph nodes are not palpably enlarged and the frozen section demonstrates no microscopic metastases then the performance of a node dissection may cure some of these patients with limited nodal metastases. Pelvic lymphadenectomy does not increase the morbidity of the procedure. (Dretler 1973; Skinner 1982a) and may improve local control of the disease. The information gained from this procedure may be of considerable prognostic value; it can be used to stratify patients for reporting results and may serve as a basis for planning future therapy.

Urethrectomy

The urethra is lined with urothelium, which, in bladder cancer patients, has been exposed to urine-borne carcinogens and to the trauma of instrumentation in the course of diagnosis and treatment. In patients coming to cystectomy there is a risk of further tumours developing in the urethra. In female patients the entire urethra will be removed as part of the radical cystectomy, but in males a routine, prophylactic, synchronous urethrectomy increases the operative time, blood loss and postoperative morbidity and should therefore be carried out in selected cases.

The risk of developing a tumour in the urethra following a cystectomy for bladder cancer is 6%–12% (Table 9.3). Gowing (1960) found an 18% incidence of carcinoma in situ and 15% incidence of atypical hyperplasia in an autopsy study of 33 patients dying of bladder cancer; a 19% incidence of carcinoma in situ was reported when this series was extended to 109 patients (Hendry et al. 1974). These lesions were patchy and could be separated by areas of normal urothelium. Poole-Wilson and Barnard (1971) reported urethral tumours in 33 (19%) of a

Table 9.3. Urethral carcinoma in men undergoing cystectomy for bladder cancer

Reference	Whole series	Prophylactic urethrectomy
Poole-Wilson and Barnard (1971)	33/173 (19%)	
Schellhammer and Whitmore (1977)	27/348 (7%)	14/110 (12.5%)
Raz et al. (1978)	17/174 (10%)	7/32 (22%)
Beahrs et al. (1984)	28/349 (8%)	
Zabbo and Montie (1984)	11/119 (9%)	4/11 (36%)
Ahlering et al. (1984)	19/174 (11%)	

series of 176 patients undergoing cystectomy for bladder cancer; tumour was present in the urethra at the time of cystectomy in 22 patients and subsequently in 11 patients. Schellhammer et al. (1976) found a 12.5% incidence of tumour when the urethra was removed prophylactically and 7% when the urethra was left. Most series have a policy of selective urethrectomy, which will clearly influence the secondary urethrectomy results, but in all series there is an appreciable incidence of tumours in the urethras that have been left behind.

The development of a urethral tumour may adversely affect the prognosis because, when invasion occurs, the tumour has direct access to the vascular spaces of the corpus spongiosum. All of the patients with urethral tumours reported by Poole-Wilson and Barnard (1971) died within 2 years, and other authors report a similar poor prognosis. Beahrs et al. (1984), however, reported that 34% of 28 patients with urethral involvement survived 5 years and that the development of urethral recurrences did not significantly affect the overall survival of the bladder cancer patients undergoing cystectomy. Most patients dying with urethral recurrence also have disseminated metastases. It is a matter of debate whether the urethral recurrence is the source of the metastases, though it is a clinical impression that it is so.

The risk of urethral involvement is greater when the bladder tumours are multifocal (Poole-Wilson and Barnard 1971; Hendry et al. 1974), but many urethral tumours occurred when the bladder tumour was solitary. A selection policy for urethrectomy is outlined in Table 9.4. The urethrectomy can either be performed synchronously, with two surgeons removing the bladder and urethra en bloc, or else the urethrectomy may be delayed for 6–8 weeks.

Table 9.4. Indications for urethrectomy

Primary (synchronous or delayed):
1. Concomitant tumour in the urethra
2. Metastases in urethral resection margin
3. Multifocal tumours
4. Widespread carcinoma in situ
5. Tumour in upper tracts and bladder (panurothelial disease)

Secondary
1. Tumour in prostatic urethra or ducts
2. Positive result to cytological examination of urethra
3. Bloody urethral discharge

If the urethra is left in situ it must never be forgotten. It must be sampled by urethral washings for cytological examination at 6-monthly intervals. When a urethrectomy is performed then the whole urethra should be removed, including the external meatus. Schellhammer and Whitmore (1976) reported that 7 of the 27 patients undergoing subtotal urethrectomy later developed a recurrence at the external meatus.

Urinary Diversion

Urinary diversion is an integral part of the cystectomy operation. This is usually performed as a one-stage procedure, though this can be carried out in the first stage for patients who are very high surgical risks (Crawford and Skinner 1980); however, the benefit of the lower operative mortality is offset by the prolonged hospitalisation and the need for two procedures. Much of the success of cystectomy and most of the complications can be attributed to the urinary diversion. A good result depends on the thorough preoperative assessment and examination of the patient, the correct choice of method of diversion, a careful and exact technique and good aftercare. The type of diversion has little influence on the survival after cystectomy for bladder cancer but may make an enormous difference to the quality of the patient's life. The subject of urinary diversion in malignant disease has recently been more fully reviewed by Walsh (1982). The main methods of diversion following cystectomy are the ileal conduit, the colon conduit, the ureterosigmoid diversion and the cutaneous ureterostomy. The rectal bladder and the continent ileal reservoir can also be considered as options in these patients.

Ileal Conduit

The commonest form of urinary diversion with cystectomy for bladder cancer is the ileal conduit. It has the advantages of being a standardised and simple technique with virtually no metabolic complications and a relatively low incidence of ureteroileal and stomal problems. In addition, the ileoileal anastomosis is probably the simplest and safest bowel anastomosis. Its principal disadvantages are the need for an external appliance and the late deterioration of the upper tracts.

The method of urinary diversion has a major influence on the long-term results, but in bladder cancer patients it is the behaviour of the tumour that influences the survival and not the diversion. The late follow-up has shown that 10%–20% with ileal conduit diversions will develop upper tract deterioration and up to 10% will develop stones. The aftercare is mainly carried out by specially trained stoma therapists, who have contributed enormously to the quality of life for these patients (Jones et al. 1981; Studer and Furger 1981).

Colon Conduit

The principle of the colon conduit operation is similar to that for the ileal conduit. It has the advantage over the ileal conduit in that a non-refluxing ureteral implant is possible; the prevention of reflux is now considered to be of importance in the preservation of renal function over long periods. This is not so critical in the bladder cancer patient as in younger adults and children. A large bowel anastomosis has, however, a higher complication rate than for small bowel.

One indication for the colon conduit is when the pelvis and small bowel have been heavily irradiated. The transverse colon may have escaped radiation damage and can be used more safely than an ileal loop (Beckley et al. 1982).

Ureterocolic Anastomosis

The procedure of ureterocolic anastomosis was first performed many years ago (Simon 1851) and its many complications have been well described. It is, however, one method of diversion that allows the patient to lead a near-normal life without the need for any external appliances. Previous radiotherapy, inflammatory bowel disease and doubtful anal continence are contraindications, as are any evidence of pyelonephritic damage to the kidneys and upper tract dilation. Observation of these patients must be lifelong because of the risks of reabsorption of urine causing severe hyperchloraemic hypokalaemic acidosis in 7%, pyelonephritic damage in 16%, loss of a kidney in 2% and upper tract dilation in 9% (Marberger 1977). The development of an adenocarcinoma at the site of the ureteric implantation after an interval of approximately 20 years is now well described. These patients will need regular limited colonoscopy to inspect the implantation site.

Of the patients with ureterosigmoid diversions 25% are fully continent and able to void at 3 to 5-h intervals, 30% void more frequently but are still able to return to work and lead an active life and the rest are restricted in their activities by their frequency. Incontinence is rare if the patients have been carefully selected. The selection procedure should include a trial with 500 ml of saline in the rectum to see if the patient can hold it for longer than 1 h.

Cutaneous Ureterostomy

One of the simplest and safest of the diversion procedures is cutaneous ureterostomy but it has a number of disadvantages that make it suitable for only a small and highly selected group of patients. These are the difficulty of securing a collecting appliance in place, the risk of stenosis of the stoma and the frequent need for it to be intubated, the length of ureter required for it to reach the surface and the risk of it necrosing. This method should only be considered for cases with a relatively poor prognosis and with at least one dilated ureter. If one kidney is non-functioning then that ureter can be tied off; if it is functioning then a transuretero-ureterostomy can be performed.

Rectal Bladder

In a few centres the rectal bladder is the preferred method of diversion (Bracci 1968, 1978; Tacciuoli et al. 1977). The isolated rectum is used as the urine reservoir and the sigmoid loop is brought through the sphincters alongside the rectum. In general these patients are fully continent by day, but at night there is a relatively high incidence of slight incontinence. The advantages of this procedure are that there is no external appliance and no mixing of the urinary and faecal streams. Previous radiotherapy is a contraindication.

Continent Reservoirs

A number of methods of constructing a continent urinary reservoir have been tried in recent years (Zingg and Tscholl 1977; Ashken 1982; Månsson 1984). The only method which may be a practical possibility for combining with cystectomy for cases with bladder cancer is the continent ileal reservoir described by Kock et al. (1982). The procedure is long and exacting and the problem of maintaining the reflux-preventing nipples over prolonged periods may not yet have been solved.

Table 9.5. Operative mortality for primary and salvage cystectomy

Reference	No. of patients	Mortality (%)
Burnham and Farrer (1960)	96	21.8
Riches (1960)	120	12.5
Whitmore and Marshall (1962)	230	14
Stone and Hodges (1966)	37	13.5
Cordonnier (1968)	129	4.6
Brown and Elliott (1969)	93	13
Schoenberg et al. (1973)	86	1.2
Reid et al. (1976)	135	13
Bredin and Prout (1977)	122	4.1
Johnson and Lamy (1977)	214	3.3
Freiha (1980)	50	2
Skinner et al. (1980)	165	2
Brannan et al. (1981)	129	3.9
Mathur et al. (1981)	58	3.4
Skinner et al. (1982a)	165	0.7

Postoperative Care

The reduction in the postoperative mortality for cystectomy (Table 9.5) has been achieved by a number of factors, not least among which have been the anticipation and prevention of complications and the attention to all the details of postoperative care. Patients need close monitoring during the first 5 days postoperatively, with particular attention being paid to the urine output and the care of the drains and splints; they should be nursed on an intensive therapy unit for at least the first 48 h.

Antibiotics

Postoperative wound infection and pelvic sepsis occur in 10%–30% of cases and are the commonest complications. The organisms responsible are now mainly the anaerobes of bowel origin. The cystectomy and diversion have therefore the same risks of postoperative infections as colonic surgery, and the antibiotic prophylaxis should be the same. In addition, the cystectomy patient may have a urinary infection which may be antibiotic resistant as a result of previous therapy. This should be determined before surgery and the appropriate antibiotic given, starting 1 day before the operation. Routine antibiotic prophylaxis is essential and should cover the Gram-negative organisms and the anaerobes. Prophylaxis should start with the induction of the anaesthetic and continue for 48 h. It may be continued longer if it is felt necessary to cover the risk of ascending infection while the splints remain in the ureters.

Analgesia

The large amounts of systemic opiates that the cystectomy patient requires postoperatively have numerous side effects, mainly respiratory depression, drowsiness and reduction of gut motility. The introduction of postoperative epidural analgesia using either opiates or local anaesthetics has been a major advance for the cystectomy patient. The epidural catheter should be placed preoperatively, as this may be used during the operation and reduces the blood loss (Ryan 1982).

The main advantages of epidural analgesia over systemic analgesics are that pain control is better, the patient is alert and cooperative, respiratory depression is less likely and the patient will mobilise more quickly. Prolonged ileus is less likely and bowel actions usually commence on the second or third day. Its disadvantages are that it requires the very close supervision usually only available in an intensive therapy unit. Infection is a potential hazard and the line must be fitted with a bacterial filter. The line can stay for up to 5 days, and the use of prophylactic anticoagulants is not contraindicated (Odoom and Sih 1981).

The use of intermittent epidural opiates has the advantage of being simple and effective, but has the major disadvantage that late respiratory effects may occur up to 24 h after injection. Respiratory rate must be continuously monitored and resuscitation facilities must be available (especially naloxone or levallorphan). Itching and vomiting may occur with the opiates and care must be taken not to use morphine containing any preservative. All injections into the epidural space are hazardous and should be given by fully trained staff. The advantages of the continuous infusion of local anaesthetics are that it is safer and gives equally good pain control; however, it requires an infusion pump and may cause weakness and sensory loss in the legs.

Parenteral Nutrition

The benefits of high-calorie parenteral nutrition for all patients undergoing cystectomy is disputed (Foster et al. 1978), and parenteral nutrition has a complication rate of its own (Ryan et al. 1974). Without major complications the patient should be taking adequate enteral nutrition by the end of the first week. However, if complications occur then parenteral nutrition should be started. In those patients who are severely malnourished preoperatively, parenteral nutrition should be started at least a week before surgery for the patient to benefit. Those patients who run high risk of developing complications, such as the salvage cystectomy cases, should receive parenteral nutrition; this should be started immediately postoperatively, and the calorie intake should be gradually built up.

Prophylaxis of Venous Thromboembolism

Patients with malignant disease who are undergoing major pelvic surgery run a high risk of developing postoperative deep vein thromboses and pulmonary emboli. The prophylactic effect of low-dose subcutaneous heparin (5000 units b.d.) is well established and does not significantly increase the operative blood loss. Heparin should be continued until the patient is fully mobile. This therapy should be changed to oral anticoagulants for the high-risk patients.

Management of the Gastrointestinal Tract

The upper gastrointestinal tract must be drained postoperatively; this may be done either by means of the conventional nasogastric tube or else by a gastrostomy, which may be inserted at the time of operation (Zincke 1982). Upper gastrointestinal tract bleeding caused by stress ulcers is a potential and serious hazard and can be prevented by the use of intravenous cimetidine. Hepatic and renal toxicity are rare when this drug is used for short periods.

Complications of Cystectomy

It is not possible to separate the morbidity and mortality of the cystectomy from the diversion procedure and they will therefore be considered together. The operative mortality of cystectomy for bladder cancer has been steadily declining from around 20% before 1960 down to less than 5% (see Table 9.5). This reduction of mortality has occurred for both primary and salvage cystectomy.

The major early complications specific to the cystectomy and diversion are wound infections, pelvic sepsis, urinary or intestinal anastomotic leaks, rectal fistula, intestinal and ureteric obstruction. The non-specific complications are mainly pulmonary emboli, gastrointestinal haemorrhage, pneumonia and myocardial infarcts. The most frequent complication in all series has been wound infection, occurring in 10%–30% of cases. The other complications are all less frequent and vary widely from series to series. The most serious of the early complications is the breakdown of the intestinal or ureteric anastomosis, which is associated with a high mortality (Thomas and Riddle 1982). Previous irradiation is the major factor contributing to the high complication rate. In the series reported by Skinner et al. (1980) the operative mortality was less than 1% of 128 patients undergoing primary cystectomy and 8.1% for 37 patients undergoing salvage cystectomy.

One particular late complication of cystectomy in the male is erectile impotence. This occurs in almost all patients undergoing radical cystectomy, when the pelvic nerves running alongside the prostate will be destroyed. Bergman et al. (1979) reported that 3 of 43 men still had erections after cystectomy and that 75% of the men continued to have some form of sexual activity.

Follow-up of the Cystectomy Patient

The reasons for following up the cystectomy patient are (1) surveillance of the upper tract for evidence of deterioration of function or further tumour formation, (2) supervision of the diversion and stoma, (3) to perform urethral cytological examination when the urethra has been left and (4) detection of local recurrence or distant metastases. The follow-up must be carried out in conjunction with the patient's general practitioner and should be continued indefinitely.

Second tumours occur in the upper tracts in 3%–5% of patients following cystectomy for bladder cancer (Rosenthal and Zingg 1984; Zincke et al. 1984), and patients with multifocal tumours in the bladder are at higher risks. The upper tracts should be visualised either by an IVU or a loopogram annually. Treatable local recurrence following cystectomy is rare, apart from the urethral recurrence previously discussed. The interpretation of the findings on rectal examination after cystectomy may be difficult, and a fine needle aspiration may be neccessary to differentiate pelvic fibrosis from recurrent tumour.

Combined Radiotherapy and Cystectomy

The results of cystectomy alone in the 1950s were poor; Whitmore (1981) reported a survival of 33% and a local recurrence rate of 37%. Although the survival with radical radiotherapy was equally poor, the effectiveness of radiotherapy in bladder cancer had been demonstrated and it was therefore logical to combine the two treatments to try and improve on these poor results. Several centres tried various protocols and noticed an improvement in results when compared to historical controls, usually from the previous decade. Many other things were changing in the management of bladder cancer during this period, and in particular the mortality for cystectomy was declining (see Table 9.5). Whitmore (1980), however, argues that the use of historical controls in his consecutive series is not invalid as the patients and their management have been consistent.

The aim of preoperative radiation was first to reduce the volume of the tumour and second to reduce the viability of the tumour cells at the time of surgery. The reduction in tumour volume would allow for a greater surgical clearance of the tumour by shrinking the primary and also by possibly sterilising the pelvic lymph nodes. Bloom et al. (1982) noted that although the overall incidence of nodal metastases after 4000 cGy was 20%, those patients that demonstrated downstaging of the primary tumour had only a 5.5% incidence of nodal metastases, as compared with 34% in those that did not show downstaging. The reduction in the viability of the tumour cells should reduce the risk of disseminating blood-borne metastases and also reduce the risk of implantation into the pelvis or wound should there be spillage of tumour cells. It is not possible to evaluate this separately from the effect on pelvic nodal metastases except by observing wound implantation. This is rare following cystectomy except when the bladder has been opened. Van der Werf-Messing (1978) has shown that a short course of radiation is sufficient to eliminate the risk of wound implantation when the bladder is opened for insertion of interstitial radium needles.

The effect of combined therapy can be assessed by the local recurrence rate after cystectomy. This has clearly been reduced by preoperative radiation in the series at the Memorial Sloan Kettering Cancer Center (MSKCC), New York, (Smith et al. 1982). There do not appear to be any significant differences

Table 9.6. Site of first recurrence following cystectomy. Data from the MSKCC series (after Smith et al. 1982)

	Group 1 no radiation	Group 2 4000 cGy	Group 3 2000 cGy true pelvis	Group 4 2000 cGy whole pelvis
Pelvic only	38 (28%)	19 (16%)	12 (14%)	9 (9%)
Distant only	10 (7%)	21 (18%)	17 (20%)	25 (25%)
Both	12 (9%)	10 (8%)	5 (6%)	8 (8%)
Undetermined	7 (5%)	3 (3%)	2 (2%)	4 (4%)
Total	67 (49%)	53 (45%)	36 (42%)	46 (46%)

regardless of whether 4000 cGy or 2000 cGy were given, except that the lowest pelvic recurrence rate was observed when the large field irradiating the whole pelvis was used (Table 9.6).

Preoperative irradiation may achieve downstaging of the tumour in 40%–68% of cases receiving 4000 cGy (van der Werf-Messing 1975; Whitmore 1980; Bloom 1981). Those patients showing downstaging had a considerably better survival than those that did not, but the question still remains as to whether the radiotherapy improved the results or indicated those patients who have a naturally better prognosis. Scanlon et al. (1983) compared patients receiving 2000 cGy in 1 week with those receiving 4000 cGy over the 4 weeks before cystectomy. There was no significant difference in survival and their conclusion was that the high-dose, long course of treatment was probably not worth the extra cost and morbidity as all it achieved was to identify a subset of patients with a favourable prognosis. Conversely, this treatment also identifies a set of patients with an extremely poor prognosis in whom adjuvant therapy would be justified.

The results of Whitmore et al. (1977) and Scanlon et al. (1983) show that there is very little advantage in the more prolonged course of radiotherapy; it is also costly and delays the definitive surgery. There is, however, no evidence that the longer course of delays of up to 6 weeks between radiotherapy and cystectomy are harmful (Bloom 1981).

Radwin (1980), Skinner and Lieskovsky (1984) and other authors (Studer et al. 1983) have challenged the view that preoperative radiotherapy is necessary to reduce local recurrences and achieve good survival, not on the basis of a randomised trial but on the results of contemporary series of patients treated by

Table 9.7. The 5-year survival (%) after radical cystectomy with and without preoperative radiotherapy. T and pT categories are not always distinguished. (Data from Jacobi et al. 1983)

Reference	Preoperative radiotherapy (dose Gy)	5-Year survival		
		pT2	pT3	pT4
Wajsman et al. (1975)	—	50[a]	32	—
Prout (1976)	—	47[a]	31	20
Whitmore et al. (1977)	—	63[a]	20	6
Pearse et al. (1978)	—	64	33	18
Bredael et al. (1980)	—	53	30	25
Mathur et al. (1981)	—	86	50	40
Skinner and Lieskovsky (1984)	—	—	50[b]	44[b]
Jacobi et al. (1983)	—	57	46	32
van der Werf-Messing (1975)	40	—	50	—
Prout (1976)	45	65	38	6
Wallace and Bloom (1976)	40	—	33	—
Miller (1977)	50	—	53	—
Smith et al. (1982)	40	44	38	22
	20[c]	50	58	25
	20[d]	67	43	33
Skinner et al. (1982a)	16	53	37	25

[a] Includes stages O, A and B.
[b] Three-year survival.
[c] True pelvis irradiated.
[d] Whole pelvis irradiated.

Table 9.8. Local recurrence rate after cystectomy (see also Table 9.6)

Reference	Preoperative radiotherapy	Local recurrence
Chan and Johnson (1978)	5000 cGy	8%
Skinner and Lieskovsky (1984)	1600 cGy	9%
Skinner and Lieskovsky (1984)	none	7%
Jacobi et al. (1983)	none	6.4%
Montie et al. (1984)	none	9%

radical cystectomy alone with pelvic lymphadenectomy. These show not only equally good results (Table 9.7) but also a similar low incidence of local recurrences (Table 9.8). One randomised trial has been performed comparing combined therapy with cystectomy alone (Anderström et al. 1983a). This did not show any statistically significant difference in survival between the two groups, though the results suggested that the preoperative radiotherapy may be beneficial.

The lack of such contemporary randomised trials prevents firm conclusions being drawn on the value of preoperative radiotherapy. The argument will clearly continue until the introduction of effective adjuvant systemic therapy for micrometastases obviates the need for it altogether.

Salvage Cystectomy

Salvage cystectomy and urinary diversion after definitive radiotherapy is a hazardous procedure. Dissection in the pelvis is made more difficult by the radiation-induced fibrosis, and the healing of the anastomoses may be prevented by the radiation vasculitis affecting both the ureters and the bowel. Mortality and morbidity are higher than for primary cystectomy, but the operative mortality should be below 10% with present-day surgical techniques and pre- and postoperative care (Blandy et al. 1980). Swanson et al. (1981) reported a series of 62 patients undergoing salvage cystectomy after definitive radiation therapy with no postoperative deaths and an overall 5-year survival of 43%. Bloom et al. (1982) reported an 11% operative mortality among 18 patients coming for salvage cystectomy in the T3 trial. However, these patients had a 5-year survival of 60%, which implies that they are a group that are highly selected for their low potential for developing distant metastases.

To obtain such good results from salvage cystectomy the patients must be selected with care. The assessment of the bladder late after radiation may be difficult because of the perivesical fibrosis. Radiation changes in the bladder mucosa may be difficult to interpret and a biopsy is essential (Wallace et al. 1979) and urine cytology helpful. Occasionally a tumour may take a long time to regress completely after radiotherapy, and decisions about salvage cystectomy should not be made within 3 months of completing the radiotherapy.

When performing the diversion particular attention must be paid to the presence of radiation changes in the bowel; if there is doubt a transverse colonic conduit should be used.

Squamous Cell Carcinoma of the Bladder

The pure squamous carcinoma is a rare tumour accounting for between 1.5% and 4.5% of all cases of bladder cancer, except in areas where bilharzia is endemic. The sex incidence is usually equal and the patients may have a long history of urinary infections or bladder calculi. In most cases the tumours are deeply invasive by the time that they present (Costello et al. 1984).

Results of treatment are poor and useful comparisons are hard to make because of the small numbers. Preoperative radiotherapy and cystectomy may give results equally as good as for T2 and T3 transitional tumours (Johnson et al. 1976; Costello et al. 1984). Jones et al. (1981) reported that 36% of the patients that completed radiotherapy survived 5 years. Although the majority of patients died of bladder cancer, only 8% developed distant metastases; the majority of patients die as a result of failure to control the local disease.

Adenocarcinoma of the Bladder

Pure primary adenocarcinoma of the bladder, like the squamous carcinoma, is rare. It is the most common malignancy to occur in the exstrophied bladder. An adenocarcinoma of the bladder may be primary, urachal or metastatic. The primary adenocarcinomas tend to be solitary, poorly differentiated, deeply invasive and associated with a poor prognosis. Anderström et al. (1983) reported only an 18% 5-year survival; Bennett et al. (1984) reported that the average survival was only 21 months, with 65% of the patients dying in less than 2 years, regardless of the mode of therapy. Extrapolating from the results of radiotherapy for adenocarcinomas at other sites and from the small amount of data for primary adenocarcinoma of the bladder it is likely that this tumour is radioresistant, and therefore surgery will be the treatment of choice.

The urachal tumour arises in the dome or anterior wall of the bladder and is intramural with deep ramifications into the bladder wall, cave of Retzius, abdominal wall and umbilicus. The tumour should be sharply demarcated from the surrounding normal bladder.

If small these tumours may be treated by a segmental resection, which should include the umbilicus en bloc if it is a urachal tumour; otherwise they should be treated as equally radically as the deeply invasive TCCs.

Part 2. Radiotherapy

P. N. Plowman

Radiobiology

Theory

Although the practice of clinical radiotherapy has evolved empirically, there are now adequate radiobiological data to rationalise many aspects of that practice. A typical 'survival curve' for mammalian cells exposed to X-rays is shown in Fig. 9.1. The data derive from the exposure of clonogenic cells to single radiation doses, and survival relates to the retention of clonogenic capability. The curve comprises

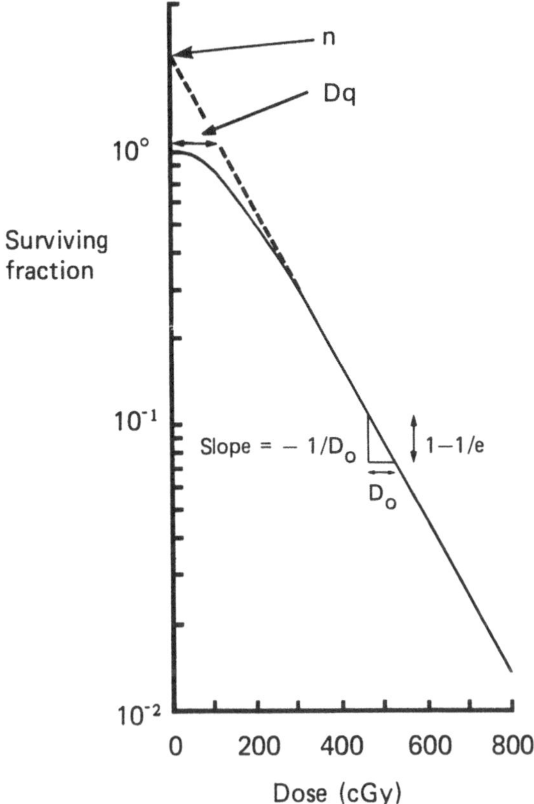

Fig. 9.1. Theoretical survival curve for mammalian cells exposed to X-radiation. *Dq* denotes the quasi-threshold dose; *Do* denotes the dose of radiation that reduces the surviving fraction to 37% of its former value; *n* denotes the width of the initial 'shoulder' and is the extrapolation number on the ordinate of the exponential part of the curve

an initial shoulder (representative of a dose range in which repair of damage by ionising radiation may occur), preceding an exponential curve, where each incremental increase in radiation dose causes a further constant fraction of cells to die. Various mathematical indices may be derived which characterise the individual cell type and its sensitivity to radiation-induced death. The Do value expresses the slope of the exponential portion of the curve, whilst the quasi-threshold (Dq) and the extrapolation number (*n*) expresses the width of the initial shoulder or the capacity for repair of sublethal ionising damage. Whilst the Do values for many mammalian cell series tested by this in vitro technique are similar, the Dq and *n* values may vary considerably (Withers et al. 1974; Hall 1978). Thus the studies of Withers on jejunal, founder crypt cells suggested high Dq and *n* values; such characteristics might be retained by slowly dividing, well-differentiated tumours derived from such epithelia. The data on *n* and Dq for human tumours are scanty, except for the compelling, albeit largely circumstantial evidence for very high Dq and *n* values in malignant melanoma. The importance of these data to clinical radiotherapy relate to the size of radiation dose per fraction required to cause significant cell kill (Fig. 9.1).

Clinical radiotherapy is based on fractionated treatment schemata (cf. the single-dose situation just described). This fractionation of treatment allows repopulation of normal tissues during the course of radiotherapy and repair of sublethal damage. The former allows an improved therapeutic ratio, as tumours are not under homeostatic control to make good a deficit in cell numbers (cf. skin and mucosa). Whether there is an improvement in the therapeutic ratio because of better repair of sublethal damage by normal tissues compared with the tumour cells is controversial as regards the commonly arising carcinomas, and may differ in different cell series (Field 1970; Withers 1970; Phillips 1972; Denekamp and Stewart 1979). These general statements from current radiobiological understanding are more difficult to apply to the bladder than most other epithelia. The normal bladder epithelium has an unusually slow turnover time of several months, and in one animal study (using an extraordinarily high single dose of 2500 cGy) there was a very delayed mitotic response to damage inflicted by radiation (Stewart et al. 1980). This delayed kinetic response contrasts with that of most epithelia in the body and brings into question the 'repopulation argument' just cited. If a tumour shrinks during the course of radiotherapy then it is less likely to contain hypoxic/radioresistant cells when later radiation fractions are given, also assisting in the local control. The likelihood of local control is higher when a high total dose is received on such fractionated radiotherapy schemes.

With regard to human tumours treated by conventionally fractionated radiotherapy (1000 cGy weekly in five daily fractions) there is evidence for a relationship between the likelihood of tumour sterilisation, total dose delivered and tumour size. Thus 5000 cGy is highly effective at sterilising microscopic carcinoma and 6000 cGy cures the majority of small tumours (2–4 cm); however, tumours of diameter greater than 5 cm are less easily controlled, and increases in dosage beyond 6000–6500 cGy do not substantially increase the control rate (Cancer 1976). There is now little doubt that a high total dose of fractionated radiotherapy achieves a higher therapeutic ratio than a course with few fractions, certainly for the cure rate of small-diameter carcinomas. Hypoxic cells may account for the resistance of larger tumours.

The therapeutic ratio is a recurring consideration in radiotherapy and we need to examine normal tissue tolerance to fractionated radiotherapy further. It has been established that the acute radiation tolerance to X-rays of normal skin lies somewhere in the region of 6000 cGy/30 fractions (F) in 42 days, and this figure is approximately correct for the acute and late tolerance of normal, adult human bladder. When doses of 7000 cGy/35 F in 42 days or more are delivered, there is a sharp rise in the early and late complication rate to the bladder and pelvic organs. There are many ways in which this tolerance dose equivalent may be reached. (The 'tolerance dose' is the radical radiation dose equivalent with an attendant incidence of major radiation complications, e.g. a 5% incidence, that is the maximum acceptable to the therapist). Thus a study at St. Bartholomew's Hospital, London, in bladder cancer patients who were treated in a hyperbaric oxygen tank (with necessarily large radiation fractions on the six occasions that they were in the tank), found that a total bladder dose of only 3400 cGy delivered as 6 × 567 cGy fractions over 19 days was beyond 'our' bladder tolerance dose equivalent, with a high incidence of late complications; the study was therefore discontinued.

Ellis (1969) derived a formula incorporating the total dose delivered, with factorial weightings to the individual fraction size (number of fractions) and the overall time of the treatment scheme to give a composite dose equivalent figure which would be comparable between different radical radiotherapy fractionation schemes, taking acute skin reactions as limiting tolerance. Although many authors writing on bladder cancer have used the Ellis formula to compare dose equivalents between radiotherapy centres, there is accumulating evidence that, for late normal-tissue morbidity, fraction size is more important than has been previously considered. By using larger individual fraction sizes the normal-tissue tolerance is approached at a lower total dose, as we found in the St. Bartholomew's hyperbaric oxygen study. An excellent study on normal human bladder tolerance at four dose equivalent levels was performed by Morrison (1975). Morrison kept the number of treatments (20) and the overall time (4 weeks) constant, but varied the individual fraction size and total dose. These data clearly demonstrate the increasing rates of major complications (approaching 40% for a bladder dose of 6250 cGy given at 20 × 313 cGy fractions) with increasing dose equivalent. Analysis of Morrison's data with regard to therapeutic ratio is difficult as the small lesions received the higher dose equivalents. A similar study was conducted in Canada, again using a range of dose equivalents for bladder radiotherapy. More complications were encountered after the high dose equivalent prescriptions; following 5000 cGy given as 15 × 333 cGy fractions in 3 weeks there was a 3% incidence of acute major complications and a 21% incidence of major late complications (Goodman et al. 1981a, b). The local control and survival data are difficult to extract from this study as the high-dose group were selected—younger, fitter, lower stage and grade of tumours.

A last factor that enters into normal-tissue tolerance equations is the volume irradiated (e.g. whole pelvis versus bladder). In general terms, for any organ or body area, a small volume of tissue will tolerate a higher dose equivalent than a large volume. When giving a high dose equivalent it is commonplace to reduce the irradiated volume after a moderate dose equivalent (e.g. to the pelvis) such that only the primary tumour bulk (e.g. the bladder) receives the highest dose equivalent.

Application for Clinical Medicine

The synthesis of all these data with regard to the scientific basis for radical radiotherapy in the treatment of human bladder cancer has, to date, led to disappointingly few advances over the empirical clinical observations. Having observed that human bladder TCC is usually responsive to conventionally fractionated radiotherapy (1000 cGy weekly in five daily fractions), and that such radiotherapy to 6000–6500 cGy is tolerated by the normal bladder with acceptable morbidity, this is usually chosen by the practising therapist—delivering daily fractions of 200 cGy for 30–32 weeks. However, deviations from this dose prescription might lead to improved therapeutic ratios and improved knowledge of the cell survival curve indices for this tumour. Morrison (1975) found evidence of increasing tumour control with increasing dose equivalents and similarly increasing complication rates; all his fractionation schemes were faster than 1000 cGy weekly, and the data do not assist in tackling the problem of therapeutic ratio. Littbrand and Edsmyr (1976) have approached the problem quite differently; they have argued that the optimal external beam radiation scheme would be one that reached a very high cumulative dose by many small fractions. In order to achieve the high total dose within normal-tissue tolerance, these workers have used small individual fractions and several fractions per day (spaced throughout the day to allow sublethal repair from the previous fraction) with a dose prescription of 8400 cGy/84 F in 8 weeks, split as follows: 3 weeks' treatment (42 F), 2 weeks' rest, 3 weeks' treatment (42 F). The Scandinavian workers claim that normal-tissue morbidity is comparable with conventionally fractionated treatment to radical dosage. They further claim improved results on the bladder cancer (Littbrand and Edsmyr 1976; Edsmyr 1981). If this low fraction size/multiple daily fractions approach is confirmed as improving the therapeutic ratio, then it suggests that the Dq and *n* for bladder cancer cells are both lower than for the normal bladder epithelial cell. Littbrand also suggests that reoxygenation during protracted radiotherapy schemes is important for optimising control; Littbrand and Revesz (1969) provided some data on the loss of the sublethal repair capacity of deeply hypoxic cells, which would then be 'unexpectedly' sensitive to small-sized radiation fractions.

Preoperative radiotherapy differs from radical radiotherapy in that it does not attempt to approach normal-tissue tolerance, its 'brief' being to sterilise the most peripheral pelvic micrometastases from the bladder cancer. This obvious but little publicised fact could be of great importance, as the therapist could here utilise large individual fraction sizes—if the tumour cell survival indices suggested this to be advantageous—without compromising the usual (radical) objective of achieving a high total dose by a well-fractionated scheme. Whether this played any part in the choosing of 5 × 400 cGy fractions versus 20 × 200 cGy fractions as preoperative prescriptions is doubtful; the difference is of theoretical interest and the results are discussed below. However, this reasoning did prompt a current preoperative radiotherapy rectal study at St Mark's Hospital, London, to examine the prescription of 3 × 500 cGy to the whole pelvis, just prior to surgery.

The rationale for the local implantation of radioisotopes into a tumour is that it is possible to deliver very high X-ray doses to the tumour whilst the dose fall-off (which obeys the inverse square law), largely spares the surrounding tissues. Implantation techniques are not appropriate for widely infiltrating cancer. Therefore, when theoretically discussing the usefulness of this technique in bladder cancer one would not expect it to prove curative as the sole radiation manoeuvre in tumours more than 4 cm diameter and more advanced than T2. As bladder cancer is now recognised as a panurothelial disease (Gowing 1960), and as individual cancers are commonly understaged clinically, there is a strong case for delivering external beam radiotherapy. Furthermore, the current widespread availability of linear accelerators has also allowed respectable, external beam bladder dosimetry—not available 20 years ago. However, a case could be made for delivering external beam radiotherapy and then boosting the dose to the primary tumour by an implant, in a manner analogous to the radiotherapy management of some oral cancers. Indeed, one group of workers is exploring combined external beam therapy and implantation (van der Werf-Messing et al. 1980).

Other methods attempting to improve radiotherapeutic results are each worthy of brief mention. The problem of hypoxic but potentially clonogenic tumour cells in bulky tumours is a potential source of radiotherapy failure as hypoxic cells are 2.5–3.0 times more resistant to X- or gamma-radiation than oxic cells. Hyperbaric oxygen treatments were not successful for many reasons (Dische 1973), and densely ionising radiation beams such as neutrons and pi-mesons (which are affected less by the hypoxia problem) are of limited availability, as well as having problems of their own (Fowler 1979). Optimised X- or gamma-ray external beam fractionated schemes are probably the best currently available means of tackling the hypoxia problem, although the new generation of the chemical, electron-affinic, hypoxic cell sensitisers (e.g. misonidiazole) are of potential importance. Such chemicals seem to diffuse into hypoxic areas of tumours (i.e. have good penetration) and selectively radiosensitise hypoxic cells (Adams 1979; Chapman 1979; Denekamp et al. 1980).

It has been appreciated for many years that hyperthermia damages cells and decreases the tolerance of normal tissues to the effects of radiation. Of more recent importance has been the recognition that hyperthermia and radiation may be complementary, in that the phase of the cell cycle most resistant to ionising radiation (late S phase) is most sensitive to hyperthermia, and that the combination of hyperthermia and radiation may be synergistic in its cytotoxic effect. The bladder is a hollow viscus and easily perfused by a heating solution; however, heating by this system would be of superficial cell layers and the major problem is with solid cancer (Hall 1978; Fowler 1979).

Other Problems Relating to Clinical Radiotherapy

There are other controversial areas in the radiation management of bladder cancer that are best discussed in a theoretical introduction. Following preoperative radiotherapy, there is an interval before surgery, which varies in length with different investigators. A conventionally fractionated, preoperative course of 4000 cGy has been followed by an interval to surgery of 'as short a time as possible' (van der Werf-Messing 1979; van der Werf-Messing et al. 1982) to 4 weeks (Wallace and Bloom 1976; Bloom et al. 1982) or longer (Whitmore 1980). From the data reported, surgery (simple cystectomy) was not more difficult or complicated after the short post-radiation interval. Following the 4-week interval before radical cystectomy there did not appear to have been significant tumour regrowth of the primary or pelvic nodal metastases. One would feel unhappy (but without scientific reason) about an interval of longer than 1 month between radiotherapy to a modest dose equivalent and surgery. Following higher preoperative radiation dose prescriptions, conventionally fractionated to 5000 cGy, a 'major complication' rate after early surgery of 48% was recorded in one large series (Miller 1977). Dose equivalents of this order should be considered as radical treatments for which surgery should be reserved as a salvage procedure—after a considerable time delay. Miller (1977) also examined post-cystectomy pelvic radiation to a radical dose equivalent (6000 cGy/30 F in 42 days). Not surprisingly, following major pelvic surgery with its attendant postoperative adhesions to bowel, a radiotherapy prescription of this order led to a 25% incidence of major complications.

The next question that arises is: If the cystectomy specimen contains downstaged tumour following preoperative radiotherapy, does this finding auger a good ultimate prognosis? The initial theoretical answer is: Not necessarily. If after radical radiotherapy (as the sole therapeutic manoeuvre) a mass of viable tumour remains in the bladder, it is not surprising that the ultimate outcome of the patient is worse than a complete responder. However, the overall situation is more complex. It is well appreciated in the radiobiological literature that tumour disappearance kinetics may be less prognostically useful than growth delay or regrowth kinetics in the assessment of the local efficacy of radiotherapy, particularly in tissues/ tumours with slow turnover and low cell loss factors (Steel 1968, 1977; Thomlinson 1982; Moore 1983). Furthermore, it is expected that mitotically active, anaplastic tumours would have faster disappearance kinetics after radiation than slowly proliferating tumours. The 'law' of Bergonie and Tribondeau [1906] is an observation that the effects of radiation on cells are inversely proportional to the cell's functional and morphological differentiation. Fast-growing anaplastic tumours, with a greater metastatic potential (perhaps already realised), might ultimately still prove to be the most lethal group, despite fast disappearance kinetics, with or without local control. However, if the metastatic potential has not been realised and the local cell kill is adequate, fast disappearance kinetics, local control and cure may go together. Several large clinical studies (discussed on p. 219) have examined the prognostic import of radiation-induced downstaging. When analysing the family of variables interconnected with downstaging, the following details should be known and reported: papillary versus solid, size, clinical classification and pathological staging. It is to be hoped that the TNM classification system will be universally accepted to facilitate the comparison of data. Most external radiation data relate to T3 cases, but the useful distinction of T2 from T3 has been questioned (Chisholm et al. 1980).

The regional lymph nodes draining the bladder are the pelvic nodes below the bifurcation of the common iliac arteries. The rationale behind preoperative radiotherapy dictates that these nodes should all be encompassed by the radiation portals. Van der Werf-Messing (1979) found no benefit from also encompassing the common iliac nodes; this further increases the large volume being treated. In radical radiotherapy also, most authors favour encompassing the pelvic nodes in the first phase of radiation before boosting the bladder to the high dose equivalent. One interesting radical bladder radiation plan and prescription takes the bladder to high dose equivalent (5000–5500 cGy/20 F in 4 weeks), whilst the 80% isodose encompasses the majority of regional nodes, thereby simultaneously treating these nodes to 4000 cGy/20 F in 4 weeks (Blandy et al. 1980; Hope-Stone et al. 1981).

Lastly, in this theoretical introduction it must be recognised that both 'survival' and 'local control' are relevant to the efficacy of radiotherapy (radical and preoperative), in the management of bladder cancer.

Radiotherapy Technique

Bratherton's first 'law' of radiotherapy states that the tumour should receive a higher radiation dose than the patient. Flouting this most fundamental objective, some authors, who have reported large numbers of patients treated for bladder cancer, have used parallel opposed, anterior and posterior portals, depositing the maximum radiation dose equally in the anterior abdominal wall and sacrum or rectum. Furthermore, in radiation treatment techniques designed to treat the bladder only, there is a possibility of geographical miss for reasons other than poor set-up technique (Goodman and Balfour 1964). With these problems in mind, a description of a modern radiation technique, as employed at St. Bartholomew's Hospital, London, is given here:

The patient is placed supine in the treatment position at simulation, with a bladder catheter in situ. Intravesical Conray (40 ml) is used to delineate superior, inferior, and posterior bladder borders, and intravesical air (10 ml) to delineate the anterior border; contrast medium in the catheter tubing outlines the urethra. The position and function of the kidneys is known, and details of the examination under anaesthetic (EUA) and staging are available on the planning table, as well as a pelvic CT scan. For the whole pelvis (Phase I) planning, the initial simulator films are taken centred (approximately at this stage) on the widest pelvic

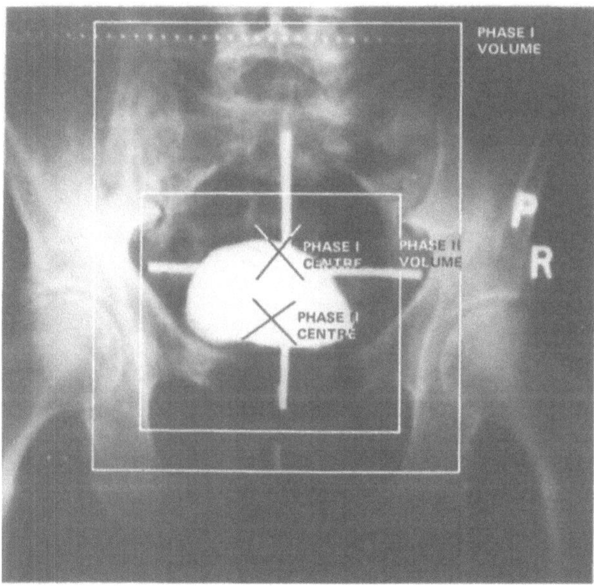

Fig. 9.2. Frontal simulator planning film depicting target volumes for Phase I (whole pelvis) and Phase II (bladder plus margins)

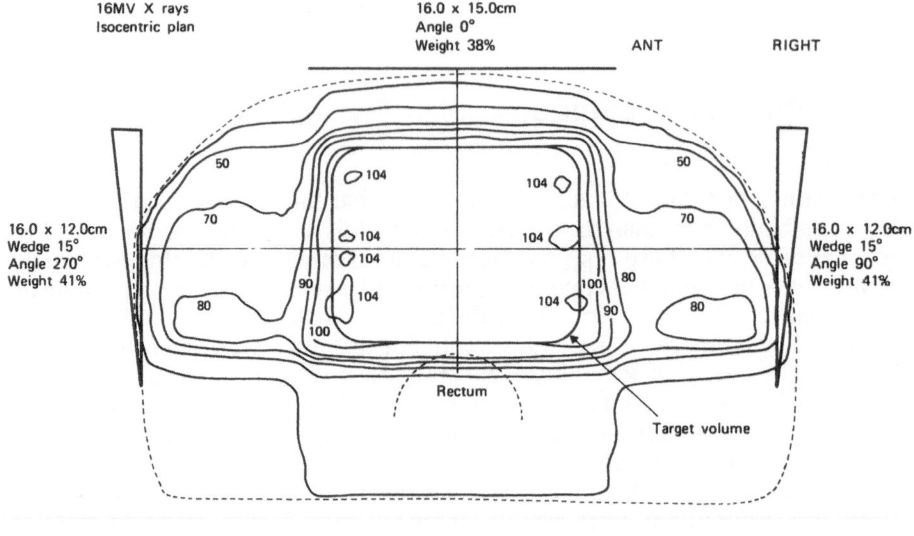

a

D_T Min (Target vol) 100%
D_T Max 104%
D_T Max (rectum) 95%
Prescription on 100% isodose

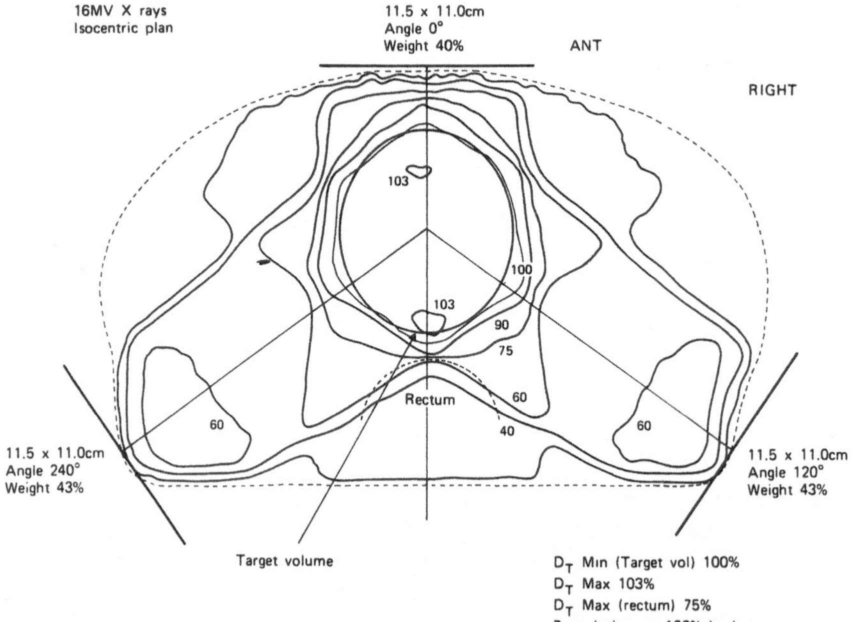

b

D_T Min (Target vol) 100%
D_T Max 103%
D_T Max (rectum) 75%
Prescription on 100% isodose

Fig. 9.3. **a** Radiotherapy treatment plan for whole pelvis (Phase I). **b** Radiotherapy treatment plan for bladder plus margins (Phase II)

diameter. The target volume is from the bottom of L-5 vertebra to the bottom of the obturator foramen, or as low as the ischial tuberosities in (many) males with possible urethral or prostatic involvement. Laterally, the target volume is 1 cm wide of the pelvic side walls or of known diseased nodes (Fig. 9.2). The volume is similarly constructed on the lateral simulator film with the anterior and posterior limits encompassing regional lymph nodes and 2 cm wide of bladder margins. An outline is taken through the accurate centre and transcribed to paper; the volume is placed on paper and computer planned for a three- or four-field pelvic 'brick' treated by a linear accelerator (8 or 16 MV X-rays) to 4000–4400 cGy tumour dose (TD)/20–22 F in 28–32 days (Fig. 9.3a) The minimum TD is usually prescribed, as with these energies the brick technique gives good dosimetry.

The second phase of treatment is also planned at the outset so that the patient is not catheterised again during therapy for this reason. Here the bladder with any known tumour extensions plus 1.5 cm margins (2.0 cm inferiorly—or lower—in males) are the target volume, and fields will be appropriately slightly larger. We change the plan for the second phase of treatment to an open anterior and two posterior oblique portals (Fig. 9.3b), and prescribe a further 2000 cGy TD/10 F in 12 days, again usually on the minimum TD. The doses given to the rectum and to the hips are known, and the change of plan for the boost again spares normal tissues.

It is in the planning of the boost to the bladder that the introduction of pelvic CT scanning has proved of great assistance to the radiotherapist. Thus, in addition to the surgeon's description of the bladder tumour at EUA and cystoscopy, we are now able to see the tumour's extravesical infiltration on the pelvic CT scan and so modify the volume boundaries for the second phase of treatment to encompass more certainly all the extensions of the primary.

Preoperative radiotherapy is given to the volume and by the technique used in Phase I. Some workers would lead off (Pb screen) the corners of the large rectangular fields if nodes were known not to lie within these regions.

Radical Radiotherapy

Clinical Results

In historical series, radical cystectomy for T3 bladder cancer produced survival rates of the order of 16%–22% (Prout et al. 1973; Whitmore 1980); this procedure is attended by a finite operative mortality (5%–10%) and loss of bladder and sexual function. If it were possible to find an alternative and effective means of local therapy this would be preferable.

In a large study of 352 patients with T2/T3 bladder cancer treated by radical radiotherapy, the overall survival at 5 years was 34% (Blandy et al. 1980; Hope-Stone 1981); the incidence of complications was inferred to be low. Of the patients that died, 23% had local recurrence, 16% local recurrence and metastases and 5% died from metastatic spread without local recurrence. Only 8% of patients came to salvage cystectomy; the operative mortality was 22%. In another UK study of 91 cases of T3 bladder cancer treated by radical radiotherapy, the corrected life table survival at 5 years was 29% (Bloom et al. 1982). Salvage cystectomy was required in 18/85 patients (with an operative mortality of 11%), and 11 of these 18 patients were alive at 5 years. In a Canadian study of 481 stage B (T2–T3a) and 186 stage C (T3b) cases treated by radical radiotherapy, the 5-year survival rates were 48% and 21% respectively. Of the survivors 68% were alive with healthy functioning bladders at 10 years. In 75/470 patients of all stages salvage cystectomy was required (giving an 11% mortality); however, the survival of this group is not reported (Goodman et al. 1981a, b). These three studies are cited in as little detail as the radiation techniques and fractionation schemes of these workers have been described in the first section of this review. Despite the relatively good survival data in the London Hospital series (Blandy et al. 1980; Hope-Stone et al. 1981), the incidence of local pelvic recurrences in this study was disquieting, and one regrets that the same local and systemic recurrence data were not analysed by the other authors.

Other authors reporting results of radical radiotherapy in T3 cases have found overall survival figures of 22% ± 5%, (Edsmyr 1975; Goffinet et al. 1975; Morrison 1975; Miller 1977; Reddy et al. 1978; Backhouse 1979). At least three groups have concluded that local control increases with increasing dose equivalent (Morrison 1975; Miller 1977; Goodman et al. 1981a, b), but there remains the caveat of the therapeutic ratio, with the normal-tissue morbidity possibly contributing differently to the fatalities from salvage surgery following different dose equivalents, and other causes of death.

Bloom et al. (1982) reported that following radical radiotherapy for T3 bladder cancer the cystoscopic and bimanual EUA 'response' at 3–6 months was complete in 40%, partial in 23% and not apparent (no response) in 37%, with 5-year survivals in these three groups of patients being 62%, 27% and 14% respectively. Similarly, Blandy et al. (1980) found a 45% 'complete' response rate and an approximately 70% 5-year survival in this group of patients, compared with an approximately 20% survival amongst the partial responders.

When discussing radical radiotherapy as the sole treatment for bladder cancer, one must also discuss the patient age range, particularly as bladder cancer incidence and operative mortality both increase with advancing years. Blandy et al. (1980) found that with radical radiotherapy alone, the 5-year survival of patients aged <55, 55–64, 65–74 and >75 years were 57%, 39%, 31% and 12% respectively. In contrast, the 5-year, disease-free survival of 34 T3 patients aged less than 60 years who were radically irradiated by Bloom et al. (1982) was only 5%, although a further 20% survived as the result of salvage surgery. However, in the age groups 60–64 years and 65–70 years, the corrected 5-year survivals were 18% and 45%. The unexpected finding of increased survival with age by these workers is extraordinary; perhaps the uncorrected survival figures would also have been meaningful when evaluating the age variable. The conclusion from both groups was that where surgery carries a higher morbidity/mortality, radical radiotherapy alone becomes a strongly competitive alternative. Bloom et al. (1982) would agree that this is the case for the elderly (patients more than 65 years); Blandy et al. (1980) argue that this is the case for all ages.

Various reasons have been expressed as to why radical radiotherapy by interstitial implantation has limited usefulness, and the clinical results discussed here will be only for T2N0M0 bladder cancer—the only patient group in which this technique might seem appropriate. Of 76 T2 patients whose tumours were radically implanted with gold-198 grains or tantalum-182 wires, 41% survived 5 years with very few radiation complications, but 38% recurred in the bladder

(Williams et al. 1981). Of 32 T2 patients radically implanted by radium needles, 3 developed local recurrences and 10 died of bladder cancer; the 5-year survival was 56% (van der Werf-Messing 1978). Of 202 T2 patients treated by pre-implant external beam bladder radiotherapy followed by an implant, 28 (14%) developed local recurrences or 'second bladder cancer'; the 5-year survival was 62% (van der Werf-Messing 1978). In this Rotterdam study, there were 8% and 1.5% incidences of fatal complications following therapy in the implant only group and external beam plus implant group respectively. Together these data suggest that a local implantation procedure, with its low incidence of radiation-induced morbidity, can be effective therapy in a selected group of T2 patients.

Complications

During the course of radical external beam radiotherapy to the bladder, it is common to encounter an acute radiation cystitis (dysuria, frequency, nocturia), at 4–6 weeks from initiation of irradiation. Microscopically, there is mucosal hyperaemia with degeneration and desquamation of epithelial cells. Clinically, the differential diagnosis is from infection, and a urine culture must be checked. Treatment of acute radiation cystitis is good oral hydration, nocturnal hypnotic, an anticholinergic and mist. potassium citrate (an alkali), perhaps with a non-narcotic analgesic. Rarely with conventionally fractionated radiation schemes the symptoms are so severe that radiotherapy must be interrupted. Also rarely the mucosal or tumour oedema may cause ureteric obstruction (or ascending infection), even to the extent of acute post-renal failure. Haemorrhage is also a rare early complication. The acute radiation cystitis subsides rapidly after the course of therapy. (This clinical human observation calls into question the extrapolation to man of the data of Stewart et al. 1980, which suggested a very delayed repopulative capability of bladder epithelium, see p. 208.).

Acute radiation reactions may also be seen in the rectum (usually presenting as tenesmus) and in the skin (usually in the intertriginous groin folds and natal cleft).

The chronic radiation-induced bladder morbidity can be divided into two major complications: contracted bladder and ureteric strictures (Rubin and Casaret 1968). The contracted bladder occurs more than a year after completion of radical radiotherapy and is multifactorial in origin. As stated above, high dose equivalent radiation (by a poorly fractionated technique) is known to be a predisposing factor, but concurrent bladder infection and extensive infiltrating bladder cancer are known to exacerbate the tendency. A 'salvage' cystectomy may be necessary for symptoms and is essential if ureteric obstruction is leading to hydronephrosis. Histologically, the contracted bladder demonstrates endarteritis obliterans and generalised vascular sclerosis; there are ever-increasing amounts of dense fibrous tissue in the subepithelial connective tissue. The loss of vascular integrity may lead to epithelial degeneration with atrophic ulcers.

Similar processes may lead to rectal mucosal ulcerations and pelvic small bowel may develop fistulae, strictures or stenosis.

Preoperative Radiotherapy

Clinical Results

Despite radical cystectomy or radical radiotherapy as definitive treatment for T3 bladder carcinoma, the majority of these patients die from this disease. Early studies of combined radiotherapy and surgery held out greater promise (Barnes et al. 1946; Emmet and Winterringer 1955; Riches 1960; Magri 1962) and prompted several large-scale clinical studies and trials. In 1966, the Rotterdam Radiotherapy Institute began a study of pelvic radiotherapy (conventionally fractionated to 4000 cGy), immediately prior to simple cystectomy for T3 bladder cancer. Their results have been continually updated (van der Werf-Messing 1975, 1979; van der Werf-Messing et al. 1982), and in the latest report on 183 patients the uncorrected 5-year survival was 52% (corrected figure 66%). As small (less than 5 cm) tumours are implanted at that centre, these figures are suggestive of an advance in treatment.

Also in 1966, the Royal Marsden/Institute of Urology Group initiated a two-armed, randomised prospective trial comparing preoperative radiotherapy (conventionally fractionated to 4000 cGy) 4 weeks before radical cystectomy (RT+C) with radical radiotherapy (Phase I—whole pelvis; Phase II—bladder boost, conventional fractionation to 6000 cGy). The subjects of the trial were patients less than 70 years with deeply infiltrating, histologically confirmed and previously untreated transitional cell carcinoma of bladder (Wallace and Bloom

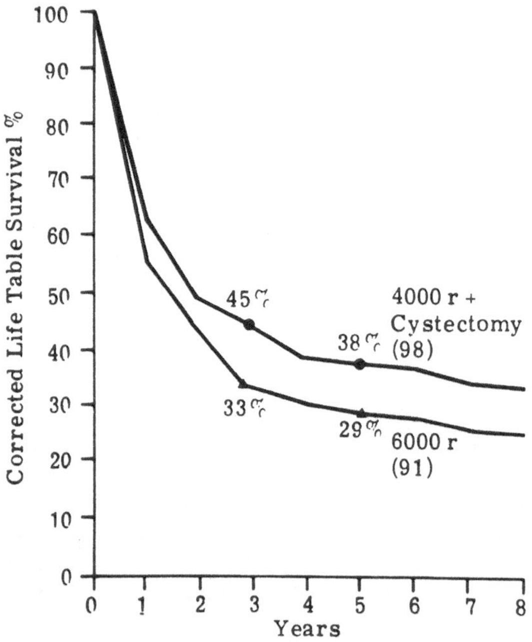

Fig. 9.4. The Institute of Urology T3 Bladder Carcinoma Trial. Survival by protocol treatment allocated. Number of patients in parentheses (P=0.2). (Bloom et al. 1982)

1976): 98 patients received RT+C and 91 had RT. The corrected 5-year survivals (Fig. 9.4a) were 38% and 29% respectively (P=0.2; Bloom et al. 1982). Eighteen patients having RT came to salvage cystectomy, and if these were excluded then the results did become significantly different; however, it is doubtful if this manoeuvre is statistically valid. Nevertheless, in this carefully conducted study there is a trend in survival advantage for RT+C over RT alone.

In the period 1959–1970, two different preoperative radiotherapy dose prescriptions were used successively (not as a two-armed clinical study), prior to radical cystectomy for invasive bladder cancer at the MSKCC (Whitmore et al. 1977). First, 119 patients were treated by pelvic radiotherapy (conventionally fractionated to 4000 cGy), 1–3 months prior to radical cystectomy. Their crude 5-year survival was 43%. From 1966 to 1970, 86 patients were treated with pelvic radiotherapy (2000 cGy in 5 × 400 cGy fractions over 1 week) immediately prior to radical cystectomy (Whitmore et al. 1977). From 1971 to 1974 101 patients were treated by pelvic radiotherapy (2000 cGy in 5 × 400 cGy fractions over 1 week) immediately prior to radical cystectomy, using, on average, slightly—but probably not critically—larger pelvic portals (Smith et al. 1982). The crude 5-year survivals of these two groups of 2000 cGy RT+C were 42% and 39% respectively, demonstrating the reproducibility of the data.

Thus, three large institutes investigating preoperative radiotherapy for invasive bladder cancer have found 5-year survival figures of 52% (corrected 66%), 38% (corrected), 43% (corrected 58%), 42% (corrected 56%) and 39% (uncorrected). All the figures demonstrate an improvement in survival of patients with invasive bladder cancer when compared with the historical treatment data base.

Further analysis of the data derived from Rotterdam, Institute of Urology/ Royal Marsden and the MSKCC suggest prognostically useful variables. First, patients with stage T3a tumours have a significantly better survival chance than those with T3b (van der Werf-Messing et al. 1982), and patients with tumours of a low histological grade have a better survival chance than those with high-grade histology (Whitmore 1980). In the Rotterdam analysis, it was found that of the patients whose cystectomy specimen was pathologically downstaged by the radiotherapy (clinical T3 becomes pT0-2), then the 5-year survival chance was greater. Approximately two-thirds of cases demonstrated downstaging, and the probability of T stage reduction could not be predicted from the histological grade of the initial biopsy (van der Werf-Messing 1975). In the larger, later analysis from this group, it was again found that T-reduction in the cystectomy specimen was neither correlated to histological grade nor to the structure of the growth (van der Werf-Messing et al. 1982). Following cystectomy, an extremely good prognostic group of patients could be defined as patients with microscopic downstaging and no vascular invasion in the cystectomy specimen; such patients had an 81% 5–year survival rate (van der Werf-Messing et al. 1982). The cystectomies at Rotterdam were simple and the node status unknown (NX).

In the Institute of Urology/Royal Marsden study, 49% of patients receiving preoperative radiotherapy demonstrated reduced pathological stage (pT) compared to the original clinical stage (T) in the cystectomy specimen. Furthermore, the 5-year survival rate for patients showing stage reduction (64%) was better than for patients not demonstrating stage reduction (27%); $P<0.01$ (Bloom et al. 1982). Although larger tumour bulk at presentation could skew the data, analysis of the nodes seemed to corroborate the conclusion (although this analysis could be similarly affected). Thus the incidence of positive pelvic nodes at radical cystectomy in downstaged patients was 6%, as compared with 34% in patients not showing downstaging.

Similarly improved survival amongst downstaged patients was observed by Prout (1976). Although there is a potential error rate in the initial clinical staging in all these studies, the risk of clinical overstaging is thought to be small and quantified as 6/136 in one study (Whitmore 1980).

The MSKCC analysis showed that in each of the preoperatively irradiated groups there was evidence of tumour downstaging, and there was improved survival amongst the patients demonstrating downstaging (Whitmore 1981). Interestingly, but not surprisingly, there was a greater incidence of tumour downstaging in the 4000 cGy (with 4-week interval to surgery) group than in the 2000 cGy (with short interval to surgery) group, although overall survival was similar for both these groups. Equally interesting is the observation that the survival rates in the non-downstaged patients in the 2000 cGy group were better than the non-downstaged 4000 cGy group. A plausible explanation for this difference relates to the time interval for cell death and absorption to become manifest.

The most interesting data on cancer recurrence patterns after preoperative radiotherapy and surgery also come from the MSKCC. Batata et al. (1980) examined the incidence of recurrent disease within the pelvis. They found that following 4000 cGy RT+C there was a 16% incidence of pelvic recurrence alone and that this figure was 14% for 2000 cGy RT+C. However, in a previous group of patients with similar invasive bladder cancer but treated by radical cystectomy the rate of pelvic recurrence was 28% (see Table 9.6). The major decrease in the pelvic recurrence rate in the irradiated patients was seen in cases with tumours of high histological grade. Using these same patient groups to analyse the incidence of extrapelvic relapse with or without pelvic recurrence, Batata et al. (1982) concluded a similar incidence of approximately 26% in all three groups. Actually, their data showed a slightly higher incidence of distant metastases in the irradiated groups. (Perhaps these patients with a clear pelvis survived longer to manifest metastases.) As the median time between cystectomy and death from these progressive extrapelvic metastases was shorter than 1 year in all groups, the authors concluded that the occult distant metastases were present at the time of cystectomy. These observations call into question some objectives of preoperative radiotherapy, and it is regrettable that other workers have not analysed their own data in this way.

The Institute of Urology/Royal Marsden trial demonstrated an advantage to preoperative radiotherapy and cystectomy over radical radiotherapy for younger patients and a higher operative mortality in the elderly; however, the unexpected survival results in the radical radiotherapy arm of this trial influenced this conclusion.

Conclusions

1. TCC of the bladder is a potentially radiocurable condition.
2. Radical radiotherapy is the treatment of choice for many elderly patients with T3 bladder cancer.

3. This author favours a conventionally fractionated radical radiotherapy prescription using daily fractions and multiple portals from a linear accelerator, over other external beam, low LET treatment plans. The multiple daily fractions of small size, to a high total dose, is of interest and the results need to be confirmed.
4. Preoperative radiotherapy schemes have shown a reduced pelvic recurrence rate as compared with surgery alone; the survival of T3 patients treated by preoperative radiotherapy and surgery is significantly better than the historical radical surgery data base.
5. Preoperative radiotherapy causes downstaging of the tumour as found in the cystectomy specimen, and in this patient group there is more compelling evidence for a survival advantage for the combined preoperative radiotherapy and cystectomy treatment.
6. This reviewer's dissension from condensed, high fraction size, radical radiotherapy treatment schemes, does not extend to condensed, high fraction size preoperative radiotherapy schemes, for the reasons argued.
7. Early and late radiation morbidity occurs. Late morbidity has a higher incidence and tends to produce more lasting sequelae in patients treated with radical condensed, high fraction size treatment schemes. Although implantation techniques are now considered to have only limited applicability, they may produce good results in T2 cases with a low incidence of morbidity.

Part 3. Primary Surgery Approach

P. C. Peters

Infiltrating bladder cancer is usually infiltrating from the start. Less than 15% of infiltrating tumours arise from tumours that were originally superficial at their onset (Barken 1983). This review is written with the assumption that the diagnosis of muscle invasion of the urinary bladder by TCC has been properly established and that the usual clinical screening studies, laboratory and radiographic, show negative results for metastatic disease. These investigations include serum alkaline phosphatase, CT scanning of the chest and abdomen, with particular attention being paid to the lymph nodes, and with enhancement techniques of the liver and the urinary bladder. CT scanning is the procedure of choice in screening for metastatic disease to the chest. These investigations can be completed in 24–36 h and then surgery can be carried out. This approach is based on the philosophy that delay in establishing the diagnosis and the employment of radiotherapy techniques of unproven value as regards survival simply give more time for metastases to occur. These diagnostic investigations are crude and extremely fallible in picking up small amounts of metastatic disease such as micrometastases (Koss et al. 1981).

The urological surgeon is faced, after the initial diagnostic study, with a current dilemma. What are the roles of adjuvant radiotherapy and chemotherapy, if any? Surgery is the current modality of choice.

I prefer surgery and start by performing lymphadenectomy from the bifurcation of the aorta to the point where the circumflex iliac vein crosses the external iliac artery anteriorly, removing external and internal iliac nodes bilaterally, including those along the course of the obturator vessels and nerves. Lower extremity oedema may be minimised by omitting the dissection of the external iliac nodes. Frozen sections are done at the time of surgery; often as many as 30 nodes are examined. If a metastatic node is encountered, surgery is abandoned at that point in those patients who are voiding well, and radiotherapy and chemotherapy are considered postoperatively. Metallic clips may be used at that point to give a general outline of the position of the tumour. Studies by W. F. Whitmore Jr. showed no increase in survival by dissecting nodes above the aortic bifurcation. In my experience, survival in patients with stage D bladder cancer approaches zero. (Six of seven patients with only one positive node were dead within 42 months.) Stage D survivors are almost anecdotal (Kaufman and Goodwin 1980). Rarely, if the patient has been noted to have considerable morbidity from a large bleeding or sloughing tumour, palliative cystectomy may be done with diversion. Occasionally a patient is returned for salvage cystectomy after radiotherapy and chemotherapy when the host has demonstrated the ability to confine the disease to the urinary bladder and no distant metastases have appeared (Johnson et al. 1977).

If no grossly metastatic nodes are encountered and no microscopic nodal metastases are discovered by frozen section, cystoprostatectomy is performed in male patients and anterior exenteration in female patients. The urethra is cut across the level of the urogenital diaphragm in the male and a section is examined at this level. If no carcinoma is seen, urethrectomy is not routinely done in the male. In the latest 100 cystectomies done by the University of Texas at Dallas, six patients have had a 'recurrence' or a clinically manifest TCC in the urethra postoperatively. Out of the six patients, four presented with the complaint of a drop of blood at the meatus and the other two were discovered on bi-monthly urine cytology done as part of the follow-up examination. In the latest 20 radical cystoprostatectomies done in male patients, 11 have had an unsuspected carcinoma of the prostate. In one patient with a T3 carcinoma of the bladder, a tumour was found in one of 30 nodes—an adenocarcinoma, metastatic, from an unsuspected prostate cancer.

After completing the lymphadenectomy, I perform urinary diversion. Ureterosigmoidostomy has been the preferred procedure as the patient has no stoma to care for. It is being supplanted in the USA by the Koch pouch or Camey procedure. The ureters must be of normal calibre and the serum creatinine less than 250 μmol/litre. Otherwise I advocate the use of a non-refluxing ileal conduit (Sagalowsky 1984) or Camey procedure or Koch pouch. Three cases of severe pyelonephritis have been encountered in the latest 30 ureterosigmoidostomies. The low incidence is attributed to efforts to create a lengthy submucosal tunnel for the ureter with a water-snug mucosa-to-mucosa anastomosis using fine chromic gut. The tunnel need not necessarily be made in one of the teniae coli and should be at least 3.5 cm in length. Also advocated is the use of forced hydration to 2 litres minimum intake daily and supplemental oral potassium citrate solution, approximately 8 mEq every 8 h, accompanied by the use twice daily of sulphatrimethroprim as a suppressant of urinary tract infection. Disadvantages of the ureterosigmoidostomy include a tendency to systemic acidosis, especially if renal function is reduced (creatinine approximating 250 μmol/litre). This is seen after ileal diversion as well if the serum creatinine is greater than 250 μmol/litre at the time of diversion. When the ureterosigmoidostomy technique is used, the patient must be informed of the increased risk of colonic tumour and a colonoscopy and barium enema every 2 years should be part of the follow-up to protect against colon neoplasms. I have not encountered a single case with a colon neoplasm developing at the site of a ureterosigmoidostomy to this date. Such tumours have been reported from the Dallas area by Spence et al. (1979). The role of the faecal flora in the production of this tumour has been beautifully demonstrated in the animal work of Crissey et al. (1980).

In patients who have had ureterosigmoidostomy and who have become bedfast because of injury, illness or subsequent surgery, I prefer to use a large indwelling 34-40 F Malecot-type catheter in the rectum until the patient is again ambulatory. This simplifies nursing care and minimises acidosis.

It is anticipated that the non-refluxing ileal conduit will have long-term advantages over a refluxing anastomosis as regards the incidence of renal calculi and the preservation of renal function and will have lesser incidence of pyelonephritis (Skinner 1982b). Also, colonoscopy in ureterosigmoidostomy patients who have excellent renal function and no evidence of clinical pyelonephritis clearly shows the anastomosis in these patients to be incapable of preventing the passage of gas which may be seen bubbling up the ureter after having been introduced by the colonoscope. (In fact, this is a very good way of locating the ureteric orifice in the thoroughly cleansed colon.)

Role of Radiation Therapy in the Management of Infiltrating Tumours

Doubt as to the efficacy of preoperative radiotherapy in enhancing survival of bladder carcinoma patients has been eloquently raised by Radwin (1980). An excellent review of the controversial subject of the role of radiotherapy has been completed by Droller (1983). I do not currently use radiation therapy in the primary preoperative plan of management for infiltrating TCC of the urinary bladder. Reasons for this are:

1. A dose of 4500–5500 cGy to the tumour is necessary for a total kill in those tumours which are comprised completely of sensitive cells (Droller 1983).
2. Time required for administration of this dose does not enhance survival predictably and postpones the date of the definitive surgery.
3. A dose of 2000 cGy, which has been advocated and shown by van der Werf-Messing and associates (1969) to diminish local wound recurrence, is treatment for a problem which is very infrequently encountered clinically with modern surgical techniques.
4. I have not had a local recurrence in the operative wound in 100 consecutive radical cystectomies done without preoperative radiotherapy, and pelvic recurrence in only 7 patients, 4 of which were really bone metastases already present at the time of surgery and not soft tissue recurrence.

Three patients died in the postoperative period within 30 days of surgery; two of these died following acute myocardial infarction and the third patient died of sepsis and peritonitis. It has been my experience that those individuals succumbing after this early postoperative period usually die of metastatic disease present at the time of surgery but undetected because of the current lack of sensitivity of staging tests.

Studies at the University of Texas M.D. Anderson Hospital by Miller and Johnson have shown the 5-year survival of patients with infiltrating carcinoma treated by radiation therapy alone to be 22%—inferior to the results of radical cystectomy alone in the same institution of 46% (Miller and Johnson 1973). Studies at the Institute of Urology in London by Bloom et al. (1982) have shown 5-year survivals of 49% for tumours showing a complete response to radical radiotherapy and 14% in those that did not respond, figures less satisfactory than the treatment by surgery alone at major centres in the USA today.

Bladder tumours, like many malignant neoplasms, represent a heterogeneous population of cells (Slack and Prout 1980). A given dose of irradiation will kill many but not all the cells in a given neoplasm each time. At present, I am unaware of any method of selecting preoperatively those patients in whom the cell population of the tumour is completely radiosensitive to a curative dose, i.e. 4000–5000 cGy to the tumour. Such tests are sorely needed and would greatly enhance the position of the radiotherapist, as most studies have shown that those patients with tumours that are radiosensitive, so that down-staging is achieved, have a much higher survival rate than those in whom the effect of radiotherapy is less apparent. It has been a frequent disappointment to me, however, to encounter a case in which no viable tumour could be detected postoperatively in a radical cystectomy specimen, but the patient still succumbed within a 2-year period to distant metastases not detected at the time of the initial diagnostic study.

A major disadvantage of adjuvant therapy in treating patients with carcinoma of the urinary bladder is simply that most of these are elderly patients, and the time required to deliver a curative dose of radiation plus the general systemic effects of chemotherapy create an arduous regimen which many patients refuse to continue. This fact has caused major patient loss and slow build-up of patient numbers in many current protocols; it is simply more treatment for the disease than the patient can sometimes bear (Prout 1976).

Chemotherapy of Bladder Tumours

Several studies have shown efficacy of *cis*-platinum as a single agent and in combination with doxorubricin and cyclophosphamide (CISCA) in the management of infiltrating and metastatic carcinoma of the urinary bladder (Yagoda et al. 1978; Yagoda 1980; Soloway et al. 1981). I have reported a series of 11 patients with stage D TCC of the bladder treated with *cis*-platinum as a single agent (Peters and O'Neill 1980). Although 3 of the 11 had dramatic temporary objective partial remissions as defined by the National Bladder Cancer Project criteria, none of the patients survived for 2 years after establishment of the diagnosis. At present an adjuvant treatment programme is under way at the University of Texas at Dallas in which patients with metastatic nodes at surgery receive either CISCA or *cis*-

platinum, and patients with non-metastatic nodes receive *cis*-platinum or observation. Although small numbers have accumulated, three of nine patients with negative nodes succumbed within 2 years after receiving adjunctive *cis*-platinum in a dosage of 1.6 mg/m^2 for a minimum of four doses. Six of seven patients with one (only) positive node are dead within 29 months. Clearly, there are no agents for treating bladder cancer with the therapeutic efficacy of those available for testis cancer.

In my experience to date overall 5-year survival results with essentially an initial surgical management and reserving chemotherapy or radiotherapy for palliation or adjuvant measures are 60% for T2 tumours, 33% for T3a tumours and 18% for T3b tumours.

Summary

Surgery alone is currently the best single treatment for infiltrative carcinoma of the urinary bladder. Current staging methods to distinguish regional from systemic disease preoperatively or at surgery are inadequate. Curative systemic therapy is seldom realised, or, expressed in another manner, adjuvant radiotherapy and chemotherapy are not predictably effective at this time in the management of infiltrating TCC of the bladder. Furthermore, they have little role in the management of squamous carcinoma or adenocarcinoma of the urinary bladder. Surgery appears to be reaching its limits as a means of patient cure. Sorely needed are radiological methods to predict sensitivity of a heterogeneous population of cells in a given tumour and effective chemotherapeutic agents to make truly effective adjuvant therapy a reality.

Part 4. Primary Radiotherapy Approach

J. P. Blandy

Every urologist knows that surgical excision can cure cancer of the bladder when it is well differentiated and has not penetrated the muscular wall. The entire bladder may be lined with multiple pT1 tumours, but, once cleared by patient resection, may remain clear for decades. This observation, however banal, is important because it confirms that it is possible to cure some cancers of the bladder by resection alone, given the right circumstances. Unfortunately, it was the universal experience that once cancer had invaded the muscle of the bladder wall, surgical excision gave very disappointing results (Barnes et al. 1967).

In the same way, although it had been known for 50 years that radiotherapy could cure some bladder tumours, either with interstitial implantation of radioactive material, or with external beam therapy, the results of attempting to cure invasive cancer of the bladder by radiation alone were notably dismal (Goffinet et al. 1975).

Thirty-five years ago in the London Hospital the only endoscopic instruments were the Bugbee electrode or Kidd's bigball cystoscope. We had no skills in TUR. When a cancer was too big for coagulation, the bladder was opened, and radium needles were placed through and across the tumour. They were left in situ for a measured time, to give the tumour a certain calculated dose. It was my duty as a student to remove the needles when the time was up. The patient suffered agonies while the needles were in position, and worse when they were pulled out. The infected, persistent radionecrotic slough in the bladder gave rise to distressing spasms. It was a memorably cruel method.

The next phase was the introduction to the London Hospital of the technique of open diathermy and interstitial implantation of radioactive radon seeds. The method was quick, painless and easy. It could be delegated safely to relatively inexperienced assistants, and in the late 1950s Hope-Stone and I together performed hundreds of these operations. The postoperative course was uncomplicated and comfortable. The 5-year survival rate for well-differentiated tumours was just as good as any then being achieved with cystectomy. It was an excellent technique, but was replaced when growing skill with the resectoscope made it possible to resect many of the tumours hitherto needing open cystodiathermy. When improvements in external beam therapy made it possible to give a well-localised dose without the need for interstitial implantation, 20 years later, it is interesting how few of the radon patients developed subsequent superficial tumours, as if exposure to radiation from the radon seeds implanted in the base of the original tumour protected the rest of the bladder against the development of further tumours. The same has been observed in the long-term follow-up of patients treated with interstitial radium needles.

When it became obvious that neither radiotherapy nor surgery by themselves were effective in the treatment of invasive bladder cancer, it was logical to try to combine them. Several centres devised regimens in which preoperative radiation was followed by cystectomy. The dose of radiation varied from one centre to another, as did the technique of cystectomy. Some removed the lymph nodes en bloc with the bladder: others performed only a simple cystectomy. At first it seemed that a combination of preoperative radiation with cystectomy was useful, for there was a steady improvement in the survival figures (Miller 1977). Some surgeons interpreted this as signifying that the addition of radiation to surgery had been useful. Others pointed out that the improvement coincided with major advances in surgery, anaesthesia and postoperative care, and perhaps these were just as likely to be responsible for the improved survival as adjuvant radiotherapy. The catch was the old one, inherent in the interpretation of all 'historical controls'.

Some surgeons had never been impressed by the evidence in favour of adjuvant preoperative radiotherapy (Jacobi et al. 1983): others began tentatively to omit it from their schemes of treatment, relying instead upon a meticulous and radical dissection of the bladder en bloc with its regional lymph nodes (Skinner 1982a). Their results were no worse than those of adjuvant radiation and surgery.

To avoid the errors that arise from 'historical controls' one requires a randomised prospective study that will compare one method with another. Such a study was conceived some 20 years ago and carried out under the auspices of the Institute of Urology in London (Wallace and Bloom 1976; Bloom et al. 1982).

Patients with T3 tumours of the bladder who were under 70 and fit enough to undergo cystectomy were assigned to one of two treatment schedules. Patients in one group were given 4000 cGy, followed by total cystectomy. Those in the other group were given 5500 cGy and were followed up; they underwent cystectomy if recurrent disease or symptoms demanded it—a procedure which came to be called, somewhat unfortunately, 'salvage cystectomy'.

The results distilled the experience of all the major teaching centres in London. There was an overall 5-year survival rate of 39%, but no significant difference between the two groups. Much was made of minor differences between them, and when the patients were broken down into smaller subgroups—statistically an even more dubious exercise—it was claimed that there was a marginal advantage in 4000 cGy followed by cystectomy, but even then only in patients under 65.

At the London Hospital, although we did participate in this multicentre controlled trial, it was never with much enthusiasm. Once the trial was over we returned to our former ways and continued to use radiotherapy as the first line of treatment, reserving cystectomy for patients in whom the cancer failed to disappear or relapsed, or in whom haemorrhage or a contracted bladder were seen as complications of radiation. When Oliver carried out a careful retrospective survey of this experience, he found, somewhat unexpectedly, that the overall results were no worse than the combination of cystectomy and radiation then in vogue: The 5-year crude survival for the entire group, which included men and women of all ages, was 38%—identical to that obtained in the Institute trial, and similar to what, a decade ago, was the norm elsewhere (Blandy et al. 1980).

This was gratifying, but of less importance than the discovery that within this overall average figure there were hidden two very different survival rates of two quite different populations of tumours. This was only recognised when Oliver, an experienced oncologist, reviewed the results in terms of 'complete' and 'partial response' to therapy.

He reviewed 220 T3 carcinomas that had been treated in the London Hospital, with the aim of curing the tumour by radiation therapy using Hope-Stone's technique (Hope-Stone et al. 1981). The tumour disappeared completely after the initial course of radiation therapy—a 'complete response' in oncological terminology—in 42% of patients. This group had an unprecedented survival rate of 70% (corrected). In contrast, there was a 'partial' or 'nil' response in 58% of patients, and in this unhappy group the survival rate was very poor indeed—only 17% (Blandy et al. 1980). If we removed the bladder without delay once it was clear that the tumour was not completely radiosensitive, then the 5-year survival was raised from the dismal 17% (of the whole group of non-responders) to 31%. At first glance, one might draw the obvious conclusion that the bladder ought to be removed as soon as it becomes clear that the tumour is radioresistant.

However, these figures concealed another fact of which we were unaware until Oliver again reviewed the results with the eye of an oncologist. Out of 16 non-responders, 5 had shown no response whatever to radiation treatment, and none of them survived 5 years after cystectomy. In contrast, in the 11 patients who showed some, but less than 50% response, 5 lived for 5 years (45%) after cystectomy.

These retrospective studies from our institution have been misinterpreted as if implying that the London Hospital team were committed to a rigid policy and determined to defend it by the customary exchange of salvoes of statistics between one centre and another. Not so. We are well aware that our retrospective study was full of faults. It was historical; it was not randomised; it incorporated no controls; and it was virtually impossible to compare our findings with those of other centres.

But this is nothing new. Comparing figures from one centre with another is always bound to be fraught with error. In centre A, the wards are modern and well-equipped. The staff are well trained. There is no such thing as a waiting list. Excellent intensive care facilities are available for every total cystectomy. It is hardly surprising that the mortality for cystectomy is a fraction of that achieved in hospital B, whose patients are old, undernourished and poor, and who may have waited several months to get into a hospital which cannot spare intensive care beds for such mundane procedures as cystectomy.

No less important are the skills and equipment available for radiotherapy. There are centres in which lack of facilities or expertise forces urologists to use cystectomy as the first treatment for invasive cancer of the bladder. Without taking all these factors into account it is impossible to make a useful comparison between one centre and another. Who will admit in print that his surgical skill is less than outstanding, or accuse his radiotherapist of being inept?

In discussing the role of surgery versus radiotherapy in the management of invasive bladder cancer, one must pay attention to the inherent limitations of any method that aims only to destroy the cancer in the pelvis. In most large series about 25% of patients die from distant metastases (Whitmore 1980). The best 5-year survival rate that can be hoped for is only 75%, and this again assumes that we can control the local disease completely.

In fact, none of the available methods of treatment offers 100% control of the local disease. Combinations of radiation therapy and total cystectomy are followed by recurrence of disease in the pelvis in about 20% of patients, i.e. the best that can be hoped for is a 5-year survival of about 55%. This is almost exactly what has been achieved by Jacobi et al. (1983) and Skinner (1982a) by means of radical cystectomy without adjuvant radiotherapy, and in our own centre by using radiotherapy first and removing the bladder if the tumours fail to respond.

Although our results would suggest that about 40% of these patients could be spared a cystectomy, it is essential in order to apply this method safely that the radioresistant tumours are detected early and removed by cystectomy. Here there are some practical difficulties. It is not always easy to be sure that a tumour is regressing, even as late as 3 months after the end of the course of radiotherapy. One may see a slough in the bladder, surrounded with angry oedema that in every way resembles a cancer, and a biopsy of this tissue may still show malignant cells, albeit of questionable viability. By 6 months the bladder may be entirely free from disease. If the tumour is insensitive to radiation, and if one defers the decision about cystectomy for as long as 6 months, the patient may be throwing off metastases from the still-living primary tumour. No surgeon, brought up in the tradition of Virchow and Halstead, finds it easy to play the part of a passive observer. We all feel the urge to do something, and our fears may be shared by the patient, who detests the idea of an undead cancer lurking inside him.

By no means all of the patients in our centre whose bladder cancers failed to go away after radiation therapy were offered total cystectomy. There were several reasons for this: some patients were unfit for cystectomy; others refused; and a small number developed distant metastases in the interval. We are, however, all conscious that there is a fourth group of patients over whom we undoubtedly dragged our feet, by failing to insist on an operation in which—at that time—we had little faith. Today we feel confident that cystectomy should be offered to every patient whose tumour fails to regress with radiotherapy. Although the patient has nothing to lose by being given radiotherapy as the first step in his treatment, it is only recently that this necessary caveat has been firmly implemented.

It is unlikely that any combination of radiation therapy and surgery will yield much more improvement than the 70% survival rate that was obtained in those of our patients who were radiosensitive, and even in this group there is no room for complacency: 30% of them still died, mainly from distant metastases. Clearly we need another adjuvant—one that will act upon micrometastases that have spread by veins or lymphatics. It is in this direction that we should now be directing our efforts.

References

Adams GE (1979) Radiation sensitisers for hypoxic cells: problems and prospects. In: Abe M, Sakramoto K, Phillips TC (eds) Treatment of radioresistant cancers. Elsevier North Holland, pp 3–9

Ahlering TE, Lieskovsky G, Skinner DG (1984) Indications for urethrectomy in men undergoing single stage radical cystectomy for bladder cancer. J Urol 131: 657–659

Anderström C, Johansson S, Nilsson S, Unsgaard B, Wahlquist L (1983a) A prospective randomized study of pre-operative irradiation with cystectomy or cystectomy alone for invasive bladder carcinoma. Eur Urol 9: 142–147

Anderström C, Johansson SL, von Schultz L (1983b) Primary adenocarcinoma of the urinary bladder: a clinopathologic and prognostic study. Cancer 52: 1273–1280

Ashken MH (1982) Urinary reservoirs. In: Ashken MH (ed) Urinary diversion. Springer, Berlin Heidelberg New York, pp 112–139

Backhouse TW (1979) A rotation technique for irradiation of the bladder and the results obtained. Clin Radiol 30: 259–262

Barken M (1983) Bladder cancer symposium. Cont Surg 23: 114

Barnes RW, Turner CL, Bergman RT (1946) Treatment of bladder tumours. California Med 65: 95–98

Barnes RW, Bergman RT, Hadley HL, Love D (1967) Control of bladder tumours by endoscopic surgery. J Urol 97: 864–868

Barnes RW, Dick AL, Hadley HL, Johnson OL (1977) Survival following transurethral resection of bladder carcinoma. Cancer Res 37: 1895–1897

Batata MA, Whitmore WF, Chu FCH, Hilaris BS, Unal A, Chung S (1980) Patterns of recurrence in bladder cancer treated by irradiation and/or cystectomy. Int J Radio Oncol Biol Phys 6: 155–159

Batata MA, Chu FCH, Hilaris BS, Kim YS, Lee MZ, Chung S, Whitmore WF (1981) Factors of prognostic and therapeutic significance in patients with bladder cancer. Int J Radiol Oncol Biol Phys 7: 575–579

Beahrs JR, Fleming TR, Zincke H (1984) Risk of local urethral recurrence after radical cystectomy for bladder cancer. J Urol 131: 264–266

Beckley S, Wajsman Z, Pontes JE, Murphy G (1982) Transverse colon conduit: A method of urinary diversion after pelvic irradiation. J Urol 128: 464–468

Bennett JK, Whetley JK, Walton KN (1984) 10-year experience with adenocarcinoma of the bladder. J Urol 131: 262–263

Bergman B, Nilsson S, Petersen I (1979) The effect on erection and orgasm of cystectomy, prostatectomy and vesiculectomy for cancer of the bladder: a clinical and electromyographic study. Br J Urol 51: 114–120

Blandy JP, England HR, Evans SJW, Hope-Stone HF, Mair GMM, Mantell BS, Oliver RTD, Paris AMI, Risdon RA (1980) T3 bladder cancer—the case for salvage cystectomy. Br J Urol 52: 506–510

Bloom HJG (1981) Preoperative intermediate-dose radiotherapy and cystectomy for deeply invasive carcinoma of the bladder: rationale and results. In: Oliver RTD, Hendry WF, Bloom HJG (eds) Bladder cancer: principles of combination therapy. Butterworths, London, pp 151–174

Bloom HJG, Hendry WF, Wallace DM, Skeet RG (1982) Treatment of T3 bladder cancer: controlled trial of preoperative radiotherapy and radical cystectomy versus radical radiotherapy. Br J Urol 54: 136–151

Bracci U (1968) Urinary diversion by the Heitz-Boyer-Hovelacque procedure. Technique and experience. Urol Int 23: 63–73

Bracci U (1978) Rectal bladder. In: Mayor G, Zingg EJ (eds) Urologic surgery. Thieme, Stuttgart, pp 557–575

Brannan W, Fuselier HA, Ochsner M, Randrup ER (1981) Critical evaluation of 1-stage cystectomy—reducing morbidity and mortality. J Urol 125: 640–642

Bredael JJ, Croker BP, Glenn DF (1980) The curability of invasive bladder cancer treated by radical cystectomy. Eur Urol 6: 206–210

Bredin HC, Prout GR (1977) One-stage radical cystectomy for bladder carcinoma: operative mortality, cost/benefit analysis. J Urol 117: 447–451

Brown MH, Elliott JS (1969) Bladder cancer: an evaluation of diagnosis and treatment of 93 patients. J Urol 106: 63–66

Burham JP, Farrer J (1960) A group experience with uteroileal cutaneous anastomosis for urinary diversion: results and complications of the isolated ilial conduit (Bricker procedure) in 96 patients. J Urol 83: 622–629

Cancer (1976) Special supplement: Tumour dose—time—volume. Cancer 37: 67–75

Chan RC, Johnson DE (1978) Integrated therapy for invasive bladder carcinoma: experience with 108 patients. Urology 12: 549–552

Chapman JD (1979) Hypoxic cell sensitisers—implications for radiation therapy. N Engl J Med 301: 1429–1432

Chisholm GD, Hindmarsh JR, Howatson AG, Webb JN, Busuttil A, Hargreave TB, Newsam JE (1980) TNM (1978) in bladder cancer: use and abuse. Br J Urol 52: 500–505

Clark PB (1978) Radical cystectomy for carcinoma of the bladder. Br J Urol 109: 414–416

Cordonnier JJ (1968) Cystectomy for carcinoma of the bladder. J Urol 99: 172–173

Costello AJ, Tiptaft RC, England HR, Blandy JP (1984) Squamous cell carcinoma of bladder. Urology 23: 234–236

Crawford ED, Skinner DG (1980) Salvage cystectomy after irradiation failure. J Urol 123: 32–34

Crissey MM, Steele GD, Gittes RF (1980) Rat model for carcinogenesis in ureterosigmoidostomy. Science 207: 1079

Daughtry JD, Susan LP, Stewart BH, Straffon RA (1977) Ileal conduit and cystectomy: a 10-year retrospective study of ileal conduits performed in conjunction with cystectomy and with a minimum 5-year follow-up. J Urol 118: 556–557

Denekamp J, Stewart FA (1979) Evidence for reduced repair capacity in mouse tumours relative to normal tissues. Int J Radiol Oncol Biol Phys 5: 2003–2010

Denekamp J, McNally NJ, Fowler JF, Joiner MC (1980) Misonidazole in fractionated radiotherapy: are many small fractions best? Br J Radiol 53: 981–990

Dische S (1973) The hyperbaric oxygen chamber in the radiotherapy of carcinoma of the bladder. Br J Radiol 46: 13–17

Dretler SP, Ragsdale BD, Leadbetter WF (1973) The value of pelvic lymphadenectomy in the surgical treatment of bladder cancer. J Urol 109: 414–416

Droller MJ (1983) Controversial role of radiation therapy as adjunctive treatment of bladder cancer. J Urol 129: 897–903

Edsmyr F (1975) Radiotherapy in the management of bladder cancer. In: Cooper EH, Williams LE (eds) The biology and clinical management of bladder cancer. Blackwell Scientific, Oxford, pp 229–254

Edsmyr F (1981) Radiotherapy in the management of bladder carcinoma. In: Oliver RTD, Hendry WF, Bloom HJG (eds) Bladder cancer: principles of combination therapy, Butterworths, London, pp 139–149

Ellis F (1969) Dose, time and fractionation: a clinical hypothesis. Clin Radiol 20: 1–7

Emmet JL, Winterringer JR (1955) Experience with implantation of radon seeds for bladder tumours: comparison of results with other forms of treatment. J Urol 73: 502–515

Field SB (1970) Discussion on repair of sublethal damage in cell systems. In: Time and dose relationship in radiation biology as applied to radiotherapy. Proceedings of the NCI–AEC Conference, Carmel, Calif, 1970. Brookhaven National Laboratory Report BNL 50203 (C-57), pp 54–65

Foster KJ, Alberti KGMM, Allen N, Jenkins AJJ, Maciver J, Smart CJ, Karran VJ (1978) The influence of early postoperative intravenous nutrition upon recovery after total cystectomy. Br J Urol 50: 319–323
Fowler JF (1979) New horizons in radiation oncology. Br J Radiol 52: 523–535
Freiha FS (1980) Complications of cystectomy. J Urol 123: 168–169
Goodman GB, Balfour J (1964) Local recurrence of bladder cancer after supervoltage irradiation. J Can Assoc Radiol 15: 92–98
Goodman GB, Balfour J, Hislop TG, Elwood JM (1981a) Carcinoma of the bladder: Results and experience with irradiation and selective cystectomy. In: Connoly JG (ed) Carcinoma of the bladder. Raven, New York, pp 227–234
Goodman GB, Hislop TG, Elwood JM, Balfour J (1981b) Conservation of the bladder function in patients with invasive bladder cancer treated by definitive irradiation and selective cystectomy. Int J Radiol Oncol Biol Phys 7: 569–573
Goffinet DR, Schneider MJ, Glatstein EJ, Ludwig H, Ray GR, Dunnick NR, Bagshaw MA (1975) Bladder cancer: results of radiation therapy in 384 patients. Radiology 117: 149–153
Gowing NFC (1960) Urethral carcinoma associated with the bladder. Br J Urol 32: 428–439
Hall EJ (1978) In: Radiobiology for the radiologist. Harper and Row, New York, pp 29–62, 324–348
Hendry WF, Gowing NFC, Wallace DM (1974) Surgical treatment of urethral tumours associated with bladder cancer. Proc R Soc Med 67: 304–307
Hewitt J, Rigby J, Reeve J, Cox AG (1973) Whole-gut irrigation in preparation for large-bowel surgery. Lancet II: 337–340
Hope-Stone HF, Blandy JP, Oliver RTD, England H (1981) Radical radiotherapy and salvage cystectomy in the treatment of invasive carcinoma of the bladder. In: Oliver RTD, Hendry WF, Bloom HJG (eds) Bladder cancer: principles of combination therapy. Butterworths, London, pp 127–138
Jacobi GH, Klippel FF, Hohenfellner R (1983) 15 Jahre Erfahrung mit der radikalen Cystektomie ohne praeoperative Radiotherapie beim Harnblasenkarzinom. Aktuel Urol 14: 63–69
Johnson DE, Lamy SM (1977) Complications of single stage radical cystectomy and ileal conduit diversion: review of 214 cases. J Urol 117: 171–173
Johnson DE, Lamy SM, Bracken RB (1977) Salvage cystectomy after radiation failure in patients with bladder carcinoma. South Med J 70: 1279–1281
Johnson DE, Schoenwald AG, Ayala AG, Miller LS (1976) Squamous cell carcinoma of the bladder. J Urol 115: 542–544
Jones MA, Breckmann B, Hendry WF (1981) Life with an ileal conduit: results of questionnaire surveys of patients and urological surgeons. In: Oliver RTD, Hendry WF, Bloom HJG (eds) Bladder cancer: principles of combination therapy. Butterworths, London, pp 183–190
Kaufman JJ, Goodwin WE (1980) Survival of a patient with bladder cancer with one positive node for 19 years. Presented at the meeting of the Western Urologic Forum, Santa Barbara, Calif, 1980
Kock NG, Nilson AE, Nilson LO, Norlen LJ, Philipson BM (1982) Urinary diversion via a continent ileal reservoir: clinical results in 12 patients. J Urol 128: 469–475
Koss JC, Arger PH, Coleman GB, Mulhern CB Jr, Pollack HM, Wein AJ (1981) CT staging of bladder carcinoma. Am J Radiol 137: 359–362
Laplante M, Brice M (1973) The upper limits of hopeful application of radical cystectomy for vesical carcinoma: does nodal metastases always indicate incurability. J Urol 109: 261–264
Littbrand B, Edsmyr F (1976) Preliminary results of bladder carcinoma irradiated with low individual doses and a high total dose. Int J Radiol Oncol Biol Phys 1: 1059–1062
Littbrand B, Revesz L (1969) The effect of oxygen on cellular survival and recovery after radiation. Br J Radiol 42: 914–924
Magri J (1962) Partial cystectomy: a review of 104 cases. Br J Urol 34: 74–87
Månsson W, Colleen S, Sundin T (1984) Continent caecal reservoir in urinary diversion. Br J Urol 56: 359–365
Marberger M (1977) Erfahrungen mit der Harnleiter-Darmimplantation. In: Zingg EJ, Tscholl R (eds) Die Supravesikale Harnableitung. Huber, Bern, pp 210–222
Mathur VK, Krahn HP, Ramsey E (1981) Total cystectomy for bladder cancer. J Urol 125: 784–786
Miller LS (1977) Bladder cancer. Superiority of preoperative irradiation and cystectomy in clinical stage B2 and C cancer. Cancer 39: 973–980
Miller LS, Johnson DE (1973) Megavoltage irradiation for bladder cancer: alone, postoperative or preoperative? In: Proceedings of the 7th National Cancer Conference. Lippincott, Philadelphia, pp 771–782
Montie JE, Straffon RA, Stewart BH (1984) Radical cystectomy without radiation therapy for carcinoma of the bladder. J Urol 131: 477–482

Moore JV (1983) Cytotoxic injury to cell populations of solid tumours. In: Potten CS, Hendry JH (eds) Cytotoxic insult to tissue. Churchill Livingstone, Edinburgh, pp 368–404
Morrison R (1975) The results of treatment of cancer of the bladder—a clinical contribution to radiobiology. Clin Radiol 26: 67–75
Odoom JA, Sih IL (1981) Epidural analgesia and anticoagulant therapy. Anaesthesia 38: 254–259
Pearse HD, Reed RR, Hodges CV (1978) Radical cystectomy for bladder cancer. J Urol 119: 216–218
Peters PC, O'Neill MR (1980) Cis-diamminedichloraplatinum as a therapeutic agent in metastatic transitional cell carcinoma. J Urol 123: 375–377
Phillips TL (1972) Split dose, recovery of anoxic and hypoxic normal and tumour cells. Radiology 105: 127–134
Poole-Wilson DS, Barnard RJ (1971) Total cystectomy for bladder tumours. Br J Urol 43: 16–23
Prout GR (1976) The surgical management of bladder carcinoma. Urol Clin North Am 3: 149–153
Prout GR, Slack NH, Bross ID (1971) Preoperative irradiation as an adjuvant in the surgical management of invasive bladder carcinoma. J Urol 105: 223–231
Prout GR, Slack NH, Bross ID (1973) Pre-operative irradiation and cystectomy for bladder carcinoma. IV. Results in a selected population. In: Proceedings of the 7th National Cancer Conference. Lippincott, Philadelphia, p 783
Radwin HM (1980) Invasive transitional cell carcinoma of the bladder: is there a place for preoperative radiotherapy? Urol Clin North Am 7(3): 551–557
Raz S, McLorie G, Johnson S, Skinner DG (1978) Management of the urethra in men undergoing cystectomy for bladder carcinoma. J Urol 120: 298–300
Reddy EK, Hartman GV, Mansfield CM (1978) Carcinoma of the urinary bladder: role of radiation therapy. Int J Radiol Oncol Biol Phys 4: 963–966
Reid EC, Oliver JA, Fishman IJ (1976) Preoperative irradiation and cystectomy in 135 cases of bladder cancer. Urology 8: 247–250
Riches G (1960) Choice of treatment in carcinoma of the bladder. J Urol 84:472–480
Rosenthal CH, Zingg EJ (1983) Erhötes Risiko der Tumorentwicklung in den oberen Harnwegen nach multizentrischen papillaren Blasentumoren. Urologie 22: 183–185
Rubin P, Casarett GW (1968) Clinical radiation pathology. Saunders, Philadelphia, pp 334–373
Ryan DW (1982) Anaesthesia for cystectomy. Anaesthesia 37: 554–560
Ryan JA, Abel RM, Abbott WM, Hopkins CC, McChesney T, Colley R, Philips K, Fisher J (1974) Catheter complications in total parenteral nutrition. N Engl J Med 290: 757–761
Sagalowsky AI (1984) Preliminary experience with non-reflux ileo-caecal conduit diversion. Presented at the 79th Annual Meeting of the American Urological Association, New Orleans, Louisiana, 6–10 May, 1984
Scanlon PW, Scott M, Segura JW (1983) A comparison of short-course, low-dose and long-course, high-dose preoperative radiation for carcinoma of the bladder. Cancer 52: 1153–1159
Schellhammer, PF, Whitmore WF (1976) Transitional cell carcinoma of the urethra in men having cystectomy for bladder cancer. J Urol 115: 56–60
Schoenberg HW, Gregory JG, Murphy JJ (1973) Low mortality cystectomy in bladder cancer. J Urol 110: 671–674
Schoenenberger A (1984) Radikale Zystektomie: Vorbereitende Massnahmen und postoperative Nachbehandlung. Aktuel Urol 15: 122–125
Sharma TC, Melamed MR, Whitmore WF (1970) Carcinoma in situ of the ureter in patients with bladder carcinoma treated by cystectomy. Cancer 26: 583–587
Simon J (1852) Ectopia vesicae: operation for diverting the orifices of the ureters into the rectum. Lancet II: 568
Skinner DG (1977) Current state of classification and staging of bladder cancer. Cancer Res 37: 2838–2842
Skinner DG (1982a) Management of invasive bladder cancer: a meticulous pelvic node dissection can make a difference. J Urol 128: 34–36
Skinner DG (1982b) Further experience with the ileocecal segment in urinary reconstruction. J Urol 128: 252–255
Skinner DG, Lieskovsky G (1984) Contemporary cystectomy with pelvic node dissection compared to preoperative radiation therapy plus cystectomy in management of invasive bladder cancer. J Urol 131: 1069–1072
Skinner DG, Crawford ED, Kaufman JJ (1980) Complications of radical cystectomy for carcinoma of the bladder. J Urol 123: 640–643
Skinner DG, Tift JP, Kaufman JJ (1982) High dose, short course preoperative irradiation therapy and immediate single stage radical cystectomy with pelvic node dissection in the management of bladder cancer. J Urol 127: 671–674

Slack NH, Prout GR (1980) The heterogenity of invasive bladder carcinoma and different responses to treatment. J Urol 123: 644–652
Smith JA, Whitmore WF (1981) Salvage cystectomy for bladder cancer after failure of definitive irradiation. J Urol 125: 643–645
Smith JA, Whitmore WF (1982) Regional lymph node metastases from bladder cancer. J Urol 126: 591–593
Smith JA, Batata M, Grabstaldt H, Sogani PC, Herr W, Whitmore F (1982) Preoperative irradiation and cystectomy for bladder cancer. Cancer 49: 869–873
Soloway MS, Ikard M, Ford K (1981) Cis-diamminedichloroplatinum in locally advanced and metastatic urothelial cancer. Cancer 47: 476–480
Spence HM, Hoffman WW, Fosmire GP (1979) Tumour of the colon as a late complication of ureterosigmoidostomy for exstrophy of the bladder. Br J Urol 51: 466–470
Steel GG (1968) Cell loss from experimental tumours. Cell Tissue Kinet 1: 193–197
Steel GG (1977) Growth kinetics of tumours. Oxford University Press, Oxford
Stewart FA, Denekamp J, Hirst DG (1980) Proliferation kinetics of the mouse bladder after irradiation. Cell Tissue Kinet 13: 75–89
Stone JH, Hodges CV (1966) Radical cystectomy for invasive bladder cancer. J Urol 96: 207–209
Studer UE, Furger P (1981) Die psychosoziale Reintegration des Urostomiepatienten. Schweiz Med Wochenschr 111: 1834–1836
Studer UE, Ruchti E, Greiner RM, Zingg EJ (1983) Faktoren welche die Überlebensrate nach totaler Zystektomie wegen Harnblasentumoren beeinflussen. Aktuel Urol 14: 70–77
Swanson DA, von Eschenbach AD, Bracken RB, Johnson DE (1981) Salvage cystectomy for bladder carcinoma. Cancer 47: 2275–2279
Tacciuoli M, Laurenti C, Racheli T (1977) 16 years' experience with Heitz-Boyer-Hovelacque procedure for exstrophy of the bladder. Br J Urol 49: 385–390
Thomas DM, Riddle PR (1982) Morbidity and mortality in 100 consecutive radical cystectomies. Br J Urol 54: 716–719
Thomlinson RH (1982) Measurement and management of carcinoma of the breast. Clin Radiol 33: 481–493
van der Werf-Messing B (1969) Carcinoma of the bladder treated by suprapubic radium implants: the value of additional external irradiation. Eur J Cancer 5: 277–285
van der Werf-Messing B (1975) Carcinoma of the bladder T3NXM0 treated by preoperative irradiation followed by cystectomy. Third report of the Rotterdam Radiotherapy Institute. Cancer 36: 718–722
van der Werf-Messing B (1978) Cancer of the urinary bladder treated by interstitial radium implant. Int J Radiol Oncol Biol Phys 4: 373–378
van der Werf-Messing B (1979) Pre-operative irradiation followed by cystectomy to treat carcinoma of the urinary bladder, category T3NX, 0–4M0. Int J Radiol Oncol Biol Phys 5: 394–401
van der Werf-Messing B, Star W, Menon RS (1980) T3NXM0 carcinoma of the urinary bladder treated by the combination of radium implant and external irradiation. A preliminary report. Int J Radiol Oncol Biol Phys 6: 1723–1725
van der Werf-Messing B, Friedell GH, Menon RS, Hop WCJ, Wassif SB (1982) Carcinoma of the urinary bladder T3NXM0 treated by pre-operative irradiation followed by simple cystectomy. Int. J Radiol Oncol Biol Phys 8: 1849–1855
Wajsman Z, Merrin C, Moore R, Murphy GP (1975) Current results from treatment of bladder tumours with total cystectomy at Roswell Park Memorial Institute. J Urol 113: 806–810
Wallace DM (1973) Total cystectomy. An editorial overview. Cancer 32: 1078–1083
Wallace DM, Bloom HJG (1976) The management of deeply infiltrating (T3) bladder carcinoma: Controlled trial of radical radiotherapy versus pre-operative radiotherapy and radical cystectomy (first report). Br J Urol 54: 136–151
Wallace DMA, Hindmarsh JR, Webb JN, Busuttil A, Hargreave TB, Newsam JE, Chisholm GD (1979) The role of multiple mucosal biopsies in the management of patients with bladder cancer. Br J Urol 51: 535–540
Walsh A (1982) Urinary diversion in malignant disease. In: Ashken MH (ed) Urinary diversion, Springer, Berlin Heidelberg New York, pp 75–100
Whitmore WF (1980) Integrated irradiation and cystectomy for bladder cancer. Br J Urol 52: 1–9
Whitmore WF (1981) Integrated irradiation and cystectomy for bladder cancer. In: Connoly JG (ed) Carcinoma of the bladder. Raven, New York, pp 235–249
Whitmore WF, Marshall VF (1962) Radical total cystectomy for cancer of the urinary bladder: 230 consecutive cases five years later. J Urol 87: 853–868
Whitmore WF, Grabstald H, Mackenzie RA (1968) Preoperative irradiation with cystectomy in the

management of bladder cancer. Am J Roentgenol Radium Ther Nucl Med 102: 570–576
Whitmore WF, Batata MA, Hilaris BS, Reddy GN, Unal A, Ghoneim MA, Grabstald H, Chu F (1977) A comparative study of two preoperative radiation regimens with cystectomy for bladder cancer. Cancer 40: 1077–1086
Williams G, Jones MA, Trott PA, Bloom HJG (1981) Carcinoma of the bladder treated by local interstitial irradiation. In: Oliver RTD, Hendry WF, Bloom HJG (eds) Bladder cancer: principles of combination therapy. Butterworths, London, pp 117–126
Withers HR (1970) Capacity for repair in cells of normal and malignant tissues. In: Time and dose relationship in radiation biology as applied to radiotherapy. Proceedings of the NCI-AEC Conference, Carmel, Calif., 1970. Brookhaven National Laboratory Report BNL 50203 (C-57), pp 54–65
Withers HR, Mason K, Reid BO, Dubrasky N, Barkley HT, Brown W, Smathers JB (1974) Response of mouse intestine to neutrons and gamma rays in relation to dose fractionation and division cycle. Cancer 34: 39–47
Yogoda A (1980) Chemotherapy of metastatic bladder cancer. Cancer 45: 1879–1888
Yogoda A, Watson RC, Kemeny N, Barzell WE, Grabstald H, Whitmore WF (1978) Diamminedichloride platinum II and cyclophosphamide in the treatment of advanced urothelial cancer. Cancer 41: 2121–2130
Zabbo A, Montie JE (1984) Management of the urethra in men undergoing radical cystectomy for bladder cancer. J Urol 131: 267–268
Zincke H (1982) Cystectomy and urinary diversion in patients eighty years old or older. Urology 19: 139–142
Zincke H, Garbeff PJ, Beahrs JR (1984) Upper urinary tract transitional cell cancer after radical cystectomy for bladder cancer. J Urol 131: 50–52
Zingg EJ, Tscholl R (1977) Continent cecoileal conduit: preliminary report. J Urol 118: 724–728
Zingg EJ, Bornet B, Bishop MC (1980) Urinary diversion in the elderly patient. Eur Urol 6: 347–351

Chapter 10

Chemotherapy of Bladder Cancer

E. Messing and J. B. deKernion

Treatment of Superficial Transitional Cell Carcinoma

Superficial bladder tumours (those not invading into muscle) represent by far the most common form of transitional cell carcinoma (TCC) (Koss 1975). They are usually papillary and of a low histological grade, although sessile tumours, which carry a somewhat worse prognosis, are not uncommon (deKernion and Skinner 1978).

Superficial tumours are generally amenable to local resection, either transurethrally or through open surgery. Survival is excellent (90% for 5 years), although recurrences occur in 50%–80% of patients (Cox et al. 1969; Droller 1980). According to most reports, the addition of standard external beam irradiation does not significantly reduce the recurrence rate (Caldwell 1976; Utz and DeWeerd 1978) and clearly has no bearing on survival. However, in non-randomised retrospective studies, van der Werf-Messing and Hop (1981) have shown that interstitial radium implant, with or without external beam irradiation, has reduced the rate of relapse in patients with solitary superficial TCC by 70%. Matsumoto et al. (1981) used historical controls to show that a single treatment with intraoperative electron irradiation implants, with or without external beam irradiation, markedly lowered the recurrence rate in superficial TCC. These reports require further confirmation in randomised prospective studies. However, external beam irradiation does have definite efficacy as a preoperative adjuvant for partial cystectomy; even in a very low dose (1000 cGy), it virtually eliminates suture line recurrence (van der Werf-Messing 1978).

Most recurrences of superficial TCC are of a similar low grade and stage and are readily managed by repeat local resection. However, recurrences eventually become invasive in 15%–25% of patients and therefore require more aggressive therapy. Means are not currently available to predict which patient will have a recurrence, although recently identified markers of aggressiveness, including absence of the expression of blood group antigens (Decenzo and Ledbetter 1976;

Alroy et al. 1978; Bergman and Javadpour 1978; Lange et al. 1978; Richie et al. 1980; Weinstein et al. 1979; Young et al. 1979; Sadoughi et al. 1980), expression of marker antigens detected by monoclonal antibodies (Chopin et al. 1984; Fredet et al. 1984; Messing et al. 1984) and/or T antigens (Summers et al. 1983) and frequent chromosomal aberrations (Sandberg 1980; Summers et al. 1981) may permit identification of those individuals whose superficial tumours are capable of more malignant behaviour. Furthermore, recurrences, although not of an advanced grade or stage, may be so numerous and diffusely spread as not to be amenable to local resection. Thus, chemotherapy has two applications in the management of superficial TCC: the prevention of recurrences, and the elimination of existing tumour confined to the bladder.

Prevention of Tumour Recurrence

The bladder's unique location renders its mucosa accessible to frequent inspection and biopsy, as well as to local applications and instillations of chemotherapeutic and immunotherapeutic agents. Moreover, since the bladder is the reservoir of renal excretory products, those agents which require metabolic activation (e.g. cyclophosphamide) generally achieve concentrations in the urine which far surpass those needed for efficacy when systemically administered. This assures the safe delivery of effective levels of medication to all areas of the bladder's mucosa and is of particular importance in the light of the multifocal nature of recurrences (Koss 1975). Finally, because of the superficial position of these tumours, all malignant and premalignant cells are theoretically exposed to concentrations of intraluminal medication which could not reach them without severe toxic effects if they invaded the deeper vesical layers or extravesical locations.

Patient Selection

Since 30%–50% of patients with superficial TCC never have recurrences after their original tumours are resected (Cox 1960; Droller 1980; Soloway 1980), and since most recurrences are of the same grade and stage found initially, treatment with potentially toxic intravesical agents (see below) is seldom warranted after resection of the initial tumour. Exceptions include patients suspected of being at high risk of recurrence because of exposure to carcinogens, patients whose tumours have indicators of increased aggressiveness (higher histological grade, loss of blood group antigens or presence of marker chromosomes on karyotypic analysis) or patients with large tumours or ones which penetrate into the submucosa.

Schedule of Administration of Intravesical Chemotherapy

The schedule for administering prophylactic intravesical chemotherapy has been devised more to conform with what is known about the behaviour of superficial

TCC than with the pharmacokinetics and mode of action of the agent being employed (see under individual agents). Recurrences are most frequent within the first 6 months of the most recent resection (Malling and Sorenson 1980). Hence, treatments are given frequently during the period (weekly or every other week for 6–12 weeks) and are followed by monthly maintenance instillations.

The first treatment is usually given 2–4 weeks after TUR. By this time much of the bladder wall has healed, thus reducing systemic absorption, patient discomfort and the risk of bladder perforation. However, some investigators believe that the denuded surfaces exposed during the resection and other technical features of the resection favour implantation of malignant cells (Boyd and Burnand 1974; Soloway 1980). These authors prefer to instill medication at the time of, or immediately following, the TUR (Burnand et al. 1976). Although the efficacy of this regimen has not been confirmed, two small clinical studies using thiotepa (Burnand et al. 1976; Gavrell et al. 1978), one short-term (3–4 month follow-up) controlled prospective trial comparing thiotepa or doxorubicin with placebo (Zinke et al. 1983) and an experimental study in rodents (Soloway 1980) have motivated the National Bladder Cancer Project (NBCP) Collaborative Group A to compare the efficacy in preventing tumour recurrence of a single post-resection (within 36 h) instillation of thiotepa with that of a standard course of weekly instillations of this medication. Theoretically, immediate post-resection instillations could result in systemic absorption of the agent and possible sensitisation to the drug. Experience with this schedule is still insufficient for determining whether these are practical problems, although some evidence attests to the relative safety of administering the agent at the time of TUR (Gavrell et al. 1978; Zinke et al. 1983). Still, anecdotal reports by Veenema (1978) describe the occurrence of complications such as simultaneous urosepsis and leucopenia with administration of thiotepa immediately after resection. It therefore may be wiser to give the agent after catheter removal (or several days later), although patient discomfort may prevent the retention of the medication for 60–90 min.

Chemotherapeutic Agents

Thiotepa (Triethylene Thiophosphamide). The standard intravesical chemotherapeutic agent is still the alkylating agent thiotepa (Veenema et al. 1962). It can be administered by either of the schedules discussed, and randomised studies indicate that doses of 30 mg and 60 mg are equally effective in reducing the incidence of recurrences (Koontz 1979). Toxic effects include severe irritative cystitis, febrile allergic episodes, leucopenia and thrombocytopenia (which seem to be more severe in elderly patients who have received higher cumulative doses; Hollister and Coleman 1980), bladder fibrosis, and renal failure when vesicoureteral reflux is present. If high-grade vesicoureteric reflux is suspected, blocking arterial balloon catheters can be placed in either ureter, with the patient in the 'reverse Trendelenburg' position. To prevent reflux to the kidneys, the bladder is then emptied by catheter drainage rather than through spontaneous voiding. While not all authors agree (Byar 1980; Asaki et al. 1980; Schulman 1980), thiotepa has reduced the frequency and number of recurrences in one-half to two-thirds of patients with a history of multiple recurrences (Malling and Sorenson 1980; Koontz et al. 1981). There is currently no way to predict which patients' tumours will respond to this therapy, although vigorous work with in vitro tumour stem cell (i.e. clonogenic) assays by a variety of investigators (Stanisic et al. 1980; von Hoff 1981) may prove fruitful in predicting this in the near future (see below).

Epodyl (Triethylene Glycol di-Glycerol Ether). The original studies utilising this agent (Riddle and Wallace 1971; Riddle 1973; Robinson et al. 1977; Nielsen and Thybo 1979; Colleen et al. 1980; Colleste et al. 1980) were not designed to determine its efficacy in preventing recurrences. However, by extrapolation one can probably expect an efficacy rate for prophylaxis similar to that of thiotepa. Epodyl's ability to prevent tumour recurrence is a current subject of investigation by the EORTC Urological Group, whose preliminary findings show it to have a role in prophylaxis approximately equal to that of thiotepa or Adriamycin (Kurth et al. 1983). A dose of 100 ml Epodyl is instilled as a 1% solution for 1 h in the same schedule as that usually used for thiotepa. Although its major toxic effect is severe vesical irritability (Nielson and Thybo 1979), occasional myelosuppression has occurred in patients with diffuse carcinoma in situ (Robinson et al. 1977). That this drug's systemic toxicity is lower than that of thiotepa may be due to Epodyl's higher molecular weight (262, as compared with 189 for thiotepa) and therefore lower systemic absorption. Larsen (1980) has emphasised the importance of not mixing this agent in an aluminium foil cup, which will result in a 50% reduction in its effective concentration within 5 min.

Mitomycin C. As with Epodyl, no studies have yet been reported which estimate the efficacy of this alkylating agent in preventing recurrence of superficial bladder tumours, although several are being conducted. However, evidence derived from its use against existing superficial tumours (Mishina et al. 1975; DeFuria et al. 1980; Soloway et al. 1981a) suggests results similar to, or better than, those reported for thiotepa. A preliminary report by the NBCP Collaborative Group A (Koontz et al. 1983) indicates that this agent may also have a beneficial role in managing thiotepa failures. Bracken et al. (1980) found that weekly instillations of at least 30 mg must be given; systemic toxicity has not been reported at this dosage. Chemical cystitis is rare (Koontz et al. 1983) and has occurred at our institution only in individuals with significant post-micturition residual urines. We now recommend catheter drainage in such patients when Mitomycin C is instilled. Murphy et al. (1981) have demonstrated that an irritant effect of this agent on urothelium occurs with exfoliation, degeneration and necrosis of bladder mucosal cells when it is administered to mice fed with the carcinogen FANFT. These changes are similar to those induced by thiotepa. The considerable expense of Mitomycin C currently inhibits its widespread use.

Adriamycin (Doxorubicin Hydrochloride). Monthly instillations of Adriamycin in 40–50 mg doses have been found to prevent the recurrence of TCC following resection of all visible tumour in over 70% of patients with short-term follow-up (Banks et al. 1977). In a prospective controlled study, doxorubicin reduced the recurrence rate from 86% in controls to 33% in treated patients with a mean follow-up of 24 months (Jacobi et al. 1979). When this agent was instilled at the end of TUR of all visible tumours in individuals with a history of recurrent tumours, Zincke et al. (1983) found a reduction of tumour recurrence 3–4 months after instillation from 81% (placebo) to 38% in patients receiving Adriamycin.

The efficacy of this agent in destroying existing tumours seems to be enhanced by the prior administration of low-dose (200–800 cGy) external beam irradiation (Uyama 1980). It induces generalised superficial inflammatory changes and squamous metaplasia in the human bladder. Severe vacuolation and keratinisation are also seen in the urothelium of FANFT-fed rats who are given Adriamycin intravesically (Banks et al. 1977). Analysis of biopsy tissue of patients receiving intravesical Adriamycin in 60 mg doses shows that only the superficial layers of the mucosa receive effective levels (10.3 μg Adriamycin/g tissue; Nagata 1980). The major toxic effects are local (haematuria and/or irritative voiding) and occur in more than 50% of patients when doses of 75–100 mg are instilled weekly (Gammelgaard et al. 1980; Melloni and Pavone-Macaluso 1980).

Cis-Platinum (DDP). The agent DDP has demonstrated its efficacy when used systemically for metastatic TCC (see below). In a limited non-randomised trial (Phase I) with short-term follow-up reported by Schulman et al. (1980), only 7% of patients with superficial tumours who had all visible tumours resected endoscopically experienced recurrence over a 6-month period after receiving three 1-h, monthly intravesical instillations of 50–100 mg DDP. All patients received 20 mg intravenous furosemide at the end of each treatment. DDP was well tolerated, although 2 of 14 patients experienced transient high-tone hearing loss. No renal or marrow toxicity was noted. Confirmation of these promising results with longer follow-up and suitable controls is warranted before the utility of this agent can be completely evaluated. However, preliminary findings by Needles et al. (1981) suggest that it is not likely to prevent recurrences in patients with completely resected aggressive tumors (T_1 or Tis).

Other Intravesical Agents. Several other chemotherapeutic agents, including 5-fluorouracil (Esquivel et al. 1965), carboquone (Ogawa, et al. 1980; Ono et al. 1980), actinomycin D (Esquivel 1965), VM-26 (Schulman 1980) and Bleomycin, both with and without hyperthermia (Moriyama and Ito 1980; Nakajima et al. 1980), have been used either in treating existing superficial TCC and/or preventing recurrences. To date, none of these agents or regimens has demonstrated significant advantages over those already discussed.

Systemic Chemotherapy for Superficial TCC

Several systemically active chemotherapeutic agents, including those administered orally, have been studied for the primary treatment of existing superficial bladder tumours. Methotrexate given weekly in a 50 mg oral dose has reduced the size of superficial tumours in over 75% of patients. After all tumour was resected, however, only 30% of patients remained tumour free for over 6 months with further oral therapy (Hall 1980b). Cyclophosphamide has been effective in treating carcinoma in situ (see p. 153; England et al. 1980) at 1 g/m^2 intravenously every 3 weeks for 6 months, and then every 6 weeks for 6 months. However, since this agent has been reported to induce bladder malignancies (Chasko et al. 1980; Glucksman 1980; Chodak et al. 1981), its use is probably not warranted in the patient with superficial bladder tumours. In a study with limited controls, neocarzinostatin given intravenously also caused reduction in superficial tumours in 75% of patients. After all residual tumour was resected, further therapy prevented tumour recurrence in 14 out of 19 patients followed for 2 years (Sakamoto et al. 1980). However, many of these patients had newly diagnosed tumours, of which up to 50% would be expected never to recur. Thus, the role of this agent in preventing tumour recurrence remains unclear.

Hyperthermia

Hyperthermia has been used in the treatment of several malignancies because tumour cells seem to be more sensitive to the destructive effects of heat than non-neoplastic cells (Storm 1982). While explanations for this phenomenon vary, most implicate the tumour's abnormal vascularity. This causes sluggish circulation within neoplasms and thus reduced ability to dissipate heat. Moreover, through both its variable effects on membranes and stimulation of metabolic processes, hyperthermia seems to enhance the effect of several chemotherapeutic agents. Recent studies examined the beneficial effects of this treatment, either alone or in combination with chemotherapeutic agents. Moriyama and Ito (1980) and Nakajima et al. (1980) independently reported tumour reduction in 30%–80% of patients treated with intravesical Bleomycin in warm saline. Best results were obtained when temperatures of 45–46°C were maintained during each treatment. A separate study using hyperthermia alone (42–45°C for 3 h for 5–14 days) reported marked tumour reduction in 38 out of 76 patients, while only 14%–28% of controls (treated with non-heated saline for 5–14 days) had similar reponses. Since treatment was not continued after tumours disappeared, it is not surprising that 80% of patients who experienced initial successes had recurrences within 1 year (Hall 1980a). Hyperthermic (45°) saline has also been instilled with urokinase resulting in tumour disappearance in 50% of patients (Okada et al. 1980). Toxic effects of hyperthermia primarily consist of local irritative symptoms, which have occurred in none (Hall 1980) to 67% of patients (Okada et al. 1980).

Immunotherapy

A variety of immunomodulators have been utilised for the prevention of superficial bladder tumour recurrence. The mechanisms of action of these agents vary, but there is little evidence that any effect attributed to them is due to specific stimulation of host immunity to tumour antigens. For example, polyiosinic acid-polycytidelic acid (poly I:C) polymer of double-stranded RNA is an interferon inducer in vitro (Young 1971). Interferon's major anticancer activity appears to be due to stimulation of non-antigen-specific effector cells, natural killer (NK) cells (Herberman 1980) or a direct antitumour effect (Billiau 1981). Similarly, while there is good evidence that bacillus Calmette-Guérin (BCG) treatments induce specific cellular and humoral immunity to mycobacterial antigens (Winters and Lamm 1981), and boost the cellular immune response to other antigens (Martinez-Piñeiro 1980; Antonaci et al. 1981), the boosted immune response, either generalised or specific, has not consistently correlated with the clinical response to the therapy (Winters and Lamm 1981). Other possible explanations for the efficacy of these agents include antigenic cross reactivity (I. Lovrekovich

1982, personal communication) or destruction of the tumour cells along with much of the normal vesical mucosa by an inflammatory reaction to BCG.

Systemic Immunotherapy. As reported by Kemeny et al. (1981), treatment with the interferon inducer poly I:C slightly reduced the rate of recurrence of superficial tumours 3 months after complete resection. Continued treatment had no effect thereafter, and recurrences had equalised between treated and control patients by 6 months. Surprisingly, while this treatment did not reduce the likelihood of developing higher grade or more invasive recurrences, it may have provided some protective effect which manifested itself in the significantly better survival of patients with carcinoma in situ treated with poly I:C who subsequently underwent cystectomy (Kemeny et al. 1981). Another systemic immunomodulator, levamisole, was ineffective in preventing recurrences in patients with superficial tumours who had undergone resection of all visible disease (Brosman 1980; Martinez-Piñeiro 1980).

BCG. Intravesical BCG instillations, with (Morales and Ersil 1979; Camacho et al. 1980; Lamm et al. 1981) or without (Brosman et al. 1981) intradermal inoculations, prevented recurrences in 60% (Morales and Ersil 1979) to 100% (Brosman et al. 1981) of patients in randomised prospective trials with more than 2 years' follow-up. The usual regimen consists of 90–120 mg of the various strains of live vaccine suspended in 60 ml instilled for 1 h weekly or biweekly for 6–12 weeks, followed by monthly instillations for 1–2 years.

The inclusion of intradermal injections at the time of intravesical treatments has not had added benefit. This finding is consistent with those of Stober and Peter (1980), who recently showed that intradermal BCG alone, while able to induce some humoral immunity to BCG in 94% of patients, did not prevent recurrence among patients in a randomised prospective study. Moreover, Brosman et al. (1981) reported the development of cellular immunity by conversion to positive PPD skin test in all patients treated with intravesical instillations of 120 mg Tice strain BCG alone. While these results fail to clarify its mechanism of action, they imply that intravesical instillation of BCG is immunogenic and sufficient for achieving this agent's maximum benefit.

BCG's major toxic effects have been irritative cystitis in virtually all patients and systemic symptoms (malaise, fever and chills) in many (Camacho et al. 1980). In our experience, severe systemic reactions can be avoided if instillations are not performed at the time of cystoscopy or bladder biopsy, or in the presence of vesicoureteric reflux. As yet untested is the possibility that the prophylactic use of antituberculosis medication may reduce toxicity.

Systemic Preventive Therapy

Because of epidemiological (Howe et al. 1980; Morrison et al. 1984) and experimental (Peterson et al. 1974; Cole 1975; Gowa et al. 1980) evidence linking TCC to environmental pollutants and chemical carcinogens, the use of ingested and parenteral agents which may interfere with the fundamental steps of malignant transformation has particular appeal in the chemoprevention of bladder cancer. Randomised human studies have focused on the retinoids, which have marked effects on proliferation and differentiation of epithelial tissues

Table 10.1. Chemo- and immunotherapy for superficial TCC

Agent	Route of administration	Prophylaxis	Total eradication of existing tumour	Carcinoma in situ
Thiotepa	Intravesical	56% (Koontz et al. 1981)	47% (Koontz et al. 1981)	20% (Koontz et al. 1983)
Epodyl	Intravesical		56% (Ek and Colleen 1980)	
Mitomycin C	Intravesical		45% (DeFuria et al. 1980)	90% (Bracken et al. 1980)
Adriamycin	Intravesical	67% (Jacobi et al. 1979)	22% (Gammelgaard et al. 1980) 31% (Duchek 1980)	67% (Edsmyr et al. 1980)
cis-Platinum	Intravesical	93%[a] (Schulman et al. 1980)		
Bleomycin (+hyperthermia)	Intravesical		40% (Moriyama and Ito 1980)	
BCG	Intravesical ±subcut.	60% (Morales and Ersil 1979) 100% (Brosman et al. 1981)	67% (Martinez-Piñeiro 1980)	77% (Morales 1980)
Urokinase (+hyperthermia)	Intravesical		50% (Okada et al. 1980)	
Interferon (human leucocyte)	Intralesional injection	?75% (Ikic et al. 1981)	75% (Ikic et al. 1981)	
Methotrexate	Orally	30% (Hall 1980)		
Cyclophosphamide	Intravenous			88%[c] (England et al. 1980)
Neocarzinostatin	Intravenous	72%[b] (Sakamoto et al. 1980)	6.7% (Sakamoto et al. 1980)	

[a] Follow-up period less than 6 months.
[b] Most patients had newly diagnosed tumours, not recurrences.
[c] One-third of patients also received external beam radiotherapy.

(Studer et al. 1984). 13-*cis*-Retinoic acid was noted to reduce the incidence of carcinogen-induced bladder cancer in rats (Sporn et al. 1977), but was found to be too toxic in humans (Soloway 1984) in a study by the NBCP Collaborative Group A. The aromatic retinoid, etretinate, at 25 mg/day, significantly reduced the number of recurrences of multiple tumours in patients with a history of recurrent superficial (Ta, T1) TCC from 48% (placebo) to 17% (treated) at 12 months. However, it did not significantly affect the overall incidence of recurrence (Studer et al. 1984). Side effects of dry mouth, skin and mucous membranes were encountered in nearly all patients started on 50 mg daily; a reduction in dosage to 25 mg effected resolution of symptoms. A cooperative study evaluating this agent is in progress.

Chemo- and Immunotherapy of Existing Superficial Bladder Tumours

While many of the agents and modalities discussed can effectively reduce or eliminate existing disease (Table 10.1), treatments should not replace complete TUR of all visible tumours. This procedure can usually be easily accomplished and provides important information to the managing physician regarding tumour grade and stage. Hence, the candidate for chemo- or immunotherapy of existing superficial tumours should be one in whom it is unlikely that resection can be performed safely and completely, usually because of the number, bulk or location of the tumour(s). A trial of intravesical therapy is certainly warranted in those patients with superficial tumours which are not manageable by repeat resection, but it is imperative that the treating physician be confident that more aggressive cancer is not present.

Since chemo- or immunotherapy for existing tumours should be viewed as an adjunct to TUR, the therapeutic goal should be the achievement of adequate regression to allow safe, complete resection. Thus, for this therapy to be considered beneficial, it is not necessary for the medication alone to make all tumours disappear completely. Most investigators agree with this concept and propose a 50% reduction in tumour size as a useful end point.

Between 40% and 70% of patients with superficial tumours can expect to have complete disappearance of all tumours following intravesical instillations of thiotepa (Koontz et al. 1981), Epodyl (Ek and Colleen 1980), Bleomycin plus warm saline (45–46°) (Moriyama and Ito 1980), Mitomycin C (DeFuria et al. 1980; Morales et al. 1981; Soloway et al. 1981a), BCG (Martinez-Piñiero 1980; Brosman et al. 1981) and Adriamycin (Garnick et al. 1984) in dosage schedules similar to those discussed for prevention of recurrences. Though these studies were not randomised and are not comparable (patients differ in number and size of tumours, inclusion of carcinoma in situ and histological grade), the results are surprisingly uniform. Tumours recur after therapy is discontinued even in patients who have had total eradication. Partial remissions account for another 15%–30% of patients, so that with any of these agents, 55%–85% of tumours are rendered manageable by combining intravesical instillations with endoscopic resection. While not as effective as the above-listed agents in accomplishing complete regression, intravenous neocarzinostatin (Sakamoto 1980) can sometimes reduce tumour size sufficiently to allow complete TUR. As occurs with more traditional forms of chemotherapy, patients who fail to respond to one regimen are often less responsive to others as well. Crossover studies examining this phenomena are rare. However, Prout et al. (1982) found that complete responses to Mitomycin C in individuals in whom attempts at tumour eradication with thiotepa had failed were significantly less common (31%) than in those who had previously had tumours eradicated with thiotepa (71%), or who had never received prior intravesical chemotherapy (80%).

In an intriguing recent study, Ikic et al. (1981) reported complete disappearance of all tumours in 6 of 8 patients with recurrent superficial TCC who were treated with 21 daily injections of 2 million interferon units of a crude preparation of human leucocyte interferon directly into, or in the vicinity of, the tumour. While half of the patients received simultaneous intramuscular injections of interferon, and almost all required several monthly courses of this therapy, most remissions have lasted over 2 years (the extent of follow-up at the time of writing) after the cessation of therapy. Although one patient with total tumour disappearance did experience rapid recurrence, two others with only partial regression have been rendered tumour free with TUR and have remained so for over 3 years. While this agent is quite promising, the prolonged and intense courses of therapy employed make wider use of this protocol unlikely. Moreover, because of the considerable trauma inflicted on the tumours by this regimen, one must seriously question interferon's role in effecting tumour regression in the absence of adequate controls.

Summary of Management of Superficial TCC

TUR, often combined with random bladder biopsy and cytological study of specimens obtained by vesical barbotage, is still the cornerstone of management of superficial tumours. This persists, despite suggestions that this treatment may be responsible for tumour implantation and recurrence (see p. 165). Such assertions are difficult to evaluate in controlled prospective trials and rely at present upon highly imperfect animal models (Soloway 1980; A. Shapiro 1982, personal communication) and circumstantial clinical impressions for their support. Resection is a safe technique which best combines specific treatment for superficial low-grade tumours with detection of more aggressive lesions while they are still at a treatable stage. For these reasons there appears to be little purpose in utilising a less definitive diagnostic step (e.g. transurethral biopsy rather than resection of tumours) followed by either radiation or chemotherapy as the primary mode of eradicating existing tumours.

The addition of radiation therapy in the primary treatment of these lesions may well be effective (van der Werf-Messing and Hop 1981; Matsumoto et al. 1981) in reducing the number and severity of recurrences. However, it is associated with definite morbidity and mortality (van der Werf-Messing and Hop 1981), it may compromise the subsequent early detection of more invasive tumours and it may limit the use of this modality if more invasive tumours develop. Moreover, there is no indication that the addition of radiation therapy to resection for superficial tumours (of any grade) significantly reduces the likelihood of having metastatic bladder cancer or improves 5-year survival (van der Werf-Messing and Hop 1981).

Chemo- or immunotherapy also have small roles in the primary therapy of low-grade superficial tumours and should be used for prophylaxis only in those patients with high likelihood of recurrence and/or high risk of subsequently developing deeply invasive cancers (Green et al. 1984). Careful selection of such patients is warranted since intravesical therapy may be toxic, and for many agents (e.g. thiotepa, Adriamycin) this toxicity is related to cumulative doses. This must be remembered, since presumably these treatments should be administered indefinitely to provide suitable protection against the factors which create and maintain the malignant state. Chemo- or immunotherapy in the treatment of existing superficial bladder tumours should be limited to those patients who are poor surgical candidates, those with tumours too numerous to resect, or those in whom tumours are suspected to persist after TUR.

If chemo- or immunotherapy is indicated, there is usually no need to employ the more toxic and no more effective systemic chemotherapy for the management of superficial low-grade disease. Possible exceptions include concomitant upper tract tumours or atypia. The agents we currently favour are Mitomycin C or BCG, which have low toxicity and considerable efficacy against not only superficial low-grade tumours but also high-grade TCC (including carcinoma in situ) which may be present but undetected at the time therapy is initiated.

Carcinoma in situ

The considerable risk of developing invasive cancer for patients with severe urothelial atypia (carcinoma in situ), either with or without a prior or concomitant history of superficial tumours, has been acknowledged since Utz et al. reviewed the Mayo Clinic experience in 1970. Many authors have confirmed these observations (Cooper et al. 1973; Friedell 1976; Koss 1979; Utz and Farrow 1980). It can be estimated that from 42% (Daly 1976) to 83% (Althausen et al. 1976) of patients with carcinoma in situ will subsequently develop tumours with muscular invasion. While these patients can be cured by performing cystectomy at the time of diagnosis, roughly one-third of patients so treated will have been subjected to the rigors of such therapy unnecessarily. Hence, attempts have been made to detect those individuals with the more favourable form of urothelial atypia, ‘carcinoma paradoxicum’ (Weinstein et al. 1980), and to try to alter the natural course of carcinoma in situ by less radical means than total cystectomy.

It is beyond the scope of this chapter to discuss the differentiation of favourable and unfavourable forms of carcinoma in situ. It is possible that some of the more recently described markers of poor prognosis, including blood group antigen deletion (see p. 44), expression of T antigen (Summers et al. 1983) or other marker antigens (Fredet et al. 1984), and severe karyotypical abnormalities (see p. 135), will prove to be helpful. The application of bladder-sparing therapy for urothelial atypia is based upon three assumptions. First, since this lesion is often imperceptible at endoscopic examination and often occupies large multifocal areas of the bladder surface, therapy must reach all of the vesical mucosa. Second, as with superficial papillary tumours, this lesion only involves the epithelium and effective therapy need not penetrate to the deeper layers of the bladder. Third, means are available (cytological examination of exfoliated cells and histological examination of randomly selected specimens of vesical mucosa) which can reliably detect persistence of urothelial atypia if conservative therapy fails, allowing curative surgery (cystectomy) before muscle invasion actually occurs. The administration of chemo- and immunotherapy not only adheres to these precepts but has recently been shown to eliminate this lesion effectively in many patients.

In small non-randomised series with short-term follow-up, intravesical Mitomycin C (Soloway et al. 1981a) and BCG (Morales 1980; S. Brosman 1981, personal communication; Herr et al. 1983) produced disappearance of carcinoma in situ in 90% and 77% of patients respectively (see Table 10.1). In a small randomised trial comparing endoscopic resection and BCG vs resection alone for patients with papillary tumours and carcinoma in situ, Herr et al. (1983) reported complete responses of 65% in the BCG group compared with only 12% in controls (30-month follow-up). While initial reports with Adriamycin were similarly favourable (Duchek 1980; Edsmyr et al. 1980; Jakse et al. 1981) more recent studies have not been able to confirm such findings when this agent was given in a maintenance regimen (Edsmyr et al. 1984; Pontes et al. 1984) or as a single instillation (Zincke et al. 1983). We are unaware of any studies reporting this degree of effectiveness against this lesion using instillations of either thiotepa (Koontz et al. 1981; Prout et al. 1983) or Epodyl. In another series, intravenous cyclophosphamide (1 g/m^2 IV every 3 weeks for 6 months and then every 6 weeks for 6 months) eliminated this lesion in eight of nine patients, although three also underwent external beam irradiation for concomitant invasive tumours (England et al. 1980). Of interest is that Jakse and Hofstädter (1981) noted reappearance of blood group antigens on the bladder mucosa in patients who responded to intravesical Adriamycin. In those in whom the atypia persisted, ABO antigens did not reappear.

Prospective studies with suitable controls and longer follow-up will be required before one can conclude that conservative management of carcinoma in situ is effective. However, preliminary results justify the inclusion of intravesical therapy in the treatment of this disease. At the UCLA School of Medicine, Los Angeles, patients with carcinoma in situ are offered weekly instillations of either Mitomycin C or BCG for 8–12 weeks after all visible tumour is resected, if no invasive disease is encountered. Cystoscopy, random bladder biopsies and bladder lavage cytological examination are repeated 3 months after the initial resection. If persistence of carcinoma in situ is confirmed, immediate cystectomy (with or without preoperative irradiation) is recommended. If no disease is detected, intravesical instillations are continued on a monthly basis, with repeat cystoscopy and cytological monitoring every 3 months. With this management, 14 of 17 patients (Brosman 1981; P. Walther, personal communication) have been spared cystectomy.

Chemotherapy of Invasive and/or Metastatic TCC

Once TCC has invaded the muscular layers of the bladder, the patient's prognosis, regardless of therapy, falls precipitously (Skinner and Kaufman 1978). The primary therapy for invasive bladder cancer is discussed in Chapter 9. However, there can be little argument that a combination of preoperative irradiation and cystectomy offers the best likelihood of local control, with local recurrence reported at less than 10% for T2 tumours and 15%–20% for T3 (Whitmore et al. 1977; Whitmore 1980). Distant spread, therefore, causes over two-thirds of mortality in patients so treated. Therapy beyond the pelvis is obviously needed for this group as well as for those patients who present with distant metastases. Metastases are often in sites where objective measures of extent of disease and responses to treatment are impracticable (Fetter et al. 1959). Most studies, therefore, are small Phase I and Phase II trials which use only historical controls.

In the following section we will review reports on systemic chemo- and immunotherapeutic agents which have shown some efficacy in patients with metastatic disease. We will then examine the role of these and other modalities as adjuvants to primary surgical treatment of potentially curable lesions (T2, T3, N0, N1; B1, B2, C, D1). Finally, we will discuss modalities available for management of patients with extravesical inoperable recurrences apparently confined to the pelvis, and for those patients with incurable disease who have intractable local symptoms.

Metastatic Disease

Single Agents

Several chemotherapeutic agents have been used as single-drug therapy for metastatic TCC. While other medications have been the subject of studies which report favourable results, we will limit our discussion to the five single agents which appear to demonstrate the greatest objective efficacy.

Doxorubicin Hydrochloride (Adriamycin). Original trials performed with this drug over ten years ago by Middleman et al. (1971) and Bonadonna et al. (1972) reported objective response rates of approximately 35% and overall (objective and subjective) responses of up to 55% (Frei et al. 1972) in patients with metastatic TCC. However, by 1977 oncologists were less enthusiastic, with Yagoda reporting an objective response rate of 16% (27% in patients who had not received prior chemotherapy) in individuals treated with intravenous boluses of 45–75 mg/m^2 every 3 weeks (not exceeding a total dose of 550 mg/m^2) at the Memorial Sloan Kettering Cancer Center, New York and 24% in a review of the literature (Yagoda 1977). Although Higby recently reported an objective response rate of 35% lasting at least 5 months (Higby 1980), he pointed out that the drug causes considerable gastrointestinal, mucosal and haematological toxic effects even when given in a dosage and schedule similar to that employed by Yagoda. However, cardiac damage, the major potentially fatal toxic effect, has been significantly reduced over the early experience (Frei et al. 1972).

Cyclophosphamide (Cytoxan). This alkylating agent has been used more often in combination therapy (see p. 249) than as a single medication for metastatic TCC, but in small non-randomised trials Merrin et al. (1975) and deKernion (1977), using 1–1.2 g/m^2 intravenously every 3 weeks, observed objective responses in 40% and 53% respectively, although in the former study some patients did not have metastatic disease. Despite the small number of patients involved, these results are closely parallel to those with a 38% remission rate summarised from the literature by Richards (1980). Unfortunately, because of its well-known complication of haemorrhagic cystitis, its haematological toxicity and the occasional reports of cyclophosphamide actually inducing bladder tumours (see p. 11), prolonged use of this agent is often inadvisable in patients with metastatic disease who have not had urinary diversions.

5-Fluorouracil. 5-FU, a pyrimidine antagonist, was the first widely used chemotherapy for advanced bladder cancer. The drug is usually given intravenously either daily for 3 days and then twice a week, or weekly at a dose of 500–600 mg/m^2 until toxicity occurs. Reports from over 20 years ago claimed a 67% (Moore et al. 1963) to 75% (Wilson 1960) objective remission rate in small non-controlled studies, although the criteria for patient selection and response were not detailed. However, in 1968 a cooperative study comparing 5-FU with placebo in patients with non-resectable bladder cancer failed to demonstrate an advantage for 5-FU therapy (Prout et al. 1968). This finding was supported by other small studies which were not nearly as well controlled (deKernion 1977). Nonetheless, claims of long-term survival in several patients have been made (Ansfield 1973), and recently reports have appeared of efficacy in 22% (Smalley et al. 1981) to 42% (Richards 1980) of patients.

Methotrexate. Methotrexate, the folic acid antagonist, is given in doses of either 0.5–1.0 mg/kg intravenously every week, or, more recently, 250 mg/m^2 IV every third week followed by citrovorum factor rescue. It has demonstrated a 26% objective response rate lasting a median of 6 months in 42 patients with metastatic bladder cancer (Natale et al. 1981), in whom most other chemotherapeutic regimens had failed. This objective response rate rose to 38% in patients with no prior chemotherapy. These results are in agreement with previous reports (Turner et al. 1977; Richards 1980) and indicate that one may expect responses in up to 38% of patients with no prior chemotherapy. Toxicity with these dosage schedules, however, is significant, for almost 75% of patients develop mucositis and 25% experience myelosuppression (Yagoda et al. 1980). This is easily managed with leucovorin (folinic acid) therapy.

cis-Dichlordiamide Platinum: *cis*-Platinum has produced objective overall response rates of 35% and rates as high as 50% for metastatic TCC in patients not previously treated with chemotherapy (Yagoda 1977). The agent is generally administered in a 50–100 mg intravenous infusion followed by induced diuresis weekly (D'Aoust et al. 1980) or every 3 weeks (Yagoda 1977). When the criterion of at least a 5-month duration of remission was applied, Herr found a 33% objective response rate. This included a 14% rate for complete remissions, all of which have lasted more than 1 year (Herr 1980). These data coincide with the findings of others (Soloway 1978; Merrin 1979; Higby 1980; Soloway et al. 1981b) with response rates varying from 35% to 42% (Yagoda 1981). In most reports dose-limiting renal toxicity (Higby 1980) and ototoxicity (D'Aoust 1980) were not inconsequential. Interestingly, Herr found that in all responding patients improvement was noted by the third treatment, indicating that *cis*-platinum can effectively induce tumour regression, but not answering whether further therapy is necessary to sustain remission in responding patients (Herr 1980). No randomised studies have compared DDP to methotrexate, but both of these drugs are effective against TCC and should be the single agents of choice unless contraindicated.

Combination Chemotherapy

To improve efficacy without increasing toxicity, many combinations of agents have been investigated. Considerable success has been reported with the combination of Adriamycin (40 mg/m^2 IV every third week to a total of 500 mg/m^2) and 5-FU (15–30 mg/kg per day on days 1, 2, and 3 every 3 weeks). Lindholm et al. (1980) and the EORTC Urological Group (Smith 1980) independently reported complete or partial remissions in approximately 40% of patients with measurable metastatic disease. All patients in one series experienced alopecia, nausea and diarrhoea (Lindholm et al. 1980). However, in a smaller but randomised study, Smalley et al. (1981) found no benefit with Adriamycin, 5-FU and cyclophosphamide compared with 5-FU alone. Similarly, when Williams et al. (1979) added *cis*-platinum to Adriamycin and 5-FU, the response rate (45%) was not significantly better than has been reported for *cis*-platinum alone.

Probably the greatest success with combination therapy has been claimed for intravenous administration every third week, of *cis*-platinum (60–100 mg/m^2) and cyclophosphamide (400–600 mg/m^2) with (Kedia et al. 1981; Logothetis 1981) or without (Yagoda 1977) Adriamycin (40–50 mg/m^2). This is known as the CISCA combination. Response rates have ranged from 52% (Logothetis 1981) to 82% (Kedia et al. 1981). In the study by Yagoda (1977), no benefit resulted from the addition of cyclophosphamide to Adriamycin, yet considerable improvement in

Table 10.2. Chemotherapy for metastatic TCC

Agents	Objective response
Single Agents	
Adriamycin	16% (Yagoda 1977)
	35% (Higby 1980)
Cyclophosphamide	38% (Richards 1979)
5-FU	Placebo (Prout et al. 1968)
	22% (Smalley 1981)
Methotrexate	26% (Natale et al. 1981)
	38% (Richards 1980)
cis-Platinum	33% (Herr 1980)
	42% (Yagoda 1981)
Combination	
Adriamycin+5-FU	15%[a] (Smalley 1981)
	42% (Smith 1980)
cis-Platinum+cyclophosphamide+ Adriamycin (CISCA)	52% (Logothetis 1981)
	82% (Kedia et al. 1981)
cis-Platinum+cyclophosphamide	61% (Yagoda 1977)
cis-Platinum+5-FU+Adriamycin	45% (Williams et al. 1979)

[a] Cyclophosphamide added to Adriamycin and 5-FU.

objective response was observed when cyclophosphamide was combined with *cis*-platinum (61% overall response rate compared to 35% for *cis*-platinum as a single agent). The advantage for the CISCA combination has persisted in a recent update by this group (Schwartz et al. 1983), although only a 45% complete and partial response rate was found for the three-drug combination compared with 33% for *cis*-platinum alone ($P<0.05$). Conversely, in a very small series in which only 53% of patients had measurable lesions, Oliver reported no difference between CISCA therapy versus methotrexate alone or *cis*-platinum alone in patients with advanced disease (Oliver 1980).

In summary, available data support claims for moderate efficacy of several agents in this disease (Table 10.2). Although reports exist of complete remissions lasting more than 1 year in patients treated with *cis*-platinum alone or in combination (Coates et al. 1981; Kedia et al. 1981; Logothetis 1981), much longer follow-up is needed to assess total impact on survival and cure. Phase III studies involving meaningful numbers of patients which compare different drugs and schedules are essential to clarify the true value of these and other agents, either alone or in combination.

Immunotherapy

Theoretical impetus for the role of immunotherapy in advanced bladder cancer arises from a variety of sources which purport to (1) demonstrate specific cellular (Bean et al. 1974; Bloom et al. 1974; Hakala et al. 1974) and humoral (Hakala et al. 1974; Elliot et al. 1978) immunity to TCC targets in the peripheral blood of patients with various stages of bladder cancer; and (2) identify a variety of tumour-associated antigens in the serum (Bowen 1978) and urine (Hollinshead 1978; Gozzo et al. 1980; Hewitt et al. 1982) of patients with bladder cancer and on human TCC cell lines using both heterologous rabbit antisera (Bloom and Brown 1980; Boxer et al. 1981) and murine monoclonal antibodies (Wright et al. 1980; Grossman 1983; Chopin et al. 1984; Fredet et al. 1984; Messing et al. 1984). However, the efficacy of immunological approaches to the treatment of patients with advanced bladder cancer remains unconfirmed. Attempts to augment pre-existing specific or non-specific antitumour immunity, or to induce cross-reactive immunity by systemic immunisation (via scarification) with microbial agents have been largely unsuccessful (Brosman 1980). Juillard attempted to stimulate the development of specific immunity by active intralymphatic immunisation with vaccines consisting of allogeneic TCC cell lines (G. Juillard 1982, personal communication). We are unaware at present of any but the most anecdotal responses in such patients and know of no prolonged complete remission in individuals with metastatic disease. Perhaps the reason for such poor results, despite scientific evidence which supports the concept of TCC as an immunogenic tumour, lies in the findings of Herr, who demonstrated in patients with advanced bladder cancer a population of suppressor cells, both in the blood (Herr 1980) and in draining pelvic lymph nodes (Herr et al. 1978), which were capable of abrogating the normal proliferative responsiveness of these same patients' peripheral blood lymphocytes.

Interferon. Another approach to treating patients with advanced bladder cancer employs various preparations of interferon. The impressive results of Ikic et al. (1981; see p. 70), who directly injected crude human leucocyte interferon into or near the tumour in several patients (including eight with superficial bladder cancer), have led to several trials using this immunomodulator in advanced disease. We are currently conducting a Phase II trial of alpha interferon in patients with metastatic TCC. Patients receive 3×10^6 IU administered intramuscularly from Monday to Friday for 15 days. Too few patients have been entered to assess response. Toxic effects with interferon preparations include transient chills and fever, malaise and nausea in most patients, and leucopenia and thrombocytopenia in those receiving higher dosages. Serum transaminase levels are elevated in 20% (G. Sarna 1982, personal communication).

Adjuvant Therapy

From a study of 107 autopsies of individuals with TCC, Jewett and Strong (1946) concluded that 80% of patients with muscular invasion should be curable by extensive local treatment (e.g. cystectomy), compared with only one-quarter of those with perivesical fat invasion. The fact that this potential curability has never been realised, regardless of the therapy employed (Skinner and Kaufman 1978), underscores the need for adjuvant therapies. Further, it can be inferred that most patients who develop metastases have tumour dissemination prior to treatment or develop it at the time of therapy since over two-thirds of those who die of bladder cancer have distant spread, and half of those who die do so within 18 months of presentation (Caldwell 1974).

Systemic Adjuvant Chemotherapy

The chemotherapeutic agents which have some efficacy in the treatment of metastatic bladder cancer are usually employed as adjuvants to aggressive local treatment of invasive disease. Unfortunately, owing to the 30%–50% objective response rates observed for metastatic disease, the considerable toxic effects of each regimen and the advanced age of the patients involved, who have recently undergone extensive local treatment, only very large prospective controlled studies can possibly determine whether available medications have a beneficial role as adjuvants. While primary treatments vary with protocols, the Southeastern Cancer Group is now using the CISCA combination (Durant 1980), and the NBCP Collaborative Group A is employing *cis*-platinum alone in similar patients (Cummings et al. 1979). Those eligible for chemotherapy have tumour present in the post-radiation therapy cystectomy specimen and/or positive pelvic lymph nodes confined to the region below the bifurcation of the iliac vessels. These studies may represent the first randomised prospective trials with suitable controls, and results are eagerly awaited. Regrettably, patient non-compliance has delayed completion of these studies and analysis of results. This impediment raises questions about the feasibility of either regimen in non-academic clinical environments.

In non-randomised studies, patients with T3 disease treated by external beam irradiation have experienced little or no benefit from 5-FU adjuvant therapy, either alone (Duchek et al. 1980) or in combination with Adriamycin (Richards 1980). However, Hall and Turner (1980) reported 100% disease free survival of patients with T2–T3 tumours 24 months after partial cystectomy and adjuvant high dose methotrexate (2000 mg with leucovorin rescue every 3 weeks for 6 months). Based upon these findings and its efficacy in metastatic disease, we feel that an extensive trial of methotrexate adjuvant therapy is indicated.

Local Adjuvants for Invasive Cancer

Following irradiation and radical cystectomy for invasive bladder carcinoma, less than one-fifth of patients develop local recurrences (Mohiuddin et al. 1982). It is thus unlikely that extending the field or intensity of regional treatment will markedly reduce the incidence of distant metastases and favourably affect survival. Such hypotheses were recently confirmed in a Phase I study reported by Jacobs and Lawson (1982), who employed intra-arterial Adriamycin combined with intravesical hyperthermia (up to 45°) followed 3–5 weeks later by cystectomy. Of nine patients with extensive pelvic involvement, only one was alive without disease at 1 year, despite the addition of radiation therapy and/or intravenous *cis*-platinum in 3 patients. Tumour stage was reduced in only one patient. These findings are similar to those of Uyama et al. (1980), who reported stage reduction in only 15% of patients following intra-arterial Adriamycin treatment. Since pelvic recurrence is no longer the major cause of treatment failure in bladder cancer, it is unlikely that any regional adjuvant regimens will improve survival.

Conversely, intra-arterial infusions of a variety of agents, including 5-FU (Nevin et al. 1973; Confer 1977), Mitomycin C (Ogata et al. 1973), methotrexate (Sullivan 1962), and *cis*-platinum (Samuels et al. 1980), in patients with unresectable disease have effected temporary tumour regression in up to 60% of patients. This therapy, however, is not without potential complications, including necrosis of buttocks and perineal skin and transient sciatica (deKernion et al. 1978). Furthermore, because of the bladder's rich and bilateral arterial supply and venous drainage, systemic toxicity from such administration is not uncommon. Thus, we favour employing high-dose systemic chemotherapy with an agent of likely efficacy (e.g. methotrexate, *cis*-platinum) prior to resorting to local infusion (except when anatomical conditions permit truly selective administrations).

In the presence of incapacitating vesical haemorrhage from cyclophosphamide therapy, radiation-induced cystitis or non-resectable bladder tumours, intravesical instillations of 4% formalin will stop bleeding in most patients (Fair 1974). A general or regional anaesthetic is required for pain control. Complications are rare in the absence of vesicoureteric reflux, although total bladder necrosis has been observed in one patient (Bergsma and Leary 1976). Our experience has been favourable, but we have often had to repeat the instillations two or three times to control bladder haemorrhage (see Chap. 11, p. 265).

Squamous Carcinoma

Squamous carcinoma represents an uncommon form of bladder cancer. By far the largest experience with this disease has been accumulated in Egypt, where, as a result of chronic bladder infections with *Schistosoma haematobium*, it is the most common solid tumour in males (Ghoneim and Awaad 1980). Hexamethylmelamine is an inhibitor of nucleic acid synthesis structurally related to alkylating agents (Sarna 1979). In an oral dose of 8 mg/kg per day, it produced objective partial remissions in 38% of patients with locally unresectable, recurrent or metastatic disease (Gad-el Mawla et al. 1978). In similar groups, single agent trials of methotrexate, VM-26, Bleomycin and Adriamycin were far less effective (Gad-el Mawla et al. 1978; Ghoneim and Awaad 1980). Since, unlike TCC, the vast majority of patients who died did so as the result of pelvic extension of the tumour rather than distant metastases (Ghoneim and Awaad 1980), regional therapeutic perfusions may be appropriate as adjuvants to extirpative surgery as well as in the treatment of unresectable disease.

Adenocarcinoma

Adenocarcinoma of the bladder, either arising from urachal remnants or as a primary tumour, is as rare as squamous carcinoma (Kramer et al. 1979). While tumours of the urachal remnant may be manageable by partial cystectomy, considerable debate exists regarding the role of radical cystectomy. We have personally never cured a patient with this tumour by partial cystectomy, possibly because of diffuse extension of tumour cells in the lymphatics on the outer surface of the bladder. Tumours arising in adenomatous rests or metaplastic tissue are best treated by cystectomy (Jones et al. 1980). As with other forms of bladder cancer, almost all survivors have had stage A or B disease (Kramer et al. 1979; Jones et al. 1980). While systemic chemotherapy has been given to patients with advanced lesions, we are unaware of reports claiming efficacy for any particular regimen. Because of the rarity of this disease, and the absence of a unique localised reservoir of patients as is found with squamous cell carcinoma, meaningful therapeutic trials will have to be performed on a cooperative basis.

Chemosensitivity Assays

From the foregoing discussion regarding causes of treatment failure, it is clear that considerable advances in systemic therapy will have to be made before improvements in patient survival are realised. At present, the selection of chemotherapeutic agents for bladder (and virtually all other) cancers remains essentially empirical. Since 50% of patients with clinically non-metastatic invasive transitional cell carcinoma who die expire within 18 months of diagnosis, little time is available for prolonged therapeutic trials. The development of rapid methods to select the proper regimen for each individual's tumour is therefore desirable. While such methods are still experimental, a review of the more promising approaches is pertinent.

In Vitro Tumour Stem Cell (Clonogenic) Assay

The theoretical basis for the clonogenic or soft agar assay is the hypothesis that tumour cells which are capable of dividing most effectively are likely to be those which demonstrate a hallmark of in vitro malignancy: loss of anchorage dependence (Montesano et al. 1977). These cells will therefore survive and undergo mitoses when suspended in soft agar. Colony formation in such a system indeed correlates well with in vivo tumourgenicity when tumour cells are injected into immunosuppressed animals, such as nude mice (Shin et al. 1975). In the assay for leukaemic cells described by Hamburger and Salmon (1977) and subsequently modified by Stanisic et al. (1980a, b) and others (von Hoff et al. 1980; Lieber and Kovach 1981; Tannock 1981) for solid tumours including TCC, tumour cells are incubated with various chemotherapeutic agents (administered in clinically realistic concentrations) for short periods and plated in soft agar in the absence of chemotherapeutic drug and inhibition of subsequent colony formation is recorded. It has been reported that in over three-quarters of patients with TCC a sufficient specimen can be obtained to allow for statistically acceptable testing of various medications. While retrospective and non-controlled prospective studies demonstrate reasonable correlation between in vivo and in vitro findings (von Hoff et al. 1980), to date the selection of agents predicted by this assay has not resulted in improved survival rates for any tumour (D. D. von Hoff 1981, personal communication).

The assay presents many technical problems, including difficulty in accurately quantifying colonies and reliably achieving tumour growth. In addition, heterogeneity exists within each tumour and between the primary lesion and metastases (Fidler 1982). Other problems include formation of colonies by non-malignant cells (D. D. von Hoff 1981, personal communication) cell-cycle dependence and need for metabolic activation of some drugs (Tannock 1978), and the confounding fact that the cells which are capable of dividing best (and hence presumably grow best in agar) are not necessarily those which preferentially metastasise (Hanna 1981).

In Vivo Assay

Owing to the difficulties cited, efforts have been made to develop in vivo assays which, while being far more cumbersome and costly, more closely approximate the clinical situation. Since these systems require survival of xenogeneic (human) tumour cells in rodent hosts for from several days to weeks, some form of immunosuppression is required to determine which chemotherapeutic agents impede tumour growth. These methods have ranged from use of (relatively) immunologically protected sites for implantation (Bogden et al. 1982) to employing very young mice who are functionally athymic (i.e. nude mice; Hanna 1982), or have been thymectomised (Tannock 1981). The first model permits direct inspection of solid tumour xenografts, thus avoiding artefacts produced by creating single-cell suspensions. The last two are particularly promising for detecting agents which inhibit vascular metastases, and thus may be useful in the selection of adjuvant systemic chemotherapy following cystectomy.

Acknowledgement

The authors wish to thank Ms. Julie Hayward for her editorial research and assistance, which greatly facilitated the writing of this chapter.

References

Alroy J, Teramura K, Miller AW, Pauli B, Gottesman JE, Flanagan M, Davidsohn I, Weinstein, RS (1978) Iso-antigens A, B, and H in urinary bladder carcinoma following radiotherapy. Cancer 41: 1739–1745

Althausen AF, Prout GR, Jr, Daly JJ (1976). Non-invasive papillary carcinoma of the bladder associated with carcinoma in situ. J Urol 116: 575–580

Ansfield F (1973) Treatment of tumours of the urinary tract. In: Ansfield F (ed) Chemotherapy of malignant neoplasms. Thomas, Springfield, Ill, pp 289–290

Antonaci S, Piccinno A, Lucivero G (1981) Effect of BCG cell-mediated cytotoxicity in bladder cancer patients following surgical treatment. Tumori 67: 177–182

Asaki T, Matsumura Y, Takahashi T, Yoshimoto J, Kaneshige T, Fujita Y, Ohmori H (1980) The effects of intravesical instillation of thiotepa on the recurrence rate of bladder tumours. Acta Med Okayama 321: 43–49

Banks MD, Pontes JE, Izbicki RM, Pierce JM (1977) Topical instillation of doxorubicin hydrochloride in the treatment of recurring superficial transitional cell carcinoma of the bladder. J Urol 118: 757–760

Bean MA, Pees H, Fogh J, Grabstald H, Oettgen HF (1974) Cytotoxicity of lymphocytes from patients with cancer of the urinary bladder. Detection by 3H-proline microcytotoxicity test. Int J Cancer 14: 186–197

Bergman S, Javadpour N (1978) The cell surface antigens A, B, O(H) as an indicator of malignant potential in stage A bladder carcinoma: a preliminary report. J Urol 119: 49–51

Bergsma CJ, Leary FJ (1976) Total bladder necrosis following intravesical formalin. In: Proceedings of the Annual Meeting of the American Urological Association, North Central Section, Annual Meeting, Palm Beach, Florida, 1976

Billiau A (1981) The clinical value of interferon as antitumor agents. Eur J Cancer Clin Oncol 17: 949–967

Bloom ET, Brown DE (1980) Detection of antigenic differences and similarities between human transitional cell carcinoma cell lines using rabbit antisera. Urol Res 8: 5–13

Bloom ET, Ossorio RC, Brosman SA (1974) Cell mediated cytotoxicity against human bladder cancer. Int J Cancer 14: 326–332

Bogden AE, Cobb WR, LePage DJ (1982) An in vitro method for testing chemotherapeutic agents against first transplant generation human tumor xenografts. In: Fidler IJ, White RJ (eds) Design of models for testing cancer therapeutic agents. Van Nostrand Reinhold, New York, pp 175–184

Bonadonna G, Monfardini S, deLena M, Fossati-Bellani F, Baretta G (1972) Trials with Adriamycin. Results of 3 years study. In: Carter SK, DiMarcos A, Ghione M et al. (eds) International symposium on Adriamycin. Springer, Berlin Heidelberg New York, pp 139–152

Bowen JG (1978) Transitional cell carcinoma: circulation tumor antigen correlated with presence/absence of tumor (leukocyte migration assay). Natl Cancer Inst Mongr 49: 245–247

Boxer RJ, Sofen H, Saxon A (1981) The detection of transitional cell bladder cancer antigen on established cell lines. Invest Urol 19: 70–74

Boyd PJR, Burnand KG (1974) Site of bladder tumor recurrence. Lancet II: 1290–1292

Bracken RB, Johnson DE, Von Eschenbach AC, Swanson DA, DeFuria D, Crooke S (1980) Role of intravesical Mitomycin C in the management of superficial bladder tumors. Urology 16: 11–15

Brosman S (1980) Immunotherapy in bladder cancer. In: Pavone-Macaluso M, Smith PH, Edsmyr F (eds) Bladder tumors and other topics in urological oncology. Plenum, New York, pp 166–170

Brosman S, Dorey F, Fahey J (1981) Intravesical BCG in superficial bladder cancer. In: Proceedings of the 7th Annual NBCP Investigator's Workshop. Hershey, Pennsylvania, June 1981

Burnand KG, Boyd PJR, Mayo MF, Shuttleworth KED, Lloyd-Davies RW (1976) Single dose intravesical thiotepa as an adjuvant to cystodiathermy in the treatment of transitional cell carcinoma. Br J Urol 48: 55–59

Byar DP (1980) The Veterans Administration study of chemo prophylaxis for recurrent stage I bladder tumors: comparisons of placebo, pyridoxine and topical thiotepa. In: Pavone-Macaluso M, Smith PH, Edsmyr R (eds) Bladder tumors and other topics in urological oncology. Plenum, New York, pp 363–370

Caldwell WL (1974) Carcinoma of the urinary bladder. JAMA 229: 1643

Caldwell WL (1976) Radiotherapy: definitive, integrated and palliative therapy. Urol Clin North Am 3: 129–148

Camacho F, Pinsky C, Kerr D, Whitmore W, Oettgen H (1980) Treatment of superficial bladder cancer with intravesical BCG. Proc Am Soc Clin Oncol 21: 359

Chasko SB, Keuhnelian JG, Gutowski WT, Gray AF (1980) Spindle cell cancer of the bladder during cyclophosphamide therapy for Wegener's granulomatosis. Am J Surg Pathol 4: 191–196

Chodak GW, Straus FW, Schoenberg HW (1981) Simultaneous occurrence of transitional, squamous and adenocarcinoma of the bladder after 15 years of cyclophosphamide therapy. J Urol 125: 424–426

Chopin DK, Bubbers JE, deKernion JB, Fahey JL (1984) Tumor associated antigens (TA A) on human bladder cancer defined by monoclonal antibodies. In: Proceedings of 10th Annual NBCP Investigators' Workshop, Sarasota, Florida, 4–7 January, 1984

Coates AS, Golovsky D, Freedman A (1981) Prolonged remission in recurrent bladder cancer after chemotherapy with *cis*-platinum. Med J Austr 1: 533–534

Cole P (1975) Lower urinary tract. In: Schottenfeld D (ed) Cancer epidemiology and prevention. Thomas, Springfield, Ill, pp 233–262

Colleen S, Hellsten AE, Lindholm CE (1980) Intracavitary Epodyl for multiple, non-invasive, highly differentiated bladder tumors. Scan J Urol Nephrol 14: 43–45

Collste L, Berlin T, Gronberg-Ohman I, Von Garrelts B, Wijkstrom H (1980) Long-term intracavitary Epodyl in multiple or extensive papillary tumors of the urinary bladder. In: Pavone-Maculoso M, Smith PH, Edsmyr R (eds) Bladder tumors and other topics in urological oncology. Plenum, New York, pp 335–336

Confer D, Smith RB, Gillespie L (1977) Dramatic palliation for painful fixed bladder squamous cell carcinoma with 5-fluorouracil. J Urol 118: 483–484

Cooper PH, Waisman J, Johnston WH, Skinner DG (1973) Severe atypia of transitional epithelium and carcinoma of the urinary bladder. Cancer 31: 1055–1060

Cox CE, Cass AS, Boyce WH (1969) Bladder cancer: a 26 year review. J Urol 101: 550–558

Cummings KB, Shipley WU, Einstein AE et al. (1979) Current concepts in the management of patients with deeply invasive bladder carcinoma. Semin Oncol 6: 220–228

Daly JJ (1976) Carcinoma in situ of the urothelium. Urol Clin North Am 3: 87–105

D'Aoust JC, Archambautt WA, Merrin CE, Rosenbaum PF, Crook ST (1980) Analysis of toxicities associated with long-term administration of *cis*-platinum to patients with urogenital tumors. Proc Am Assoc Cancer Res 21: 355

Decenzo JM, Ledbetter GW (1976) The interaction of host immunocompetence and tumor aggressiveness in superficial bladder carcinoma. J Urol 115: 262–263

DeFuria MD, Bracken RB, Johnson DE, Soloway MS, Merrin CE, Morgan LR, Miller HC, Crooke ST (1980) Phase I-II study of Mitomycin C topical therapy for low grade, low stage transitional cell carcinoma of the bladder: an interim report. Cancer Treat Rep 64: 225–230

deKernion JB (1977) The chemotherapy of advanced bladder carcinoma. Cancer Res 37: 2771–2774

deKernion JB, Skinner DG (1978) Epidemiology, diagnosis and staging of bladder cancer. In: Skinner DG, deKernion JB (eds) Genitourinary cancer. Saunders, Philadelphia, pp 213–231

deKernion JB, Stewart BH, Yagoda A (1978) Treatment of advanced bladder cancer. In: Skinner DG, deKernion JB (eds) Genitourinary cancer. Saunders, Philadelphia, pp 284–294

Droller JJ (1980) Transitional cell carcinoma: an overview. Urol Clin North Am 7: 731–733

Duchek M (1980) Local treatment of uroepithelial bladder tumors with Adriamycin. In: Pavone-Macaluso M, Smith PH, Edsmyr F (eds) Bladder tumors and other topics in urological oncology. Plenum, New York, pp 323–326

Duchek M, Edsmyr F, Nasland I (1980) 5-Fluorouracil in the treatment of recurrent cancer of the urinary bladder. In: Pavone-Macaluso M, Smith PH, Edsmyr F (eds) Bladder tumors and other topics in urological oncology. Plenum, New York, pp 399–400

Durant JR (1980) Phase III adjuvant chemotherapy with cytoxan-Adriamycin-*cis*-platinum for resected transitional cell bladder carcinoma. In: Proceedings of the 6th NBCP Annual Meeting

Edsmyr F, Berlin T, Boman J, Duchek M, Esposti PL, Gustavson H, Wikstrom H (1980) Intravesical therapy with Adriamycin in patients with superficial bladder tumors. In: Pavone-Macaluso M, Smith PH, Edsmyr F (eds) Bladder tumors and other topics in urological oncology. Plenum, New York, pp 321–322

Edsmyr F, Andersson L, Esposti P (1984) Intravesical chemotherapy of carcinoma in situ in bladder cancer. Urology (Suppl) 23: 37–39

Ek A, Colleen S (1980) Treatment of multiple non-invasive bladder tumours with intravesical Epodyl. In: Pavone-Macaluso M, Smith PH, Edsmyr F (eds) Bladder tumors and other topics in urological oncology. Plenum, New York, pp 337–342

Elliott AY, Dombrovski S, Fraley EE (1978) Transitional cell carcinoma: fluorescent antibody binding to tumor cells. Natl Cancer Inst Mongr 49: 23

England HR, Molland EA, Oliver RT, Blandy JP (1980) Flat carcinoma in situ of the bladder treated by systemic cyclophosphamide—a preliminary report. In: Pavone-Macaluso J, Smith PH, Edsmyr F (eds) Bladder tumors and other topics in urological oncology. Plenum, New York, pp 371–376

Esquivel EL, Mackenzie AR, Whitmore WF (1965) Treatment of bladder tumors by instillation of thiotepa, Actinomycin D, or 5-fluorouracil. Invest Urol 2: 381

Fair WR (1974) Formalin in the treatment of massive bladder hemorrhage. Urology 3: 573–577

Fetter TB, Bogaev JH, McCuskey B, Seres JL (1959) Carcinoma of the bladder: sites of metastases. J Urol 81: 746–748

Fidler IJ (1982) The role of host factors and tumor heterogeneity in the testing of therapeutic agents. In: Fidler IJ, White RJ (eds) Desig. of models for testing cancer therapeutic agents. Van Nostrand Reinhold, New York, pp 239–247

Field AK, Tytell AA, Lampson GP, Hilleman MR (1967) Inducers of interferon and h st resistance. II. Multistranded synthetic polyneucleotide complexes. Proc Natl Acad Sci USA 58: 1004–1010

Fradet Y, Cordon-Cardo C, Whitmore WF, Old LJ (1984) Definition of human bladder tumor subsets with monoclonal antibodies to tumor associated antigens. In: Proceedings of the 10th Annual NBCP Investigators Workshop. Sarasota, Florida, 4–7 January, 1984, p 37

Frei E, Luce JK, Middleman E (1972) Clinical trials of Adriamycin. In: Carter SK, DiMarco A, Ghione A et al. (eds) International symposium on Adriamycin. Springer, Berlin Heidelberg New York, pp 153–164

Friedell GH (1976) Carcinoma, carcinoma in situ and "early lesions" of the uterine cervix and urinary bladder: introduction and definitions. Cancer Res 36: 2482

Gad-el Mawla N, Muggia PM, Hamza MR, El-Morsi B, Sherif M, Mansour MA, Khafagy M, El Sebai IT (1978) Chemotherapeutic management of carcinoma of the bilharzial bladder. A Phase II trial with hexamethylmelamine and VM-26. Cancer Treat Rep 62: 993–996

Gammelgaard PA, Morgensen P, Lindbeck F (1980) Bladder instillation of Adriamycin in multiple recurrent noninvasive papillomatous bladder tumours. In: Pavone-Macaluso M, Smith PH, Edsmyr F (eds) Bladder tumors and other topics in urological oncology. Plenum, New York, pp 329–331

Garnick B, Scade D, Israel M, Maxwell B, Richie JP (1984) Intravesical doxorubicin for prophylaxis in management of recurrent superficial bladder carcinoma. J Urol 131: 43–46

Gavrell GJ, Lewis RW, Meehan WL, LeBlanc GA (1978) Intravesical thiotepa in the immediate postoperative period in patients with recurrent transitional cell carcinoma of the bladder. J Urol 120: 410–411

Ghoneim MA, and Awaad HK (1980) Results of treatment in carcinoma of the bilharzial bladder. J Urol 123: 850–852

Gonwa TA, Corbett WT, Schey HM, Buckalew VM (1980) Analgesic-associated nephropathy and transitional cell carcinoma of the urinary tract. Ann Intern Med 93: 249–252

Gozzo JJ, Cronin WJ, O'Brien P, Monaco AP (1980) Detection of tumor associated antigens in the urine of patients with bladder cancer. J Urol 125: 804–807

Glucksman MA (1980) Bladder carcinoma after cyclophosphamide therapy. (Letter to the Editor). Urology 16: 553

Green DF, Robinson MRG, Glashan R, Newling D, Dalesio O, Smith PH (1984) Does intravesical chemotherapy prevent invasive bladder cancer? J Urol 131: 33–35

Grossman HB (1983) Hybridoma antibodies reactive with human bladder carcinoma cell surface antigens. J Urol 130: 610–615

Hakala TR, Lange PH, Castro AB, Elliott A, Fraley EE (1974) Antibody induction of lymphocyte mediated cytoxicity against human transitional cell carcinomas of the gentitourinary tract. Cancer 34: 1929–1934

Hall RR (1980a) Intravesical hyperthermia for transitional cell carcinoma of the bladder. In: Pavone-Macaluso M, Smith PH, Edsmyr F (eds) Bladder tumors and other topics in urological oncology. Plenum, New York, pp 267–270

Hall RR (1980b) Methotrexate therapy for multiple T1 category bladder carcinoma. In: Pavone-Macaluso M, Smith PH, Edsymr F (eds) Bladder tumors and other topics in urological oncology. Plenum, New York, pp 337–380

Hall RR, Turner AG (1980) Methotrexate treatment for advanced bladder cancer. A review after 6 years. Br J Urol 52: 403

Hamburger AW, Salmon SE (1977) Primary bioassay of human tumor stem cells. Science 197: 461–463

Hanna N (1981) Preparation of tumor cells for in vivo drug sensitivity testing. In: Proceedings of the UCLA Department of Microbiology and Immunology Workshop No 33, Los Angeles, California, 14–15 May, 1981

Hanna N (1982) Nude mice as recipients for syngeneic, allogeneic and xenogeneic neoplasms. In:

Fidler IJ, White RJ (eds) Design of models for testing cancer therapeutic agents. Van Nostrand Reinhold, New York, pp 165–174

Herberman RB (1980) Summary—augmentation of NK activity. In: Herberman RB (ed) Natural cell mediated immunity against tumors. New York, Academic, pp 707–719

Herr HW (1980) Diamminedichloride platinum II in the treatment of advanced bladder cancer. J Urol 123: 853–855

Herr HW, Bean MA, Whitmore WF (1978) Mixed leukocyte culture reactivity of lymph node cells regional to transitional cell carcinoma of the bladder. Natl Cancer Inst Monogr 49: 177–181

Herr HW, Pinsky CM, Whitmore WF, Oettgen HF, Melamed MR (1983) Intravesical BCG therapy of superficial bladder tumors. In: Proceedings of the 78th Annual Meeting of the American Urological Association, Las Vegas, Nevada, 19 April, 1983

Hewitt CW, Shultz SM, Cole J, Miller JB, Martin DC (1982) Identification of bladder-cancer associated antigens by two dimensional gel immuno-electrophoresis. In: Proceedings of the 77th Annual Meeting of the American Urological Association, Kansas City, Missouri, 1982

Higby DJ (1980) Chemotherapeutic management of bladder cancer. In: Aisner J, Chang P (eds) Cancer treatment research. Developments in oncology series, vol 2. Martinus Nijhoff, The Hague, pp 142–152

Hollinshead AC (1978) Preliminary studies of sera and urine from patients with bladder cancer. Natl Cancer Inst Monogr 49: 193–198

Hollister D, Coleman M (1980) Hematologic effects of intravesical thiotepa for bladder carcinoma. JAMA 244: 2065–2067

Howe GR, Burch JO, Miller AD, Cook GM, Esteves J, Morrison B, Gordon P, Chambers LW, Fodor G, Winsor GM (1980) Tobacco use, occupation, coffee, various nutrients, and bladder cancer. J Natl Cancer Inst 64: 701–713

Ikic D, Maricic Z, Oresic V, Rode B, Nola P, Smudj K, Knezevic M, Jusic D, Soos E (1981) Application of human leukocyte interferon in patients with urinary bladder papillomatosis, breast cancer and melanoma. Lancet I: 1022–1024

Jacobi GH, Kurth KH, Klipper KF, Hohenfellner R (1979) On the biological behavior of T1 transitional cell tumor of the urinary bladder and initial results of the prophylactic use of topical Adriamycin under controlled and randomized conditions. In: Diagnosis and treatment of superficial bladder tumors. Motedison, Stockholm, pp 83–94

Jacobs SE, Lawson RK (1982) Pathological effects of precystectomy therapy with combination of doxorubicin hydrochloride and local bladder hyperthermia for bladder cancer. J Urol 127: 43–47

Jakse G, Hofstädter F (1981) ABH antigenicity of in situ carcinoma of the urinary bladder during intracavity treatment with doxorubicin hydrochloride. Urol Res 9: 153–159

Jakse G, Hofstädter F, Marberger H (1981) Intracavitary doxorubicin hydrochloride therapy for carcinoma in situ of the bladder. J Urol 125: 185–190

Jewett HJ, Strong GH (1946) Infiltrating carcinoma of the bladder. Relation of depth of penetration of the bladder wall to incidence of local extension and metastases. J Urol 55: 366–372

Jones WA, Gibbons RP, Correa RJ, Cummings KB, Mason JT (1980) Primary adenocarcinoma of the bladder. Urology 15: 119–122

Kedia KR, Gibbons C, Persky L (1981) The management of advanced bladder carcinoma. J Urol 125: 655–658

Kemeny N, Yagoda A, Wang Y, Field K, Wrobleski H, Whitmore W (1981) Randomized trial of standard therapy with or without poly I:C in patients with superficial bladder cancer. Cancer 48: 2154–2157

Koontz WW (1979) Intravesical chemotherapy and chemoprevention of superficial, low grade, low stage bladder carcinoma. Semin Oncol 6: 217–219

Koontz WW, Prout GR Jr, Smith W, Frable WJ, Minnis JE (1981) The use of intravesical thiotepa in the management of non-invasive carcinoma of the bladder. J Urol 125: 307–312

Koontz WW, Heney N, Schmidt JD, Soloway M, Penick GD, Ahmed S, Prout G (1983) The ablative effect of intravesical Mitomycin C for thiotepa failures. In: Proceedings of the 78th Annual Meeting of the American Urological Association, Las Vegas, Nevada, 19 April, 1983

Koss LG (1975) Tumors of the urinary bladder. In: Koss (ed) Atlas of tumor pathology, fascicle 11, 2nd ser. Armed Forces Institute of Pathology, Washington DC

Koss LG (1979) Tumors of the urinary tract and prostate. In: Koss LG (ed) Diagnostic cytology and its histological basis, 3rd edn. Lippincott, Philadelphia, p 684

Kramer SA, Bredael J, Croker BP, Paulson DF, Glenn JF (1979) Primary non-urachal adenocarcinoma of the bladder. J Urol 121: 278–281

Kurth KH, Tunn U, Ay R, Debruyne F, dePauw M, Sylvester R, Tenkate FW (1983) Phase II chemotherapy with Adriamycin or ethoglucid (Epodyl) for resected Ta and T1 papillary carcinoma of the bladder. In: Proceedings of the 78th Annual Meeting of the American Urological Association, Las Vegas, Nevada, 19 April, 1983

Lamm DL, Thor DE, Winters WD, Stogdill VO, Radwin H (1981) BCG immunotherapy of bladder cancer: inhibition of tumor recurrence and associated immune responses. Cancer 48: 82–86

Lange PH, Limas C, Fraley EE (1978) Tissue blood-group antigens and prognosis in low stage transitional cell carcinoma of the bladder. J Urol 119: 52–55

Larsen J (1980) Inactivation of Epodyl in aluminium foil cups as a cause of ineffective treatment of non-invasive bladder tumors. Scan J Urol Nephrol 14: 239–242

Lieber MM, Kovach JS (1981) Soft agar clonogenic assay for primary human renal carcinoma: in vitro chemotherapeutic drug sensitivity testing. In: Proceedings of the 76th Annual Meeting of the American Urological Association, Boston, Maryland, 1981

Lindholm CE, Mattson W, Langeland P, Gunning I (1980) 5-Fluorouracil and Adriamycin in locally recurrent and/or metastatic bladder cancer. In: Pavone-Macaluso M, Smith PH, Edsmyr F (eds) Bladder tumors and other topics in urological oncology. Plenum, New York, pp 391–394

Logothetis CT (1981) CISCA chemotherapy for bladder cancer. Cancer Bull 33: 79–80

Malling N, Sorensen SS (1980) Adjuvant thiotepa in the treatment of bladder papillomata. A prospective randomized experiment (Abstr). Ugeskr Laeger 142: 1678–1679

Martinez-Piñeiro JA (1980) Introduction to immunology and immunotherapy of bladder tumors. In: Pavone-Macaluso M, Smith PH, Edsmyr F (eds) Bladder tumors and other topics in urological oncology. Plenum, New York, pp 131–134

Matsumoto K, Kakizoe T, Mikuriya S, Tanaka T, Kondo I, Umegaki Y (1981) Clinical evaluation of intraoperative radiotherapy for carcinoma of the urinary bladder. Cancer 47: 509–513

Melloni D, Pavone-Macaluso M (1980) Intravesical treatment of superficial urinary bladder tumors with Adriamycin. In: Pavone-Macaluso M, Smith PH, Esmyr F (eds) Bladder tumors and other topics in urological oncology. Plenum, New York, pp 317–320

Merrin CE (1979) Treatment of genitourinary tumors with *cis*-dichlorodiammineplatinum (II): experience in 250 patients. Cancer Treat Rep 63: 1570–1584

Merrin CE, Cartagena R, Wajsman Z, Baumgartner G, Murphy GP (1975) Chemotherapy of bladder carcinoma with cyclophosphamide and Adriamycin. J Urol 114: 884–887

Messing EM, Bubbers JE, Whitmore KE, deKernion JB, Fahey JL (1984) Murine hybridoma antibodies to human transitional cell carcinoma. J Urol (in press)

Middleman E, Luce J, Frei E (1971) Clinical trials with Adriamycin. Cancer 28: 844–850

Mishima T, Oda K, Murata S, Ooe H, Mori Y, Takahashi T (1975) Mitomycin C bladder instillation therapy for bladder tumors. J Urol 114: 217–219

Mohiuddin M, Strong GH, Mulholland SG (1982) Combined pre and postoperative adjuvant radiotherapy for bladder cancer. Urology 19: 135–138

Moore G, Bross ID, Ausman R, Nadler S, Jones R, Slack N, Reimm A (1963) Effects of 5-fluorouracil in 389 patients with cancer. Cancer Chemother Rep 27: 67–69

Montesano R, Devron C, Kuroki T, Saint Vincent L, Handleman S, Sanford KK, Defeo D, Weinstein IB (1977) Test for malignant transformation of rat liver cells in culture: cytology, growth in soft agar, and production of plasminogen activator. J Natl Cancer Inst 59: 1651–1658

Morales A (1980) Treatment of carcinoma in situ of the bladder with BCG: Phase II trial. Cancer Immunol Immunother 9: 69–72

Morales A, Ersil A (1979) Prophylaxis of recurrent bladder cancer with Bacillus-Calmette-Guérin in cancer of the genitourinary tract. In: Johnson DE, Samuels ML (eds) Proceedings of the University of Texas Systems Cancer Center M D Anderson Hospital and Tumor Institute, 23rd Annual Conference in Cancer, Houston, Texas, November 1978. Raven, New York, p 121

Morales A, Ottenhof P, Emerson L (1981) Treatment of residual non-infiltrating bladder cancer with Bacillus Calmette-Gúerin. J Urol 125: 649–651

Moriyama N, Ito K (1980) Light and electron microscopic changes in bladder tumor cells after intravesical instillation and hyperthermic vesical irrigation of Bleomycin (Abstr). Nippon, Hinyokika Gakkai Zasshi 71: 1371–1380

Morrison AS, Buring JE, Verhouk WG, Aoki K, Leck I, Ohno Y, Obata K (1984) International study of smoking and bladder cancer. J Urol 131: 650–654

Murphy WM, Soloway MS, Crabtree WM (1981) The morphologic effects of Mitomycin C in mammalian urinary bladder. Cancer 47: 2567–2574

Nagata K (1980) Studies on the absorption of anticancer agents through the bladder—basis of instillation therapy—III. Urinary excretion and vesical tissue concentration of instilled Adriamycin in patients with bladder cancer (Abstr). Hinyokika Kiyo 26: 983–988

Nakajima K, Hisazumi H, Uchibayashi T, Naito K, Misaki T, Kuroda K, Miyazaki K, Fujita Y, Taya T, Kameda K (1980) A combination therapy of hyperthermia and Bleomycin for bladder cancer

(Abstr). Hinokika Kiyo 26: 1153–1161

Natale RB, Yagoda A, Watson RC, Whitmore WF, Blumenreich M, Braun DW (1981) Methotrexate: an active drug in bladder cancer. Cancer 47: 1246–1250

Needles B, Blumenreich M, Yagoda A, Sogani P, Whitmore WF (1981) Intravesical *cis*-platinum for superficial bladder cancer. Proc Am Assoc Cancer Res 22: 158, 625

Nevin JE, Melnick I, Baggerly JT, Hoffman A, Landes RR, Easley C (1973) The continuous arterial infusion of 5-fluorouracil as a therapeutic adjunct in the treatment of carcinoma of the bladder and prostate. Cancer 31: 138–144

Nielsen HV, Thybo E (1979) Epodyl treatment of bladder tumors. Scan J Urol Nephrol 13: 59–63

Ogata J, Migita N, Nakamura T (1973) Treatment of carcinoma of the bladder by infusion of the anticancer agent (Mitomycin C) via the internal iliac artery. J Urol 110: 667–670

Ogawa H, Onodera Y, Watanabe M, Higaki Y, Yoshida H, Imamura K, Sugiyama Y (1980) Clinical effect of intravesical instillation with carboquone and cystosine arabinoside on superficial bladder tumors (Abstr). Hinyokika Kiyo 26: 1437–1448

Okada K, Gon H, Nogaki J, Niimura T, Saito T, Amagai T, Yamamoto T, Kiyotaki S, Sato Y, Ogawa N, Morita H, Kitajima K, Kishimoto T (1980) Hyperthermic treatment for bladder tumors. Urokinase combination therapy (Abstr). Nishinippon Hinyokika 42: 967–971

Oliver RTD (1980) The place of chemotherapy in the treatment of patients with invasive carcinoma of the bladder. In: Pavone-Macaluso M, Smith PH, Edsmyr F (eds) Bladder tumors and other topics in urological oncology. Plenum, New York, pp 381–385

Peterson LT, Paulson DF, Bonar RA (1974) Response of human urothelium to chemical carcinogens in vitro. J Urol 111: 154–159

Pontes JE, Dhawbwala CB, Pierce JM (1984) Intravesical Adriamycin therapy for bladder cancer—long-term results. Urology (Suppl). 23: 35–36

Prout GR Jr, Bross ID, Slack NH, Ausman RK (1968) Carcinoma of the bladder. 5-Fluorouracil and the critical role of a placebo: a cooperative group report. I. Cancer 22: 926–931

Prout GR Jr, Griffen, PP, Nocks BN, DeFuria MD, Daly JJ (1982) Intravesical therapy of low stage bladder carcinoma with Mitomycin C: comparison of results in untreated and previously treated patients. J Urol 127: 1096–1098

Prout GR, Koontz WW, Coombs LJ, Hawkins IR, Friedell GH (1983) Long-term fate of 90 patients with superficial bladder cancer randomly assigned to receive or not receive thiotepa. J Urol 130: 677–680

Richards B (1980) Adjuvant chemotherapy following primary irradiation in T3 tumors, and other topics in urological oncology. In: Pavone Macaluso M, Smith PH, Edsmyr F (eds) Bladder tumors and other topics in urological oncology. Plenum, New York, pp 395–397

Richie JP, Blute RD, Waisman J (1980) Immunologic indications of prognosis in bladder cancer. The importance of cell surface antigens. J Urol 123: 22–24

Riddle PR (1973) The management of superficial bladder tumors with intravesical Epodyl. Br J Urol 45: 84–87

Riddle PR, Wallace DM (1971) Intracavitary chemotherapy for multiple non-invasive bladder tumors. Br J Urol 43: 181–184

Robinson MGR, Shelty MB, Richards B, Bastaple J, Glashan RW, Smith PH (1977) Intravesical Epodyl in the management of bladder tumors. Combined experience of the Yorkshire Urological Cancer Group. J Urol 118: 972–973

Sadoughi H, Rubenstone A, Misna J, Davidsohn I (1980) The cell surface antigens of bladder washing specimens in patients with bladder tumor. A new approach. J Urol 123: 19–21

Sakamoto S, Ogata J, Ikegami K, Maeda H (1980) Chemotherapy for bladder cancer with neocarzinostatin: evaluation of systemic administration. Eur J Cancer 16: 103–113

Samuels ML, Logothetis C, Trindate A, Johnson DE (1980) Cytoxan, Adriamycin and *cis*-platinum (CISCA) in metastatic bladder cancer. Proc Am Assoc Cancer Res 21: 137

Sandberg AA (1980) Tumors of the urinary tract. In: Sandberg AA (ed) The chromosomes in human cancer and leukemia. Elsevier North Holland, New York, pp 503–511

Sarna G (1979) Principles of chemotherapy. In: Skinner DG, deKernion JB (eds) Genitourinary cancer. Saunders, Philadelphia, pp 14–39

Schulman CC (1980) Adjuvant therapy of T1 bladder carcinoma: preliminary results of an EORTC randomized study. In: Pavone-Macaluso M, Smith PH, Edsmyr F (eds) Bladder tumors and other topics in urological oncology. Plenum, New York, pp 347–354

Schulman CC, Denis LJ, Wauters E (1980) Intravesical *cis*-platinum in bladder tumors: toxicity study. In: Pavone-Macaluso M, Smith PH, Edsmyr F (eds) bladder tumors and other topics in urological oncology. Plenum, New York, pp 355–359

Schwartz S, Yagoda A, Natale RB, Watson RC, Whitmore WF, Lesser M (1983) Phase II trial of

sequentially administered *cis*-platinum, cyclophosphamide and doxorubicin for urothelial tract tumors. J Urol 130: 681–684
Shin SI, Freedman VH, Risser R, Pollack R (1975) Tumorigenicity of virus transformed cells in nude mice is correlated specifically with anchorage independent growth in vitro. Proc Natl Acad Sci USA 72: 4435
Skinner DG, Kaufman JJ (1978) Management of invasive and high grade bladder cancer. In: Skinner DG, deKernion JB (eds) Genitourinary cancer. Saunders, Philadelphia, p 268
Smalley RU, Bartolucci AA, Hemstreet G, Hester M (1981) A Phase II evaluation of a 3 drug combination of cyclophosphamide, doxorubicin and 5-fluorouracil and of 5-fluorouracil in patients with advanced bladder carcinoma or stage D prostatic carcinoma. J Urol 125: 191–195
Smith PH (1980) The aims and activities of the EORTC Urological Group. In: Pavone-Macaluso M, Smith PH, Edsmyr F (eds) Bladder tumors and other topics in urological oncology. Plenum, New York, pp 35–40
Soloway MS (1978) *Cis*-diamminedichloroplatinum (II) (DDP) in advanced bladder cancer. J Urol 120: 716–719
Soloway MS (1980) Rationale for intensive intravesical chemotherapy for superficial bladder cancer. J Urol 123: 461–466
Soloway MS (1982) Editorial comment. J Urol 127: 1098
Soloway MS (1984) Editorial comment. J Urol 131: 49
Soloway MS, Murphy WM, deFuria MD, Crooke S, Finebaum P (1981a) The effect of Mitomycin C on superficial bladder cancer. J Urol 125: 646–648
Soloway MS, Ikard M, Ford K (1981b). *Cis*-diamminedichloroplatinum (II) in locally advanced and metastatic urothelial cancer. Cancer 47: 476–480
Stanisic TH, Buick RN, Salmon SE (1980a) Soft agar methylcellulose assay for human bladder carcinoma. In: Salmon SE (ed) Cloning of human tumor cells. Alan R Liss, New York, pp 75–84
Stanisic TH, Buick RN, Trent JM, Fry SE, Salmon SE (1980b) In vitro clonal assay for bladder cancer: the biological potential of urothelium and determination of in vitro sensitivity to cytotoxic agents. Surg Forum 31: 585–587
Stober U, Peter HH (1980) BCG immunotherapy for prevention of relapse in patients with bladder cancer? (Abstr). Therapiewoche 30: 6067–6070
Storm FK (1982) Hyperthermia in cancer therapy. In: Proceedings of UCLA Interdepartmental Conference—New advances in oncology, Los Angeles, California, 4 March 1982
Studer UE, Biedermann C, Chollet C, Karrer P, Kraft H, Toggenburg, Vonbank F (1984) Prevention of recurrent superficial bladder tumors by oral etretinate. Preliminary results of randomized, double-blind multicenter trial in Switzerland. J Urol 131: 47–49
Sullivan RD (1962) Intraarterial methotrexate therapy: the dose, duration and route of administration of methotrexate in clinical cancer chemotherapy. In: Porter R, Wiltshaw E (eds) First symposium on methotrexate in the treatment of cancer. Wright, Bristol, pp 50–55
Summers JL, Falor WH, Ward R (1981) A ten year analysis of chromosomes in non-invasive papillary carcinoma of the bladder. J Urol 125: 424–426
Summers JL, Coon JS, Ward RM, Falor WH, Miller AW, Weinstein RS (1983) Prognosis in carcinoma of the urinary bladder based upon tissue group ABH and Thomsen-Friedenreich antigen status and karotype of the initial tumor. Cancer Res 43: 934–939
Tannock IF (1978) Cell kinetics and chemotherapy. A critical review. Cancer Treat Rep 62: 1117–1133
Tannock IF (1981) Selection of chemotherapeutic agents. In: Proceedings of the 7th Annual NBCP Investigators' Workshop. Hershey, Pennsylvania, June 1981
Turner AG, Hendry WF, Williams GB, Bloom HJG (1977) The treatment of advanced bladder cancer with methotrexate. Br J Urol 46: 431–438
Utz DC, DeWeerd JH (1978) The management of low grade low stage carcinoma of the bladder. In: Skinner DG, deKernion JB (eds) Genitourinary cancer. Saunders, Philadelphia, pp 256–268
Utz DC, Farrow GM (1980) Management of carcinoma in situ of the bladder: the case for surgical management. Urol Clin North Am 7: 533–541
Utz DC, Hanna KA, Farrow GM (1970) The plight of the patient with carcinoma in situ of the bladder. J Urol 103: 160–164
Uyama T (1980) Intravesical instillation of Adriamycin combined with low-dose irradiation for superficial bladder cancer. Urology 15: 584–587
Uyama T, Nakamura S, Yamamoto A, Moriwaki S (1980) Treatment of advanced bladder cancer by intraarterial infusion of Adriamycin (Abstr). G an To Kagaku Ryoho 7: 1964–1970
van der Werf-Messing B (1978) Cancer of the urinary bladder treated by interstitial radium implant. Int J Radiol Oncol Biol Phys 45: 373–378
van der Werf-Messing B, Hop WCJ (1981) Carcinoma of the urinary bladder (category T1NXM0)

treated either by radium implant or by transurethral resection only. Int J Radiol Oncol Biol Phys 7: 299–303

Veenema RJ (1978) Editorial comment. J Urol 120: 1411

Veenema RJ, Dean AL, Roberts M, Fingerhut B, Chowhury RK, Tarassoly H (1962) Bladder carcinoma treated by direct instillation of thiotepa. J Urol 88: 60–63

von Hoff DD, Harris GJ, Johnson G, Glaubiger D (1980) Initial experience with the human tumor stem cell assay system: potential and problems. In: Salmon SE (ed) Cloning of human tumor stem cells. Alan R Liss, New York, pp 113–124

Weinstein RS, Alroy J, Farrow GM, Miller AW, Davidsohn I (1979) Blood group isoantigen deletion in carcinoma in situ of the human bladder. Cancer 43: 661–668

Weinstein RS, Miller AW, Pauli BU (1980) Carcinoma in situ: the pathology of a paradox. Urol Clin North Am 7: 523

Whitmore WF (1980) Integrated irradiation and cystectomy for bladder cancer. Br J Urol 52: 1

Whitmore WF, Batata MA, Ghoneim MS, Grabstald H, Unal A (1977) Radical cystectomy with or without prior irradiation for the treatment of bladder cancer. J Urol 118: 184–187

Williams SD, Einhorn LH, Donohue JP (1979) *Cis*-platinum combination chemotherapy of bladder cancer. Cancer Clin Trials 2: 335–338

Wilson WL (1960) Chemotherapy of human solid tumors with 5-fluorouracil. Cancer 13: 1230–1239

Winters WD, Lamm DL (1981) Antibody responses to Bacillus-Calmette-Guérin during immunotherapy in bladder cancer patients. Cancer Res 41: 2672–2676

Wright GL, Starling JJ, Sieg SM (1981) Monoclonal antibodies to tumor associated antigens in human prostate and bladder cancer. Fed Proc 40 (II): 995

Yagoda A (1977) Future implications of Phase 2 chemotherapy trials in 95 patients with measurable advanced bladder cancer. Cancer Res 37: 2775–2780

Yagoda A (1981) Chemotherapy of advanced bladder cancer. In: Conolly JG (ed) Carcinoma of the bladder. Raven Press, New York, pp 251–260

Yagoda A, Watson RC, Whitmore WF (1980) Phase II trial of methotrexate in urinary bladder cancer. Proc Am Assoc Cancer Res 21: 427

Young AK, Hammond B, Middleton AW (1979) The prognostic value of cell-surface antigens in low grade non-invasive transitional cell carcinoma of the bladder. J Urol 122: 462–464

Young CW (1971) Interferon inducers in cancer. Med Clin North Am 55: 721–728

Zincke H, Utz DC, Taylor WF, Myers RP, Leary FJ (1983) Influence of thiotepa and doxorubicin instillation at the time of transurethral surgical treatment of bladder cancer on tumor recurrence: a prospective, randomized, double-blind, controlled trial. J Urol 129: 505–509

Chapter 11

Palliative Treatment

K. H. Kurth

Introduction

By definition palliative therapy in patients with advanced bladder carcinoma may eliminate or reduce symptoms, but cure is rarely achieved and the prognosis is ultimately hopeless. Yet Culp (1979) has stated:

> . . . hopelessness is a state of mind and it must be avoided. It is the duty of the physician to determine from the patient how they live their remaining days and to provide them with a rewarding period of life until death. A true physician is responsible for all aspects of a patient's care, particularly during the palliative period.

However, the relief of ureteric obstruction to prolong the life of the patient who then has to face severe, untreatable bladder symptoms or painful metastases is false palliation. Reliable data on the results of purely palliative treatment are rarely recorded and the quality of life is not usually considered when describing the results of therapy in patients with advanced bladder carcinoma. Nevertheless, an attempt should be made to summarise the therapeutic possibilities and to assess their relative merits in various clinical settings.

Palliative Local Procedures

The primary goal is to eliminate symptoms and to preserve bladder function whenever possible. This cannot always be achieved, and in some cases palliative cystectomy and urinary diversion may be unavoidable. An irritable, painful, bleeding bladder is one of the most distressing problems, and a number of therapeutic manoeuvres have been developed to control these symptoms.

Hydrostatic Pressure

In 1966, Helmstein introduced the method of intravesical pressure therapy which is based on the observation that increased intravesical pressure causes a reduction of blood flow and produces anoxia. Two different techniques have been used to increase the intravesical pressure to a level close to the diastolic blood pressure: the Foley catheter method and the large rubber balloon method. In the Foley catheter method the bladder is filled with saline and the increased intravesical pressure holds the balloon of the catheter against the bladder neck and prevents the escape of fluid.

Instead of infusing saline directly into the bladder a specially designed catheter with a large rubber balloon attached may be introduced into the bladder under regional anaesthesia and the intravesical pressure increased up to the patient's diastolic blood pressure and maintained at that level for 5–6 h. The volume of instilled fluid is easy to control with the large balloon technique and so this method is preferable.

The intravesical pressure is adjusted by varying the elevation of the infusion set. When the drip rate slows down, the intravesical pressure corresponds to the vertical distance between the infusion set and the patient's bladder when the Foley catheter technique is used, but with the large balloon technique 25 cm should be subtracted from the compliance of the balloon. When a pressure of 70 cm of water has been reached the infusion set may be raised by 5 cm at a time until the intravesical pressure reaches the patient's diastolic pressure. A final intravesical pressure of 100 cm of water (approximately 75 mmHg) should not be exceeded. A rapid increase of the drip rate indicates imminent rupture of the bladder or of the balloon.

The hydrostatic pressure treatment has been recommended for patients with extensive superficial tumours (see Chap. 8, p. 171), for larger tumours in patients who are not candidates for more extensive surgical procedures and for the control of intractable haemorrhage resulting from radiation or cyclophosphamide cystitis. Complications of this treatment are rare, but bladder rupture can occur and a chronically scarred and contracted bladder may result, especially if the procedure is followed by radiotherapy.

According to Helmstein (1972), necrosis is limited to the neoplastic region because the vessels in the vascular bed of the tumour are abnormal and collapse more easily when the intravesical pressure is raised. The normal bladder mucosa is less severely affected and will easily regenerate. After technical failure of hydrostatic pressure treatment the procedure can be repeated. The interval between treatments depends on the grade of the tumour; low-grade tumours may be retreated after only 1 month, but with highly malignant tumours an interval of 2 months should elapse. A survey of the results of hydrostatic pressure treatments for bladder tumours is given in Table 11.1. Treatment has consistently failed in those tumours invading the vesical muscle.

Hydrostatic pressure treatment can, however, be used in patients with symptoms caused by very advanced, fixed and inoperable T3/T4 tumours. Many of these patients have already had radiation and pose a problem because of their symptoms of frequency, bleeding and pain. After Helmstein's treatment the exophytic part of the tumour may develop massive necrosis and, although there is still viable tumour present, the patients may lose their pain and stop bleeding. Very often their frequency is also considerably improved.

As a palliative measure hydrostatic distension can stop bleeding, especially from a radiation cystitis. In patients with large superficial tumours which are difficult to resect, distension may clear the bladder (see Chap. 8, p. 171). There is no evidence that it influences the natural history of superficial tumours. The procedure does not, as was hoped, immunise the patient against the tumour (Helmstein 1972; Hirose 1977). There is some evidence that combining hydrostatic pressure with hyperthermia may have a more pronounced effect on the bladder tumour (Ludgate et al. 1976; Newsam and Law 1982).

Intravesical Formalin

The instillation of a formalin solution into the bladder was advocated by Brown (1969) as a method of controlling vesical haemorrhage in patients with advanced carcinoma of the bladder. This technique can also be used to control the bleeding from radiation or cyclophosphamide cystitis that has not responded to other treatment. The indications, techniques, complications and results are shown in Table 11.2. The intravesical instillation of formalin for the management of intractable haematuria has several advantages which make it an attractive alternative to other modes of therapy. Formalin is universally available and can be made in the required concentration by any pharmacy. It should be noted that a saturated solution of formaldehyde contains 37% formaldehyde and this is known as formalin. A 10% solution of formalin therefore contains 3.7% formaldehyde. These two concentrations should not be confused.

The instillation is simple and requires no special apparatus, but an anaesthetic is required as it is extremely painful. The procedure may take up to 48 h to arrest the bleeding but it can be repeated after this interval. The probable mode of action is the precipitation of cellular proteins in the bladder mucosa and the thrombosis of the submucosal vessels. Intravesical formalin therapy is generally free of systemic toxicity but may have some serious complications. Total bladder necrosis has been reported (Bergsma and Leary 1976), and hydronephrosis secondary to vesicoureteric reflux or obstruction also occurs (Fair 1974; Kumar et al. 1975). The possibility of vesicoureteric reflux must be excluded by the evidence of a cystogram before formalin instillation. A Fogarty catheter can be used to prevent reflux into the upper tracts during treatment (Bright et al. 1977). Suprapubic pain and urge incontinence may result from the bladder fibrosis induced by the formalin. Merimsky and Jossiphov (1980) described a case of tubular necrosis caused by the systemic absorption of formalin after intravesical treatment of a patient with profuse bleeding from a recurrent bladder tumour. Capen et al. (1982) reported a case of intraperitoneal spillage of formalin which caused extensive medical problems.

Nearly all the complications have been associated with the use of 10% solutions of formalin. Fair (1974) reported that a 1% solution is as effective as the 10% solution and is free of the complications. It is therefore recommended that only a 1% or 4% solution is used and that the contact time is only 15 min.

Intravesical phenol, alcohol and silver nitrate have also been reported to be of benefit in the control of intractable bladder haemorrhage, but these solutions do not appear to be as effective as formalin.

Table 11.1. Hydrostatic pressure treatment for malignant lesions of the bladder and for control of bleeding from the bladder mucosa

Reference	Indication	No. of patients	Complications	Results successful/total no. of patients
				Total tumour necrosis:
Helmstein (1972)	T1 bladder carcinoma	14	Total bladder rupture (2)	11/14
	T2 bladder carcinoma	12	Partial bladder rupture (5)	5/12
	T3 bladder carcinoma	9	Perforation (1)	5/9
	T4 bladder carcinoma	8	Haemorrhage (1)	2/8
			No mortality	Partial tumour necrosis:
	Total	43		T1 2/14
				T2 4/12
				T3 2/9
Holstein et al. (1973)	Cyclophosphamide cystitis		Septicaemia	1/1
	Radiation cystitis		—	3/4
	Exophytic bladder Ca		—	1/1
Debré and Steg (1981)	Ta bladder carcinoma (11 patients had more than one distension)	57	From 105 treatments: Balloon rupture 1; Bladder rupture 4; Septicaemia 3	Ta: Tumour disappeared 12/57; Reduced tumour size 31/57; Slight or no tumour reduction 14/57

Table 11.1 (*continued*)

Reference	Indication	No. of patients	Complications	Results successful/total no. of patients
	Tis bladder carcinoma	3		Tis: Normal cytology 1/3
	T1 bladder carcinoma	8		T1: Reduced tumour size 6/8
	T2 bladder carcinoma	8		T2: Tumour disappeared 1/8 No effect 7/8
Hirose et al. (1977)	Bladder carcinoma <T2 (50 patients)		Bladder fissure (23) in 70 distensions 'Slight fever for a few days'	Tumour disappeared 12/50 Marked regression 20/50 Fair response 18/50
England et al. (1973)	Ta, T1 bladder carcinoma	23	Death (myocardial infarct; 1)	Total necrosis: Ta, T1 6/23 T2 1/3
	T2 bladder carcinoma	3	Bladder rupture (conservative therapy; 1)	Substantial necrosis: Ta, T1 10/23
	T3 bladder carcinoma	8	Urinary tract infection (4)	T3 1/8
	T4 bladder carcinoma	11		T4 5/11 No improvement: Ta, T1 7/23 T2 2/3 T3 7/8 T4 6/11
	Radiation cystitis	3		Haemorrhage stopped 3/3

Table 11.2. Formalin instillation

Reference	Indication	Technique	Complications	Results: successful/total no. of patients (%)
Brown (1969)	Ca bladder	10% formalin for 15 min to limit of bladder capacity	None	22/24 (91.5)
Firlit (1973)	Primary or secondary Ca bladder	10% formalin for 15 min to limit of capacity. Bladder irrigated with saline	Transient tachycardia in all	6/6 (100)
Fair (1974)	Radiation or cyclophosphamide cystitis	10% formalin (4 patients) for 10 min	Hydroureteronephrosis (2), ureterovesical reflux (3), diminished bladder capacity (2) and fibrosis of ureter (1), bacteraemia	4/4 (100)
Barakat et al. (1973)	Radiation or cyclophosphamide cystitis	150–300 ml 10% formalin for 10 min	Bil. hydronephrosis	5/5 (100)
Kumar et al. (1975)	Primary or secondary Ca bladder	10–30 ml 10% formalin for 15 min	Vesicocutaneous fistula (1), vesicoureteric reflux and hydronephrosis (1) (neither complication definitely proved to be caused by formalin per se)	8/10 (80)

Table 11.2. *(continued)*

Reference	Indication	Technique	Complications	Results: successful/total no. of patients (%)
Likourinas et al. (1979)	Ca bladder, radiation cystitis	100–150 ml 10% formalin for 15 min	Transient tachycardia in 16/17 Stroke 1/17 UTI 1/17	12/77 (71)
Jorest et al. (1977)	Ca bladder, radiation cystitis	50–100 ml 10% formalin for 10–15 min	Transient tachycardia in 11/28 Extravasation of formalin 3/28 UTI 23/28	13/28 (46)
Shah and Albert (1973)	Ca bladder (some had radiotherapy and cytotoxic drugs)	100–150 ml 4% formalin by gravity for 30 min. Bladder is rinsed with 10% alcohol and saline	None	10/12 (83.3)
Fair (1974)	Radiation or cyclophosphamide cystitis	500–1000 ml 1% formalin (14 patients) irrigated into bladder for 10 min. Bladder washed with 1 litre distilled water	None	14/14 (100)
Godec and Gleich (1983)	Ca bladder, Ca cervix with radiation	Bladder filled to capacity with 3%–10% formalin for 5–15 min	Bil. hydronephrosis (1), vesicovaginal fistula (1)	5/5 (100)

Local Hyperthermia for Bladder Cancer

The effectiveness of hyperthermia for the treatment of cancer has been demonstrated both clinically and experimentally. The heat can be administered either by raising the body temperature or by local application. This has been regarded with suspicion by many oncologists, but it has been shown experimentally that tumour cells, both in vivo and in vitro, are more susceptible to heat than normal tissues (Cavaliere et al. 1967; Dickson 1977) and may be killed when subjected to temperatures over 40° C. The urinary bladder is exceptional in being readily treatable by local hyperthermia.

Method of Hyperthermia by Irrigation

Hall et al. (1974) heated the bladder by irrigation through a three-way catheter with normal saline heated by passage through a heating coil and waterbath. The flow was approximately 2 litres/h and was adjusted so that the outflow temperature was about 45° C. This temperature was tolerated by all patients; higher temperatures tended to cause discomfort. Irrigation was carried out for 1–3 h per day for 12 days. Vesicoureteric reflux was not considered to be a contraindication to therapy, but urinary tract infections were treated prior to hyperthermia. They recommended that a second catheter is placed in the rectum to irrigate the rectum with cold saline if the temperature of the anterior rectal wall rises, in order to avoid the possibility of producing a rectovesical fistula by thermal necrosis. The temperature of the irrigating fluid is measured at both the inflow and outflow. If the procedure is done at laparotomy, needle thermocouples may be placed in the bladder lumen, beneath the peritoneum over the dome of the bladder and in the mucosa of the anterior rectal wall to measure the gradient across the bladder wall.

Results. A total of 52 patients with multiple Ta and T1 tumours and 8 patients with invasive bladder cancers were treated: 9 patients with superficial tumours were completely clear of tumour on follow-up cystoscopy; 23 patients had more than a 50% reduction in tumour size; 10 patients had minimal regression and 10 patients had no visible change in the tumour up to 8 weeks after treatment. The invasive carcinomas showed necrosis of the visible tumour in four cases (Hall 1978). Cystoscopy the day after treatment showed changes ranging from moderate congestion of the mucosa to oedematous cystitis. After an interval of 2 weeks the mucosa generally looked normal. Biopsy specimens, taken from the tumours persisting after hyperthermia, showed the same morphological pattern as those obtained before treatment. Biopsies of normal bladder mucosa also showed varying degrees of hyperplasia both before and after therapy. This experience showed that hyperthermic irrigation can produce necrosis of superficial transitional cell carcinoma without damaging the bladder mucosa, provided that the intravesical temperature is kept between 41° and 45° C.

Four other patients were treated with high-temperature bladder irrigation as an alternative to cystectomy because of their age and frailty (Hall et al. 1976). Three had T3 bladder carcinomas and one had widespread urothelial atypia with carcinoma in situ and a contracted bladder. At laparotomy the bladder was isolated from the other viscera by a dry pack pushed well into the rectovesical fossa and was then covered with aluminium foil. Bladder heating was maintained for 25–70 min while the ileal conduit diversion of the urine was performed. The irrigating fluid was heated to between 63° and 82° C. In three cases the bladder tumour was not destroyed even after hyperthermia to 82° C for 25 min. Apparently viable tumour cells were found in the muscle layer 6 weeks after hyperthermia. The treatment caused necrosis of the anterior wall of the rectum in one patient. The patient with carcinoma in situ developed further bladder contracture and 6 years later developed a recurrent invasive bladder cancer.

As yet hyperthermia has been assessed as palliative therapy only in small series of patients with severe local symptoms of invasive and inoperable cancer (Ludgate et al. 1976; Newsam and Law 1982). Further experience and data will be necessary before the results of this type of therapy can be evaluated. Hyperthermic irrigation of the bladder at 60°–80° C is not recommended as it is hazardous.

High-Frequency Hyperthermia

Hyperthermia irrigation of the bladder may cause non-uniform heating of the bladder wall. An alternative is transurethrally applied local high-frequency hyperthermia as described by Harzmann et al. (1978). These authors have developed an optically controlled system for local high-frequency hyperthermia (Fig. 11.1). Temperature regulation is made possible by using a thermocouple thrust into the bladder wall and another sensor registering the temperature in the bladder lumen. The method was first tested in rabbits who had received a transplant of the Brown-Pearce carcinoma into the bladder wall. The temperature in the tumour was found to be 7° C higher than in the tumour-free bladder wall, demonstrating the higher thermosensitivity of tumour tissue. After hyperthermia the healthy urothelium showed reversible oedema over a period of 70 days. Tumours treated to 43° C for 30 min were smaller than untreated ones and showed

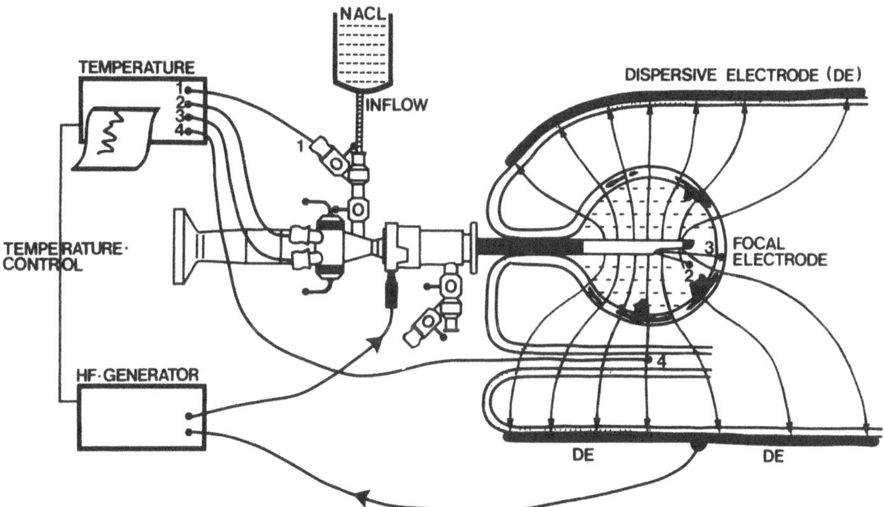

Fig. 11.1. Optically controlled system for local high-frequency hyperthermia of the bladder. (Harzmann et al. 1978)

haemorrhagic necrosis. Later this method was tested on dogs and again subtotal tumour necrosis was seen.

In 1980 Harzmann et al. described their first clinical experience in 28 patients with advanced carcinoma of the bladder who were unfit for extensive surgery and who were treated under local anaesthesia by high-frequency hyperthermia. The hyperthermia was produced by an active internal electrode with an inactive belt-shaped external electrode. A modified high-frequency apparatus[1] which produced 30 to 300 W at a frequency of 500 kHz (in the long wave region) was used. These conditions were chosen to ensure more homogeneous heating of the tissue, which is not achieved by bladder irrigation. The temperature of the tumour-free bladder wall rose quickly to 43° C and was maintained for 60 min. The patients were treated three times by this procedure. Macroscopic haematuria disappeared within 48 h and endoscopic checks performed at weekly intervals showed oedema and a reduction of the tumour volume. The histological late findings were stromal hyalinisation without any permanent side effects on the tumour-free areas of the bladder. This treatment should be considered as palliation because complete destruction of the tumour was not observed. Combination of this therapy with radiotherapy or chemotherapy may lead to an improvement in the treatment of advanced carcinoma of the bladder, if synergism can be demonstrated (Jacobs et al. 1982).

The results obtained with local hyperthermia alone are not convincing and the palliative effect is doubtful. High-frequency hyperthermia should be superior to irrigation with heated saline because homogeneous heating of the tissue can be guaranteed. Further experience is needed to define the value of this treatment, either alone or in combinations with other therapies, in the palliation of locally advanced bladder cancer.

Cryotherapy

Urological cryosurgery was initiated by Gonder et al. (1964), though de Quervain (1927) first reported the freezing of a bladder cancer. Cahan et al. (1970) reported on five patients with uncontrolled bladder haemorrhage treated by cryosurgery after palliative radiotherapy. In three of the patients the bladder was filled three times with liquid nitrogen, and in the other two an all-purpose cryoprobe was brought into contact with the bleeding area and consecutive freeze-thaw cycles were completed with probe tip temperatures of −130° and −140° C. In three out of five cases the bladder was not excluded from urine during and after the cryosurgical procedure. The postoperative evacuation of the cryonecrotic slough required 3–5 weeks. Haematuria did not reappear after cryosurgery. One patient was well and had no bleeding 2½ years after cryosurgery.

In a subsequent report from the same institute (Memorial Hospital, New York) MacKenzie (1972) presented the results of 15 patients treated for carcinoma of the bladder by topical liquid nitrogen and 7 additional patients treated by segmental cryotherapy. All tumours were deeply infiltrating and one had metastases. Two patients had T3 tumours at laparotomy and no recurrence was evident when these patients died of cardiac and pulmonary disease. Three patients died of metastases,

[1] Manufactured by Firma Erbe Elekromedizin, 7400 Tübingen, Federal Republic of Germany.

one patient was well following a cystectomy and one patient with recurrence died of myocardial infarction. Thus 2 out of 15 patients treated by liquid nitrogen remained free of recurrence, and 5 out of 7 patients treated with the cryoprobe for deeply infiltrating bladder carcinoma developed recurrences.

The adjuvant use of a cryoprobe prior to open excision of bladder tumours and also as an adjuvant after palliative TUR of deeply infiltrating tumours has been reported (Reuter 1978). In 1974 Haschek stated:

> I have not yet found any paper giving results of cryosurgery in the management of bladder tumours. It is not logical that one go deeper with cryosurgery than with transurethral resection. There is a need for research demonstrating the advantage of cryosurgery in the management of cancer of the bladder and prostate.

Such reports, with stage-related results and an adequate follow-up, are still lacking. Therefore cryotherapy remains unproven and is not suitable for routine use.

Transurethral Laser Irradiation

A laser is a high-intensity light source which emits a nearly parallel beam of electromagnetic radiation of given wavelength, generated in a suitable atomic or molecular system by means of quantum-optical processes. In medicine the CO_2 laser (wavelength 10.6 μm), the neodymium-YAG (Nd-YAG) laser (wavelength 1.06 nm) and the argon laser (wavelengths between 485 and 515 nm) are employed (Hall 1982; see also Chap 8, p. 177). For endoscopic application flexible light conductors have been developed. Argon and Nd-YAG lasers have been used experimentally in rabbits to examine the morphological and histological changes produced in the healthy bladder and in bladder tumours and also to obtain technical safety data (Staehler and Hofstetter 1979).

Hofstetter (1981) treated 302 bladder tumours up to thumb-tip size with the Nd-YAG laser; 196 larger bladder tumours were removed by TUR followed by laser irradiation 1 week later. All tumours were staged Ta to T3N0M0. The later results of this treatment are not reported, but at the first cystoscopy 2 months after the irradiation a recurrence was seen in 9.9% of the tumours treated by irradiation alone and in 8.1% of the tumours resected transurethrally prior to laser irradiation. In the group treated by laser irradiation alone, the recurrence was seen in the irradiated area in 3.6% and at the border of the irradiated area in 6.3%. In the group having the combined treatment these figures were 2.5% and 5.6% respectively.

It is too early for a definitive assessment of laser therapy in patients with bladder tumours. It is not clear whether this method has any advantages over the standard TUR. However, the Nd-YAG laser is able to destroy bladder tumours. In this laser the lasting element is a synthetic diamond (YAG being an acronym for yttrium aluminium garnet) treated with neodymium. The radiation from this element is carried along a 2-m length of quartz fibre set into the shaft of a 21 F cystoscope specially constructed for this purpose. The fibre extends beyond the end of the cystoscope and the radiation beam can be directed by an Albarran lever. During treatment the bladder is filled with 0.9% sodium chloride and the tip of the light guide is brought within 2–5 mm of the tumour, which creates a focal point of 2–3 mm diameter. With a power of 40–50 W the radiation is delivered to the tumour in a series of doses each lasting not more than 3 s. The appearance of white discoloration shows that the treatment is effective; the appearance of carbon deposits is a sign that the energy has been absorbed by blood on the surface of the tumour and the energy is insufficient to destroy tumour in the deeper layers of the bladder wall.

The thermal effects of the forward scattering on organs adjacent to the bladder must be considered. Kronester et al. (1981) concluded that intestinal damage, which has a risk of perforation, can be avoided if the laser radiation has a power of no more than 42 W and is applied for maximum periods of 3 s with a focus of at least 2 mm diameter onto areas of the bladder that are at least 3 mm in thickness. Lower powers (less than 40 W) and much longer periods of application may be preferable for achieving necrosis of tumour infiltrating the bladder wall.

Laser irradiation therefore has the ability to destroy up to 8 mm in depth of tissue; this may be useful for the palliative treatment of infiltrating bladder tumours with known metastatic disease. To what extent patients with local disease can be cured by lasers must be the subject of future reports.

Transcatheter Embolisation in the Management of Intractable Bladder Haemorrhage

Transcatheter haemostasis is used to treat genitourinary haemorrhages with a variety of causes. Techniques of selective catheterisation of pelvic arteries make transcatheter embolisation of bleeding vessels in the bladder possible, with results that are equal to those of ligation of the hypogastric arteries. A variety of materials may be placed in the artery to achieve occlusion, and the results of embolisation have been greatly improved by refinements in angiographic techniques and the development of new embolic materials such as the smaller steel coil/wool thread combination, small detachable balloons and liquid tissue adhesives. Superselective occlusions can be performed in almost every area.

Gel foam used to be the principal agent for embolisation. It can be delivered through standard 5 or 6.5 F catheters into the selected position. However, the occlusion is not always permanent and reflux of gel foam fragments into the systemic circulation is a serious potential complication. Insertion of the Gianturco-Wallace steel coil into a major artery following embolisation with gel foam gives more permanent occlusion. The gel foam slows down the blood flow enough to allow the formation of a solid thrombus at the site of the coil. Use of the Gianturco coil requires an intact clotting system; the procedure is limited to larger vessels and requires a 7 F catheter for delivery. Anatomical variations or vascular tortuosity increase the difficulty of the procedure. Permanent occlusion of larger

Table 11.3. Complications of pelvic embolisation

Mild febrile reaction
Gluteal discomfort (one-third of the patients)
Transient buttock claudication (minimised by passing the catheter beyond the superior gluteal artery)
Impotence after bilateral hypogastric embolisation in men
Gangrene (necrosis) of the bladder
Paralysis of a leg (spinal cord damage)
Accidental occlusion of other arteries
Unplanned vessel damage

Table 11.4. Transcatheter embolisation in the management of haemorrhage from the bladder

Reference	Aetiology	No. of patients	Site of embolisation	Material for embolisation	Results
Huguet et al. (1980)	Bladder carcinoma (and other malignancies)	43	Bilateral embolisation	Gel foam, IBCA	Haemostasis achieved in 36 patients (duration not listed); 7 failures (1 for technical reasons)
	Radiation cystitis	2			
Günther et al. (1981)	Bladder carcinoma	5	Superselective embolisation (no further details)	IBCA plus lipiodol	Successful in all patients (duration of haemostasis not listed); 2 patients with recurrent haemorrhage 3, 5 months later
	Prostatic carcinoma	1			
	Cervix carcinoma	1			
Bush and Freeny (1980)	Bladder carcinoma		Unilateral hypogastric artery occlusion	IBCA	Successful
	Bladder carcinoma		Bilateral hypogastric artery occlusion	IBCA	Successful
	Cervix carcinoma		Bilateral hypogastric artery occlusion	IBCA	Successful
Hermanowicz et al. (1980)	Bladder carcinoma	17	13 patients—bilateral occlusion of hypogastric artery; 5 patients—unilateral occlusion of hypogastric artery	Gel foam	Successful in 15 patients (duration of haemostasis not listed)
	Cervix carcinoma	1			

vessels can also be accomplished by detachable balloons. Isobutyl-cyanoacrylate (IBCA) is an acrylic resin that polymerises quickly upon contact with blood and becomes a firm mass that occludes the arterial tree by forming a cast. It is a non-reabsorbable embolic material (Günther et al. 1981). The use of Pantopaque instead of the usual tantalum for opacification of the acrylate slightly retards polymerisation. The technical difficulties, the possibility of revascularisation and the fear of bladder necrosis or distal embolism have hindered the development of bilateral internal iliac embolisation. Selective catheterisation of the internal iliac arteries by an experienced angiographist is nearly always possible; the transaxillary, ipsilateral or contralateral femoral approaches may be used. The superselective catheter techniques permit selective engagement of branch vessels, such as the superior vesical artery, and thus limit embolisation to the area supplied by that branch (Lang et al. 1979). In patients with multiple demonstrable bleeding points supplied from different branch vessels the infarcting substance may be channelled by the midstream of the appropriate division of the hypogastric artery, relying on the syphoning effect of the bleeding lesion to direct them into the appropriate branches. To limit embolisation to the desired region and to preclude inadvertant regurgitation into the main vessels, fluoroscopic monitoring and fractional embolisation are imperative. The excellent collateral network in the bladder musculature ensures sufficient capillary flow to any segment in which the principal vascular supply has been embolised so that tissue necrosis is prevented. In cases with haemorrhage from the bladder resulting from carcinoma, specific bleeding points may not be identifiable on the arteriogram. If superselective embolisation cannot be performed, or if a specific bleeding source is not evident, then the main branches of one or both hypogastric arteries can be infarcted using a combination of gel foam and steel coils or liquid tissue adhesive. Revascularisation of an embolised arterial tree has been described when clots or gel foam were used as the embolic material. Acrylate or Gianturco coils may therefore be preferable. The effectiveness of embolisation is in contrast to the experience with surgical ligation. This may be due to the occlusion of the small vessels on the bleeding side which would otherwise function in the development of a collateral blood supply (Schuhrke and Barr 1976). After embolisation the patient may suffer from transient post-embolisation upper thigh and gluteal pain related to the post-infarction syndrome. Further complications are listed in Table 11.3 and the indications and results of transcatheter embolisation in the management of haemorrhage from the bladder are listed in Table 11.4.

From these results we can conclude that bleeding from unresectable bladder cancer can be controlled by hypogastric artery embolisation. In the hands of experienced radiologists this procedure offers an attractive method for palliative treatment. A variety of embolic devices is available, each offering certain advantages for specific genitourinary problems; most radiologists develop their expertise with a limited number of methods. Bilateral hypogastric artery occlusion has been performed by many investigators without untoward effects (Lang et al. 1979; Günther et al. 1981). Recanalisation or revascularisation of the embolised artery may be avoided by using a non-reabsorbable embolic material such as isobutyl-2-cyanoacrylate.

Hypogastric Artery Infusion

Intra-arterial chemotherapy may offer advantages over intravenous chemotherapy by delivering active drugs in much higher concentrations to the tumour without any increase in the systemic toxicity. The ideal agent would be a drug that is extremely toxic to cancer cells but is quite innocuous to the adjacent normal tissue, or is completely inactivated during its passage through the venous circulation. The goal of synthesising compounds that are able to produce regional damage during a single transit through the capillary bed after intra-arterial infusion and which are rapidly inactivated in the venous circulation has not yet been achieved. Nevertheless, regional perfusion remains an attractive approach for the following reasons (Goodman et al. 1982):

1. The bone marrow and immune system are protected from the toxic action of the drug.
2. A higher concentration in the tumour circulation can be achieved, usually 4–12 times the level attained by intravenous use.
3. Alkylating effects are potentiated by increased tissue oxygenation.
4. Potentiation by local hyperthermia.
5. Removal by washout of excess therapeutic agent and toxic products of the treatment.

The complications of regional chemotherapy include:

1. Local oedema
2. Haemorrhage and tissue necrosis
3. Skin sloughs occurring in perfusion of extremities
4. Local, irreversible vascular changes which may occur as a direct effect of the drug on the vessel wall, depending on its concentration, the flow in the vessel, the calibre of the vessel and the anatomical configuration
5. Gastrointestinal symptoms
6. Nerve damage
7. Infection, which is always a hazard when indwelling catheters remain in a blood vessel for a long period of time

After a report by Sullivan in 1962, Ogata et al. (1973) and Nevin et al. (1974) confirmed the technical feasibility of pelvic infusion therapy in patients with unresectable bladder cancer and in patients who refused radical surgery. Nevin's protocol consisted of arterial infusion with 5-FU, or a combination of 5-FU with Bleomycin and Adriamycin, as the sole treatment for patients with bladder cancer recurring after radiotherapy. Patients who were not previously irradiated were first treated by arterial infusion with these three drugs, followed by supervoltage irradiation. Patients with metastatic disease outside the pelvis were not excluded. All patients selected for treatment underwent laparotomy and partial iliac lymphadenectomy for staging, followed by insertion of infusion catheters into both internal iliac arteries. After wound healing the patients were able to be discharged from hospital with the infusion catheters in place and the chemotherapy was continued in the outpatient department. The infusion was

Table 11.5. Treatment of advanced carcinoma of the bladder using hypogastric infusion

Reference	Indication	No. of patients	Infusion drug	Results
Kato et al. (1981)	Advanced bladder carcinoma Cervical carcinoma involving the urinary bladder	6 2	Preoperative Mitymocin-C micro-capsule infusion in 5 patients, followed by radical surgery	4 patients alive NED at 7, 13, 20, 21 months; 1 patient alive with tumour 19 months; 1 patient died at 10 months; 1 patient alive with NED at 9 months; haemorrhage stopped in 7 patients
Nakazono and Iwata (1980)	Infiltrating bladder carcinoma	11	70–170 mg Adriamycin over 7–10 days, followed by total cystectomy (8 cases) or partial cystectomy (1 case)	5 tumours disappeared; partial destruction in 3 cases; 3 low-grade tumours showed no significant changes
Wallace et al. (1982)	T4 bladder carcinoma (9 patients had previous radiation therapy) or, local recurrence after cystectomy	15	*cis*-Platinum 80–120 mg/m^2 over 24-h intra-arterially, 3 or fewer courses; 2 patients received after failure of *cis*-platinum 5-FU intra-arterially 1000 mg/m^2 for 5 days, Adriamycin 20 mg/m^2 for 3 days and Mitomycin-C 5 mg/m^2 for 2 days through a subclavian venous line	NED 8 patients at 6, 8, 9, 10 13, 13, 13, 19 months); alive with tumours (6, 13 17 months); 4 patients dead with tumour (8, 13, 17, 17 months). Median survival in all patients, 12 months

Table 11.5. (*continued*)

Reference	Indication	No. of patients	Infusion drug	Results
Jacobs et al. (1982)	T3 (3n) and T4 (3n) bladder carcinoma	6	Precystectomy intra-arterial *cis*-platinum together with local bladder hyperthermia; 4 patients underwent cystectomy, 2 patients exploratory laparotomy	2 patients pT0; 4 patients had viable tumours on the bladder serosal surface; 2 patients NED 34, 36 weeks; 2 patients alive with local tumour or bone metastases 34, 34 weeks; 2 patients died with metastases 11, 20 weeks
Harada et al. (1982)	TCC bladder carcinoma:		Bilateral internal iliac artery catheterisation: 50 or 80 mg Adriamycin, 10 mg Mitomycin or 60 mg Bleomycin infused over 3 h	3 patients alive 4, 7, 12 months; 2 patients died after 4, 7 months
	Stage A	1		
	Stage C	1		
	Stage D	2		
	Squamous cell bladder carcinoma stage D	1		
Logothetis et al. (1982)	Loco-regional pelvic recurrences of malignant urothelial tumour:		5-FU (1 g/m^2) daily for 5 days via bilateral, hypogastric catheters, combined with intravenous Adriamycin (25 mg/m^2) and Mitomycin-C (5 mg/m^2). Three courses of combined intra-arterial and systemic chemotherapy were followed by systemic chemotherapy only	17/29 achieved an objective response (data on CR/PR not given). Median survival 52 weeks in responding patients and 28 weeks in non-responding patients
	after cystectomy	8		
	after radiation therapy	16		
	Distant metastases	2		
	Rectal invasion	5		

provided by a battery-operated sigmamotor portable infusion pump. This regimen was continued for 3 months in those patients who were to receive megavoltage radiation, unless the patients experienced severe toxic reactions to the drug. Those patients who had previously received megavoltage radiation were continuously infused until the catheter failed to function or toxic reaction to the drug terminated the treatment. The infusions were maintained for as long as 1 year. Those patients who were irradiated after infusion tended to have fewer complaints during the irradiation than those who were treated before infusion therapy or who received no infusion therapy. None of the patients developed complications as the result of the insertion of the catheter, and no arterial or venous thromboses, bleeding or septic complications were seen. More recently, intra-arterial infusion of chemotherapeutic drugs has been used as an adjuvant to surgical therapy combined with local hyperthermia (see Table 11.5).

From the limited experience with intra-arterial chemotherapy one can conclude that intra-arterial infusion is more effective than intravenous treatment, as judged by the survival and remission rates that are reported. Combined treatment with radiotherapy, hyperthermia and surgery may enhance the response. *cis*-Platinum, currently the most effective chemotherapeutic agent for metastatic bladder cancer, has a short plasma half-life owing to its high affinity for tissue proteins. Intra-arterial infusion should increase the local concentration and its gradient across the tumour cell membranes. Side effects, such as nausea and vomiting, are remarkably low after intra-arterial infusion of *cis*-platinum. The interaction of hyperthermia with chemotherapeutic agents frequently results in a greater cytotoxicity than would be expected from a purely additive effect. Marmor (1979) showed that local hyperthermia to 42° C can potentiate the activity of *cis*-platinum in animal models. The delivery of *cis*-platinum intra-arterially can cause a 5.4 times greater uptake in the bladder tumour, as compared with normal bladder muscle (Jacobs et al. 1982). In addition to its favourable effect on tumour size intra-arterial infusion can control haematuria and relieve pain (Confer et al. 1977; Wallace et al. 1982).

The use of percutaneous catheter systems may be complicated by the presence of infection at the exit site. Recently a system has been developed which allows drug infusion without the need for chronic skin penetration or multiple vena punctures. The Port-A-Catheter[2] is an implantable catheter system consisting of an implantable silicone catheter and a stainless steel portal with a self-sealing septum for hypodermic needle entry. The portal is positioned in a subcutaneous pocket and can be repeatedly accessed by percutaneous needle puncture. First experiences with this system were reported by Niederhuber et al. (1982). A ten times more expensive implantable infusion pump[3] was used and had no complications such as arterial thrombosis, catheter sepsis and dislodgement, pump infusion variation and pump failure (Barone et al. 1982). Another way to avoid continuous infusion may be chemo-embolisation, as described by Kato et al. (1981). These authors used microspheres of ethylcellulose containing Mitomycin-C. When injected into the hypogastric artery the spheres block the small branches and the ethylcellulose is enzymatically degraded to release the Mitomycin-C slowly.

---

[2] Manufactured by Pharmacia Nu Tech, Piscataway, New Jersey.

[3] Manufactured by Infusaid Corp., Norwood, Massachusetts.

Table 11.6. Results of radical and palliative irradiation in patients with advanced bladder carcinoma (number of treated patients shown in parentheses)

Reference	Indication	Therapy		Survival % (5 years)
Green and George (1974)	T4b	45 patients received 4000 cGy or more	(52)	Median survival 10 months
	TXN3, N4		(12)	
	T4a	27 patients received 4000 cGy	(8)	Median survival 5 months
Fish and Fayos (1976)	D1 (pT4N0-3)	*Group I*: 6000 cGy in 6 weeks to a volume of 1.050 cm^3	(20)	0
		Group II: 6542 cGy in 6 weeks to a volume of ±1.700 cm^3	(40)	11.4
Rider and Evans (1976)	T4 palliative treatment	22 MEV Betatron 5×/5 days (a few with Cobalt 60 units; dose not reported)	(284)	8/201 alive at 5 years; median survival 0.5 years
	T4 radical treatment	3000 cGy 16 ×/3 weeks to pelvis and lymph nodes and bladder 1500 cGy 5 ×/5 days	(74)	26
Morrison (1978)	T4	5250 cGy (including primary tumour, extravesical tissue, external iliac nodes) in 4 weeks, an additional 1000–1250 cGy in 1 week	(52)	6.5
van der Werf-Messing (1978)	TXNXM1	6000 cGy	(124)	0
	T4	6000 cGy (external mega-voltage irradiation)	(396)	5
Hübener and Voss, (1979)	T4	Cobalt 60 units 6000 cGy	(21)	29 (3 years) 22 (4 years) 0 (5 years)

As a method of local treatment for advanced bladder carcinoma intra-arterial drug infusion warrants further use and study. The techniques should be familiar to urological oncologists.

Palliative Radiotherapy

Palliative radiotherapy has been advocated for control of intractable haemorrhage, pain and bladder irritability. Some of the results are summarised in Table 11.6. Green and George (1974) examined 74 patients with proven localised advanced bladder cancer who were treated by radiotherapy and found no difference in the response according to histological type or extent of tumour spread. In 12 of 35 patients with haematuria palliation lasted until death. Pelvic pain was usually alleviated, but bladder irritability was not often affected. Ten per cent of the patients were free of local symptoms at death. The duration of survival was longer in patients treated with higher tumour doses than in those treated with lower doses.

A new approach for palliative control of haematuria or ureteric obstruction was presented by Chan et al. (1979). They treated seven patients with carcinoma of the bladder whose medical condition or disease status prevented radical surgery; five had intractable vesical haemorrhage and two had progressive azotaemia caused by ureteric obstruction. The patients received single fractions of 1000 cGy pelvic irradiation delivered with 25 MeV X-rays using parallel opposed anteroposterior 12 × 12 portals. Four patients completed three fractions of 1000 cGy at 3–4 weekly intervals. Bleeding subsided promptly in the five patients treated for bladder haemorrhage, and one patient had complete relief of pelvic pain. The duration of responses ranged from 2 to 8 months, with a median of 5 months. Severe bleeding recurred in only one patient 12 months after completion of irradiation. Both patients with ureteric obstruction received only a single dose of 1000 cGy and improvement was noted in the blood nitrogen levels in both patients. Acute reactions consisted of diarrhoea, nausea and vomiting for 3–4 days after irradiation. The authors concluded that 'radiobiologically the use of a single or a few massive doses generally is inferior to more conventional fractionation, but the therapeutic ratio may be reversed when used palliatively in patients with short survival'.

In attempting palliation of an inoperable primary tumour one should have limited aims. Palliative irradiation may be considered for patients with unresectable advanced bladder carcinomas when haematuria is present. Symptomatic improvement can occur within a relatively short time because of obliteration of the blood supply to the tumour. Dysuria may also be improved, but frequency may become worse. In any clinical situation the time factor for palliative therapy should be as short as possible. This is of special importance in advanced bladder cancer, where the life expectancy may be short. The treatment plan should therefore be simple and short; the goal is homogeneous irradiation of the entire bladder and perivesical region, including the iliac lymph nodes and, in males, the prostatic urethra. A dose of 4000 cGy seems to be equally good for relief of symptoms and is better tolerated than a higher dose. The decision to treat only with a palliative dose is certainly easy to take in the elderly. In a young patient or a patient in good physical condition and with no distant metastases, radical radiotherapy is justified, even though the probability of cure is relatively small.

Urinary bypass procedures are not indicated prior to palliative radiotherapy in patients with unilateral obstruction. The bypass procedure may increase the patient's comfort during and after treatment, but a major surgical procedure is not the best approach in patients who are in poor general condition. Urinary diversion is indicated in patients in good general condition who have bilateral obstruction prior to radiotherapy. The decision to perform urinary diversion must be taken only after considering carefully each individual case, and one has to be aware that the patient will probably die of cachexia instead of uraemia. Greiner et al. (1977) showed that ureteric obstruction has the same prognostic importance as a positive lymphogram (only 3 patients out of 61 showed significant improvement in the obstruction after irradiation with 7000–7500 cGy). The insertion of a percutaneous nephrostomy tube into the obstructed upper tracts is now a standard procedure which obviates the need for major surgery to divert the urine and its use has greatly facilitated the decision as to whether the patient should be diverted before radiotherapy (see p. 287).

Palliative Operative Procedures

TUR of Bladder Tumours

TUR is the standard treatment for superficial bladder tumours (Ta and T1). It is generally accepted that tumours infiltrating the deeper muscle layers of the

Table 11.7. Bladder carcinoma treated by TUR

Reference	Clinical stage	No. of patients surviving for 5 years (%)
Flocks (1951)	T2, T3	68/142 (47)
Milner (1954)	T2	51/89 (57)
	T3	20/86 (23)
	T4	1/13 (7)
Nichols and Marshall (1956)	T2, T3	3/20 (15)
Barnes et al. (1967)	T2/T3	46/114 (40)
	T4	2/36 (5)
	TXM1	1/20 (5)
Marberger et al. (1972)	T3-4	10/69 (14)
	T4NX or M1	0/38 (0)
O'Flynn et al. (1975)	T2	101/181 (56)
	T3	21/109 (20)
	T4	0/49 (0)
Hohenfellner (1978)	T2–T4 (combined irradiation)	8/44 (19)
	T2–T4 (TUR only)	6/32 (19)
Kenny et al. (1972)	C	13/23 (1 year)
		3/23 (2 years)
		2/23 (5 years)
	D	33/96 (1 year)
		13/96 (2 years)
		4/96 (5 years)

Table 11.8. Survival (5-year) after cystectomy for advanced or metastatic bladder carcinoma

Reference	Pathological stage	Therapy	Survival no.
Cordonnier (1968)	D (pT4)	Simple cystectomy	0/11
Long et al. (1972)	D (pT4)	Simple cystectomy	0/12
	D (pT4 or Npos)	Cystectomy + node dissection	2/11
Whitmore et al. (1977)	D1	Radical cystectomy + node dissection	2/16
	D2	Radical cystectomy + node dissection	0/18
	D1	(1 year later, after 6000 cGy)	1/11
	D2	(1 year later, after 6000 cGy)	1/14
	D1	Preoperative irradiation with 4000 cGy; radical cystectomy + node dissection	2/9
	D2	Preoperative irradiation with 4000 cGy; radical cystectomy + node dissection	1/16
	D3	Preoperative irradiation with 4000 cGy; radical cystectomy + node dissection	0/13

Table 11.8. *(continued)*

Reference	Pathological stage	Therapy	Survival no.
	D1	Preoperative irradiation with 2000 cGy; radical cystectomy + node dissection	3/12
	D2	Preoperative irradiation with 2000 cGy; radical cystectomy + node dissection	1/16
Daughtry et al. (1977)	D (pT4NX)	Simple and radical cystectomy	0/11
Kursh et al. (1977)	D (6 patients T4N0M0)	Simple cystectomy	3/6 living; mean survival 20 months
Clark (1978)	pT4N0	Radical cystectomy + node dissection	1/13
	pTXN1-3 (D1)	Radical cystectomy + node dissection	3/12
Vinnicombe and Abercrombie (1978)	pT4	Radical cystectomy + node dissection	3/6
Camey and Le Duc (1979)	pT4N0	Radical cystectomy + node dissection (preoperative irradiation)	2/8 (4 years)
Mathur et al. (1981)	D1 (pTXN1-3)	Radical cystectomy	2/5
Kutscher et al. (1981)	D (pTXNpos)	Partly irradiation	0/13 (2/18 survived 3 years)

bladder cannot be radically removed by TUR. However, in patients with known metastatic disease, the bulk of the tumour can be removed and the patients' symptoms can be controlled by TUR and coagulation, which can be repeated. Further palliation can be obtained by combining the TUR with local external radiotherapy and systemic chemotherapy (Jackse et al. 1983). Reuter (1978) combined TUR of infiltrating tumours with cryotherapy and cobalt irradiation. In rapidly growing and recurring tumours repeated operations are impracticable. Reduction of the tumour bulk and removal of the necrotic intravesical portion of the tumour may improve the results of radiotherapy and moderate the intensity of the radiation reaction. The results of TUR of invasive bladder tumours are listed in Table 11.7.

If simple endoscopic surgery can control local symptoms in patients with metastatic disease then this form of therapy is preferable to more extensive extirpational or diversionary procedures.

Palliative Cystectomy

The survival of patients treated by cystectomy for tumours invading adjacent organs or lymph nodes have been reported by several authors and are set out in Table 11.8. The results are extremely poor, and this cure cannot be expected in patients with tumours fixed to the pelvic wall or invading adjacent organs (category T4), or in patients with lymph nodes invaded above the bifurcation of the common iliac artery (stage D2 or category N4). If urinary diversion has already been performed and a local procedure to stop massive haemorrhage or local pain has failed, then cystectomy may be the only way to relieve the patient's symptoms. Morbidity and mortality are high in those patients who have had previous local palliative procedures (TUR, formalin, radiotherapy etc.). Brown et al. (1977) reported a mortality of 39% and a median survival of only 3.1 months in patients who had received radiotherapy or systemic chemotherapy prior to the palliative cystectomy. Thus palliative cystectomy in patients with advanced disease is very rarely justified. Understaging, especially of lymph nodes, may result in the surgeon being confronted with the decision as to whether to proceed with a cystectomy when positive lymph nodes are found above the common iliac bifurcation at the time of surgery. Schröder and Jellinghaus (1975) reported that the indication for cystectomy should be limited to stages B, C and D1 (TNM categories T2–3, N1–3). Approximately 80% of patients with stage D bladder cancers died in the first year following cystectomy (Kenny et al. 1972).

Partial Cystectomy

Partial cystectomy is usually reserved for patients who have localised disease which cannot be resected adequately transurethrally (Grossman 1979). If the lesion is locally resectable and the remainder of the bladder is normal, and neither regional nor distant metastases are present, then partial cystectomy offers an effective form of therapy. Most patients who undergo partial cystectomy for tumour invading the muscle layer and who have a resectable lesion attain a satisfactory bladder capacity (Novick and Stewart 1976). Very few patients are suitable for segmental resections because the vast majority of tumours are situated on the base of the bladder near the ureteric orifices or they are multifocal (see Chaps. 8 and 9, pp. 174 and 191). The morbidity after partial cystectomy is significantly lower than after a total cystectomy; therefore, if surgery is unavoidable, a suitable localised lesion can be treated by a partial cystectomy. Bladder carcinomas invading the anterior abdominal wall can sometimes be excised with either a partial or total cystectomy and produce effective palliation or even long-term survival (Bracken and Grabstald 1975).

Urinary Diversion

Palliative urinary diversion may be considered in patients with advanced metastatic bladder cancer if haematuria, pain, obstruction and frequency cannot be controlled by conservative means. Diversion of the urine can occasionally reduce severe haemorrhage and the discomfort associated with the local lesion by excluding the urine from the bladder and by removing the urinary enzymes that perpetuate the bleeding (Kirk et al. 1982). The patient's prognosis must justify the initial morbidity and mortality of the surgery. Brin et al. (1975) reported 47 cases in which palliative urinary diversion was performed for ureteric obstruction secondary to advanced pelvic malignancy. The average survival time was 5.3 months, with 50% of the patients alive at 3 months and only 22.7% alive at 6 months; 38% of the survival time was spent in hospital. Thus palliative diversion is rarely justified in the management of advanced pelvic malignancies. Urinary diversion may, however, increase the effectiveness of local procedures such as radiotherapy, formalin instillation or arterial embolisation. Over the age of 70 years the mortality of the surgery increases, and, if urinary diversion is unavoidable, a simple method is preferred. If the ureters are dilated then a cutaneous ureterostomy can be carried out rapidly and with less morbidity than a colonic or ileal conduit (Stewart and Novik 1977).

Ortlip and Fraley (1982) reviewed the results of palliative diversion performed in patients with obstruction secondary to cancer. In eight retrospective clinical studies conducted at different institutions with a variety of primary malignant diseases the survival after diversion was found to be only 3–6 months, with very few exceptions. Open procedures for urinary drainage are fraught with complications. Although an accurate assessment of operative morbidity and mortality is severely limited by the complexity of the underlying disease, the reported complication rates lie between 45% and 60% (Sharer et al. 1978; Holden et al. 1979). Only 31% of patients recovered uneventfully. In an analysis of 218 consecutive cases in which the patients underwent open nephrostomy insertion because of pelvic genitourinary malignancies or non-pelvic retroperitoneal metastases, 99 patients had some complications including septicaemia, cardiovascular, respiratory and gastrointestinal problems. Between 3% and 8% died as a direct result of the diversion procedure (Sharer et al. 1978; Holden et al. 1979). Approximately half of the patients reported by Kohler et al. (1980) returned to a useful life after the urinary diversion.

The percutaneous insertion of a nephrostomy tube has, in constrast, a very small operative risk. Performed under local anaesthesia this procedure is well tolerated by the patient and is simple to perform, provided that the upper tracts are dilated and easily visualised by ultrasound or radiological screening.

Complications such as transient sepsis, extravasation of urine or serious haemorrhage are rarely seen. An antegrade approach to the ureter and insertion of a double pigtail stent allows conversion to internal drainage in patients where endoscopic insertion of a stent is impossible.

Percutaneous nephrostomy is easy to perform, and therefore a rational policy must be based on an accurate assessment of the prognosis. Consistent predictors are difficult to indentify, but rapid progression of obstruction usually indicates a poor prognosis. Neurological pain caused by direct infiltration will not be influenced by urinary diversion.

Suitable candidates for palliative percutaneous diversion include those patients with localised disease in whom further therapy holds the promise of prolongation of a useful life. Patients who are to receive nephrotoxic drugs such as *cis*-platinum or methotrexate may require diversion even for partial obstructions. Other criteria for the selection of patients for diversion are stable neoplasms, obstruction complicated by fistula or septicaemia, young patients (<60 years), and patients with the potential for an independent existence who are optimally provided for by their families and for whom the quality of life offered is acceptable. None of these criteria is absolute but all should be considered.

One cannot expect patients with advanced bladder cancer who have not responded to conventional therapy to benefit from a urinary diversion. Serious consideration must be given to each individual case before diversion is undertaken. Allowing the patient to die peacefully from uraemia may be the better decision than trying to prolong an already painful existence.

Treatment of Metastatic Disease

Radiotherapy

Localised metastases causing symptoms can be effectively treated by irradiation. The treatment is completed in as short a time as possible. The time taken depends on two factors: (1) the tolerance of the surrounding tissues, which is important if the field is large and covers radiosensitive areas such as the abdomen; and (2) whether swelling of the tumour after a single large dose could adversely affect the nervous or circulatory systems, in which case the treatment must be started slowly and be gradually built up to a standard dose level (Kligerman 1982). Swelling of the tumour is especially important when treating tumours in the brain, tumours impinging on or within the spinal cord, or those causing superior mediastinal compression. In managing the patient with advanced cancer, the presence of a mass is not necessarily an indication for active treatment. Asymptomatic, superficial metastases in soft tissues or bone need not be treated if they are not causing,pain, are not about to ulcerate, are not compressing vital structures and are not threatening to cause a pathological fracture. In patients with known threatening metastases the size should be regularly assessed by physical examination or X-rays films to estimate the rate of growth. Patients should be irradiated if the metastasis is growing rapidly or if the presence of the mass is psychologically disturbing to the patient. Lesions in weight-bearing bones, such as the femur or vertebral bodies, should be treated early to prevent pathological fractures. Cases with increased intracranial pressure should be treated as emergencies. When cord compression is accompanied by urological symptoms, laminectomy may be indicated for decompression before starting radiotherapy. In patients with multiple metastatic lesions in bone, the treatment should be directed only to the area presenting the greatest symptoms or the greatest threat to the patient. Often a second area not painful enough to be important to the patient initially, is subsequently found to require treatment. Localised radiotherapy does not interfere with starting treatment with chemotherapy.

Even early carcinomas of the bladder may metastasise through the lymphatics to involve the retroperitoneal lymph nodes. Pelvic bones, particularly the ischium and pubis, may become involved through local extension, and involvement of the lumbosacral spine may result from tumour extension via the lymphatics to the retroperitoneal nodes or via the venous plexus. Involvement of distant bones is presumably the result of haematogenous spread. In patients who have undergone cystectomy, distant metastases are seen more often than local recurrence (Whitmore et al. 1977).

Fitzpatrick and Rider (1976) reported on 'half body' irradiation for palliation in patients with symptomatic widespread metastases. Doses in the range of 500–1000 cGy as a single fraction were used. This irradiation was followed by a period of 1 month to allow for haematological recovery before a further dose of 800–1000 cGy was delivered to the second half of the body. The acute radiation syndrome was rarely severe and did not cause a major clinical problem. It was always more marked with upper body irradiation. No patients showed signs of renal impairment and haematological tolerance was good. Pain relief frequently occurred within 24 h of treatment.

Pain Relief

The evaluation and treatment of pain is a matter of major concern to the medical profession in general and to the oncologist in particular. Pain appears to be related to a group of emotional states and is subject to influences stemming from the cultural background, expectations and fear. Pain in the cancer patient is not usually an early complaint. Its appearance often implies advanced disease, with all the attendant problems of variable degrees of deterioration in different organ systems. The treatment of such cases is to make the patient's last few months as comfortable as possible. The need for pain relief may dominate the clinical picture. In many centres oncologists, anaesthetists, radiotherapists and other experts all work together in a pain relief clinic, and this arrangement has many advantages. Patients will benefit from a careful assessment and therapy based on the consideration of all available treatment modalities.

Pain perception was once thought to be the result of a direct and unmodifiable connection between the pain perceptor and a 'pain centre'. The gate control theory introduced by Melzack and Wall (1965) allowed for modification by local events at the level of the spinal cord and modification by impulses descending from above.

A new dimension is added when one considers that the central levels of neurotransmitters and their release, availability and metabolism may modulate the responses to stimuli. Of these compounds the endorphins have excited the greatest interest (Guillemin 1977).

Clinical Aspects

Pain may be classified into four general categories: superficial pain, deep pain, neurological pain and psychological pain. Superficial pain is not a major problem in the cancer patient. Deep pain arises from the viscera and is characteristically dull and poorly localised; it leads to autonomic nervous system activity causing nausea, sweating, restlessness and tachycardia. Pain of visceral or deep origin is of major importance in patients with cancer. The most effective treatment for deep pain is the removal of the cause. Palliative surgical procedures may be the most effective form of pain relief. Neurological pain is produced by damage to the peripheral nerve or nerve roots. It has usually a burning or searing quality and may be the most difficult to treat. Pain of psychological origin is difficult to diagnose and also to treat. It is observed mainly in patients with primary or reactive depression and is of hypochondriacal origin.

Treatment of Pain

The removal of the cause of the pain is by far the most useful manoeuvre, even in patients in whom long survival is not anticipated. The chronic use of medication is always associated with side effects which may interfere with physical or mental function. The first step in the treatment of cancer-related pain is to evaluate the relationship between tissue damage and pain perception using the available diagnostic methods (X-ray films, CT scans, bone scans etc.). The second step is to assess the pain itself. The patient is required to rate pain intensity by means of graphic or verbal scales. The data on pain intensity should be supplemented by information about the patient's day-to-day life, physical performance and psychosocial state (Ventafridda 1981). Current methods of pain relief fall into three main groups:

1. Treatment aimed at modifying the pathological process
2. Modulator treatment
3. Lesion treatment

Treatment of the pathological process includes surgery, radiotherapy and chemotherapy. Palliative surgery may prove extremely effective in relieving pain caused by obstruction to hollow viscera. High-energy radiation is one of the most effective means of pain control. Well-planned radiotherapy will reduce the pain from bone metastases and may cause osteolytic lesions to regress. Pain relief results from a reduction of the mechanical pressure exerted by the tumour mass. In the case of chemotherapy, pain relief is also of an indirect type and results from the antitumoural action of the drugs (Confer et al. 1977; Wallace et al. 1982).

Modulator treatment covers the methods designed to raise the pain perception threshold by either peripheral or central inhibition of nervous pathways using analgesics, psychic and rehabilitation procedures, local anaesthetic and stimulation techniques. Analgesics should be given at fixed intervals and not on demand. Psychotropic drugs combined with other analgesics have a potentiating effect and reduce the sensation of pain caused by nerve lesions. Narcotics are most effective for the control of intense and severe pain; only in patients who have reached the advanced stages of the disease should they be used for protracted periods. Morphine hydrochloride is the most commonly used narcotic analgesic. Two similar oral preparations are known under the names 'Brompton mixture' and 'Greenwalt's solution'. Their formulae are as follows:

Brompton mixture:

10 mg morphine sulphate
10 mg cocaine HCl
5 ml ethanol
5 ml syrup
20 ml chloroform water qs

Dose: 20 ml every 4 h

Greenwalt's solution:

2 mg levorphanol
10 mg cocaine HCl
2.5 ml ethanol (95%)
5 ml syrup
20 ml water qs

Dose: 20 ml every 4 h

Both preparations have been highly effective in controlling pain in the cancer patient. Levorphanol may offer an advantage over morphine in that it is better absorbed when given orally. The quantity of morphine can be raised gradually up to 40 mg/20 ml.

The most important psychological measures are the facilitation of sleep and rest. The attention of the patient should be distracted from the disease and a constant friendly and reassuring atmosphere should be provided.

Stimulation treatment is based on the principle of counterirritation proposed by the Melzack–Wall theory. A sensation of pain may be controlled by other sensations produced by stimulation. This modulation occurs at the dorsal horns of the spinal cord. Stimulation is performed either transcutaneously or percutaneously on the nerve fibre itself by means of microstimulators. These techniques, though still experimental, are free from harmful side effects.

Repeated infiltration of local anaesthetics, both at the site of the pain and along peripheral nerves, produces a reduction of pain through attenuation of the painful input. In cancer patients with very limited survival, lesion treatment is a method of pain control. Neurophysiological findings have shown that pain is due to the excitation of several pathways and gate control systems in the vast regions of cortical and subcortical structures. New pathways may establish themselves when one specific pathway has been interrupted. The technique consists of the infiltration of neurolytic substances such as alcohol or phenol into the subarachnoid space in order to destroy the sensitive posterior roots of the spinal cord or the peripheral nerves. Such infiltration into the coeliac and lumbar sympathetic ganglia has proved effective in control of visceral pain.

According to Ventafridda (1981) this is effective in 40%–60% of cases, with a complication rate of 11%–30%. Complications usually occur in patients who are already suffering from a functional deficit. The most significant are paralysis and incontinence. Patients may be selected by trial epidural block, using an epidural catheter which is left in place for several days so that repeated blocks may be performed. By this method the patient may be made aware of the pain relief that may be achieved. Visceral pain may be relieved temporarily by a local anaesthetic block of the coeliac plexus or lumbar sympathetic chain; a neurolytic block may then be achieved with 50% alcohol or 5% phenol and water.

Chordotomy is a surgical method for the relief of cancer pain below the neck. Rosomoff et al. (1966) introduced percutaneous chordotomy by means of radiofrequency irradiation. If this technique fails or is not available, then an open chordotomy, which requires laminectomy, must be performed. For pain below the mid-abdomen a thoracic chordotomy at the level of T-2 may be employed. The success rate is of the order of 80%–90%. Percutaneous chordotomy is generally carried out at C-1 to C-2, whatever the level of the pain. Cervical chordotomy results in diminished pulmonary function on the same side. Bilateral pelvic or lower extremity pain may be treated by bilateral open thoracic chordotomy without this respiratory risk. Voluntary muscle and bladder complications occur in 4%–20% of the patients following unilateral chordotomy. Bilateral chordotomy is usually done in two steps to reduce the risk of incontinence and paralysis. Analgesia occurs in 70%–90% of the cases immediately following chordotomy, but after 6 months the level of analgesia has often diminished. Thus lasting relief cannot be assured in patients surviving for this length of time.

Hypnosis, acupuncture, biofeedback and conditioning may be of research interest, but these techniques are not readily applicable to patients with advanced cancer. All available means must be employed, however, to make this final period of life tolerable and comfortable.

Chemotherapy

In patients with advanced disease and metastases chemotherapy is clearly the major hope, not only for palliation, but also ultimately for cure. The majority of investigations on systemic chemotherapeutic agents for bladder cancer have been carried out in patients with advanced or metastatic measurable disease. The evaluation of the results of these trials are of great importance to the management of advanced bladder cancer and have been covered in Chapter 10 (see pp. 246–254).

Conclusion

The relief of symptoms and the creation of a sense of wellbeing are important criteria in evaluating the benefits of palliative treatment and have been little emphasised in many of the reports mentioned in this chapter. If cure of the advanced disease cannot be achieved, the quality of life with or without treatment becomes of the highest importance to the patient. Decisions on palliative treatment should be taken not in an attempt to cure but rather to eliminate the most burdensome symptoms, to prevent complications, to prolong useful life and to provide a psychological uplift. A high operative risk, which can reasonably be accepted when there is a prospect of cure, is not justified when the treatment is for palliation only. The same also applies to mutilating surgery. The indication for palliative surgery or radiotherapy has to be weighed up case by case, taking into account the rate of advance of the disease, the life expectancy, the seriousness of the disturbance caused by the disease and the degree of symptomatic improvement that can be expected.

Over the past 20 years regional chemotherapy of tumours has gained wide acceptance. The aim is to deliver to the tumour a high concentration of the drug, which is confined to a single anatomical region, thereby reducing the harmful effects of the drug on the rest of the body. Regional chemotherapy is reserved for malignant tumours that have no distant metastases, and regional perfusion combined with hyperthermia is beginning to produce some encouraging results.

Some forms of palliative treatment have not been discussed in this chapter (e.g. intracavitary radiotherapy), either because only a few institutes are familiar with them and results in advanced disease have not been reported, or because they have been replaced by newer methods (e.g. hypogastric artery embolisation instead of ligation). Some methods have been discussed relatively extensively, despite limited experience of their use (e.g. lasers). New developments deserve attention as they may become the accepted alternative treatments in the near future. Standard treatments, such as TUR, do not need extended discussion, though it is surprising how few reports can be found which analyse the results in advanced disease.

Acknowledgement

The author wishes to thank Karin von Alphen, who persevered through the many typings of this manuscript.

References

Barakat HA, Javadpour N, Bush IM (1973) Management of massive intractable hematuria. Urology 1: 351–353

Barnes RW, Bergman RT, Hadley HL, Love D (1967) Control of bladder tumors by endoscopic surgery. J Urol 97: 864–808

Barone RM, Byfield JE, Goldfarb PB, Frankel S, Ginn C, Greer S (1982) Intra-arterial chemotherapy using an implantable infusion pump and liver irradiation for the treatment of hepatic metastases. Cancer 50: 850–862

Bergsma CJ, Leary FJ (1976) Total bladder necrosis following intravesical formalin. Presented at North Central Section of American Urological Association, Palm Beach, Florida. Cited in deKernion JB (1976) Genitourinary cancer. Saunders, Philadelphia, p 291

Bracken RB, Grabstald H (1975) Bladder carcinoma involving the lower abdominal wall. J Urol 114: 715–721

Bright JF, Tosi SE, Chrichlow RW, Selikowitz SM (1977) Prevention of vesicoureteral reflux with Fogarty catheters during formalin therapy. J Urol 118: 950–952

Brin EN, Schiff M, Weiss RM (1975) Pallative urinary diversion for pelvic malignancy. J Urol 113: 619–622

Brown PW, Terz JJ, Lawrence W, Blievernicht SW (1977) Survival after palliative surgery for advanced intraabdominal cancer. Am. J Surg 134: 575–578

Brown RB (1969) Management of inoperable carcinoma of the bladder. Med J Austr 66: 23–24

Bush WH, Freeny PC (1980) Transcatheter vascular occlusive therapy in genitourinary problems. Bull Mason Clin 34: 1–9
Cahan WG, Adam Y, Mackenzie RA, Brockunier A, Clark DG (1970) Intractable bladder hemorrhage treated by cryosurgery: a preliminary report. J Urol 103: 606–611
Camey M, le Duc A (1979) L'entéro-cystoplastie après cysto-prostatectomie totale pour cancer de vessie. Ann Urol 13(2): 114–123
Capen CV, Weigel JW, Magrina JF, Masterson BJ (1982) Intraperitoneal spillage of formalin after intravesical instillation. Urology 19(6): 599–601
Cavaliere R, Ciocatto EC, Giovanella BC, Heidelberger C, Johnson RO, Margottini M, Mondovi B, Moricca G, Rossi-Fanelli A (1967) Selective heat sensitivity of cancer cells. Biochemical and clinical studies. Cancer 20: 1351–1381
Chan RC, Bracken B, Johnson DE (1979) Single dose whole pelvis megavoltage irradiation for palliative control of hematuria or ureteral obstruction. J Urol 122: 750–751
Clark PB (1978) Radical cystectomy for carcinoma of the bladder. Br J Urol 50: 492–495
Confer DJ, Smith RB, Gillespie L (1977) Dramatic palliation for painful, fixed bladder squamous cell carcinoma with 5-fluorouracil infusion. J Urol 118: 483–484
Cordonnier JJ (1968) Cystectomy for carcinoma of the bladder. J Urol 99: 172–173
Culp DA (1979) Palliative treatment of the patient with disseminated carcinoma of the bladder. Semin Oncol 6(2): 249–253
Daughtry JD, Susan LP, Stewart BH, Straffon RA (1977) Ileal conduit and cystectomy: a 10-year retrospective study of ileal conduits performed in conjunction with cystectomy and with a minimum 5-year follow-up. J Urol 118: 556–557
Debré B, Steg A (1981) Distension vésicale hydrostatique, technique et indications. Nouv Presse Med 10(1): 21–24
de Quervain F (1927) Le traitement du cancer de la vessie par la neige d'acide carbonique. Rev Med Suisse Romande 47: 259. Cited by Cahan et al. (1970)
Dickson JA (1977) The effects of hyperthermia in animal test systems. In: Rossi-Fanella AR, Cavaliere R, Mondovi B, Moricca B (eds) Selective heat sensitivity of cancer cells, Springer, Berlin Heidelberg New York, pp 43–111 (Recent results in cancer research, vol 59)
England HR, Rigby C, Shepheard BGF, Tresidder GC, Blandy JP (1973) Evaluation of Helmstein's distension method for carcinoma of the bladder. Br J Urol 45: 593–599
Fair WR (1974) Formalin in the treatment of massive bladder hemorrhage. Techniques, results and complications. Urology 3: 573–576
Firlit CF (1973) Intractable hemorrhagic cystitis secondary to extensive carcinomatosis: management with formalin solution. J Urol 110: 57–58
Fish JF, Fayos JV (1976) Carcinoma of the urinary bladder. Radiology 118: 179–182
Fitzpatrick P, Rider W (1976) Half body radiotherapy. Int J Radiol Oncol Biol Phys 197: 197–207
Flocks RH (1951) Treatment of patients with carcinoma of the bladder. JAMA 145: 295–301
Godec CJ, Gleich P (1983) Intractable hematuria and formalin. J Urol 130: 688–691
Gonder MJ, Soanes WA, Smith V (1964) Experimental prostate cryosurgery. Invest Urol 1: 610–619
Goodman LA, Seligman AM, Calabresi P (1982) Regional chemotherapy. In: Holland JF, Frei E (eds) Cancer medicine. Lea & Febiger, Philadelphia, pp 752–758
Green M, George FW (1974) Radiotherapy of advanced localized bladder cancer. J Urol 111: 611–612
Greiner R, Skaleric C, Veraguth P (1977) The prognostic significance of ureteral obstruction in carcinoma of the bladder. Int J Radio Oncol Biol Phys 2; 1095–1100
Grossman HB (1979) Current therapy of bladder carcinoma. J Urol 121: 1–7
Guillemin R (1977) Endorphins, brain peptides that act like opiates. N Engl J Med 296: 226–228
Günther R, Klose K, Jacobi G (1981) Superselektive Embolisation mit Gewebekleber im Urogenitaltrakt. Fortschr Roentgenstr 134(5): 536–539
Hall RR (1978) Intravesical hyperthermia for transitional cell carcinoma of the bladder. In: Bladder tumors and other topics in urological oncology. Plenum, New York, pp 267–270
Hall RR, Schade ROK, Swinney J (1974) Effects of hyperthermia on bladder cancer. Br Med J 2: 593–594
Hall RR, Wadehra V, Towler JM, Hindmarsh JR, Byrne PO (1976) Hyperthermia in the treatment of bladder tumors. Br J Urol 48: 603–608
Harada T, Ohmura H, Nishizawa O, Tsuchida S (1982) Efficacy and side-effects of the regional arterial infusion of anti-cancer drugs combined with direct haemoperfusion in malignancies of the urinary tract. J Urol 128: 524–527
Harzmann R, Bichler KH, Gericke D, Dietzel F, Erdmann D (1978) Lokale Hochfrequenz-Hyperthermie des Brown-Pearce Karzinoms der Harnblase des Kaninchens. Urologe [A] 17: 130–134

Harzmann R, Bichler KH, Fastenmeier K, Flachenecker G, Gericke D (1980) Transurethrally applied local high frequency hyperthermia for treatment of urinary bladder carcinoma. In: Argangeli G, Mauro F (eds) Hyperthermia in radiation oncology. Masson, Mailand, pp 289–293

Haschek H (1974) Cryosurgery and the 'poor risk' patient: indications for cryosurgery. In: Reuter HJ (ed) Cryosurgery in urology. Thieme, Stuttgart, pp 93–95

Helmstein K (1972) Treatment of bladder carcinoma by a hydrostatic pressure technique. Br J Urol 44: 434–450

Hermanowicz M, Serment G, Manolli P, Coulang C, Clerissa J, Pinot JJ, Richaud C, Ducassou J (1980) A propos du traitement paliatif des hématuries vésicales d'origine tumorale. J Urol Nephrol (Paris) 86: 133–135

Hirose K, Seto T, Takayasu H (1977) Re-evaluation of hydrostatic pressure treatment for malignant bladder lesion. J Urol 118: 762–764

Hofstetter A (1981) Endoskopische Zerstörung von Blasentumoren mit Laser. Urologe [A] 20: 317–322

Hohenfellner R (1978) Harnblasenkarzinom: Klinisches Referat. In: Arnoldt F (ed) Verhandlungsbericht der Deutschen Gesellschaft für Urologie, vol 29. Springer, Berlin Heidelberg New York, pp 8–11

Holden S, McPhee M, Grabstald H (1979) The rationale of urinary diversion in cancer patients. J Urol 121: 19–21

Holstein P, Jacobsen K, Pedersen JF, Sorensen JS (1973) Intravesical hydrostatic pressure treatment: new method for control of bleeding from the bladder mucosa. J Urol 109: 234–236

Hübener KH, Voss AC (1979) Ergebnisse Postoperativer Radiotherapie von Harnblasencarcinomen. Urologe [A] 18: 137–142

Huguet JF, Clerissi J, Chamant M, Serment G (1980) L'embolisation des hémorrhagies vésicales. Ann Radiol 24(5): 456–460

Jacobs SC, McClellan SL, Maher C, Lawson RK (1982) Precystectomy intra-arterial *cis*-diamminedichloroplatinum (II)/local bladder hyperthermia for bladder cancer. In: Proceedings of the 77th Annual Meeting of the American Urological Association, Kansas City, Missouri, 1982

Jakse G, Frommhold H, Marberger M (1983) Combined *cis*-platinum and radiation therapy in patients with stages pT3 and pT4 bladder cancer: a pilot study. J Urol 129: 502–504

Jorest R, Monneins F, Boccon-Gibod L, Steg A (1977) Le traitement des hématuries des cancers vésicule évolués par la formolisation vésicale. Ann Urol 12: 101–105

Kato T, Nemoto R, Mori H, Takahashi M, Harada M (1981) Arterial chemo-embolization with Mitomycin-C microcapsules in the treatment of primary or secondary carcinoma of the kidney, liver, bone and intrapelvic organs. Cancer 48: 674–680

Kenny CM, Hardner GL, Moore RM, Murphy GP (1972) Current results from treatment of simple C and D bladder tumors at Roswell Park Memorial Institute. J Urol 107: 56–59

Kirk D, Slade N, Feneley RCL (1982) The role of palliative urinary diversion in the management of bladder cancer. Br J Urol 54: 363–365

Kligerman MM (1982) Principles of radiation therapy. In: Holland JF, Frei E (eds) Cancer medicine. Lea & Febiger, Philadelphia, pp 573–595

Kohler JP, Lyon ES, Schoenberg HW (1980) Reassessment of circle tube nephrostomy in advanced pelvic malignancy. J Urol 123: 17–18

Kronester A, Staehler G, Weinberg W, Keiditsch E (1981) Gefährdung des Darmes bei endoskopischer Bestrahlung von Harnblasentumoren mit dem Neodym-YAG-Laser. Urologe [A] 20: 305–309

Kumar S, Rosen P, Grabstald H (1975) Intravesical formalin for the control of intractable bladder hemorrhage secondary to cystitis or cancer. J Urol 114: 540–543

Kursh ED, Rabin R, Persky L (1977) Is cystectomy a safe procedure in elderly patients with carcinoma of the bladder? J Urol 118: 40–42

Kutscher HA, Leadbetter GW, Vinson RK (1981) Survival after radical cystectomy for invasive transitional cell carcinoma of bladder. Urology 17(3): 231–234

Lang EK, Deutsch JS, Goodman JR, Barnett TF, Lanasa JA, Duplessis GH (1979) Transcatheter embolization of hypogastric branch arteries in the management of intractable bladder hemorrhage. J Urol 121: 30–36

Likourinas M, Cranides A, Jiannopoulos B, Kostakopoulos A, Dimopoulos C (1979) Intravesical formalin for the control of intractable bladder hemorrhage secondary to radiation cystitis or bladder cancer. Urol Res 7: 125–126

Logothetis CJ, Samuels ML, Wallace S, Chuang V, Trindade A, Grant C, Haynie TP, Johnson DE (1982) Management of pelvic complications of malignant urothelial tumors with combined intra-arterial and i.v. chemotherapy. Cancer Treat Rep 66: 1501–1507

Long RTL, Grummon RA, Spratt JS, Perez-Mesa C (1972) Carcinoma of the urinary bladder (comparison with radical, simple and partial cystectomy and intravesical formalin). Cancer 29: 98–105

Ludgate CM, McLean N, Carswell GF, Newsam JE, Pettigrew RT, Selby Tulloch W (1976) Hyperthermic perfusion of the distended urinary bladder in the management of recurrent transitional cell carcinoma. Br J Urol 47: 841–848

Mackenzie AR (1972) Cryotherapy of the bladder for cancer. J Urol 107: 387–388

Madonna HM (1981) Pain relief in terminal cancer. Urol Letter Club 91

Marberger H, Marberger M, Decristoforo A (1972) The current status of transurethral resection in the diagnosis and therapy of carcinoma of the urinary bladder. Int Urol Nephrol 4(1): 35–44

Marmor JB (1979) Interactions of hyperthermia and chemotherapy in animals. Cancer Res 39: 2269–2276

Mathur VK, Krahn HP, Ramsey EW (1981) Total cystectomy for bladder cancer. J Urol 125: 784–786

Melzack R, Wall PD (1965) Pain mechanism: a new theory. Science 150: 971–979

Merimsky E, Jossiphov J (1980) L'action toxique sur le rein des instillations endovésicales de formaldéhyde. J Urol Nephrol (Paris) 86(7): 527–529

Milner WA (1954) The role of conservative surgery in the treatment of bladder tumours. Br J Urol 26: 375–384

Morrison R (1978) Carcinoma of the bladder—radiotherapy. Urol Res 6: 225–227

Nakazono I, Iwata S (1980) Intra-arterial infusion as a preoperative chemotherapeutic treatment for bladder tumor. In: Proceedings of the 75th Annual Meeting of the American Urological Association, San Francisco, California, 1980

Nevin JE, Melnick I, Baggerly JT, Easley CA, Landes R (1974) Advanced carcinoma of bladder: treatment using hypogastric artery infusion with 5-fluorouracil, either as a single agent or in combination with Bleomycin or Adriamycin and supervoltage radiation. J Urol 112: 752–758

Newsam JE, Law HT (1982) Hyperthermic perfusion of the distended urinary bladder in the management of recurrent transitional cell carcinoma. A review after 6 years. Br J Urol 54: 64–65

Nichols JA, Marshall VF (1956) Treatment of histologically benign papilloma of the urinary bladder by local excision and fulguration. Cancer 9: 24–25

Niederhuber JE, Ensminger W, Gyves JW, Liepman M, Doan K, Cozzi E (1982) Totally implanted venous and arterial access system to replace external catheters in cancer treatment. Surgery 92: 706–712

Novick AC, Stewart BH (1976) Partial cystectomy in the treatment of primary and secondary carcinoma of the bladder. J Urol 116: 570–573

O'Flynn JD, Smith JM, Hanson JS (1975) Transurethral resection for the assessment and treatment of vesical neoplasms. Eur Urol 1: 38–40

Ogata J, Migita N, Nakamura T (1973) Treatment of carcinoma of the bladder by infusion of the anticancer agent (Mitomycin C) via the internal iliac artery. J Urol 110: 667–669

Ortlip SA, Fraley EE (1982) Indications for palliative urinary diversion in patients with cancer. Urol Clin North Am 9(1): 79–83

Reuter HJ (1978) Die Kältchirurgie von Blasentumoren. In: Arnoldt F (ed) Verhandlungsbericht der Deutschen Gesellschaft für Urologie, vol 29. Springer, Berlin Heidelberg New York, pp 113–117

Rider WD, Evans DH (1976) Radiotherapy in the treatment of recurrent bladder cancer. Br J Urol 48: 595–601

Rosomoff HF, Sheppsek P, Carrol F (1966) Modern pain relief: percutaneous cordotomy. JAMA 196: 482–486

Schröder FH, Jellinghaus W (1975) Das Blasencarcinom—Grenzen der Operabilität und Ursachen des Versagens der Radikalen Cystektomie. Urologe [A] 14: 60–64

Schuhrke TD, Barr JW (1976) Intractable bladder hemorrhage: therapeutic angiographic embolization of the hypogastric arteries. J Urol 116: 523–525

Shah BC, Albert DJ (1973) Intravesical instillation of formalin for the management of intractable hematuria. J Urol 110: 519–520

Sharer W, Grayhack JT, Graham J (1978) Palliative urinary diversion for malignant ureteral obstruction. J Urol 120: 162–164

Staehler G, Hofstetter A (1979) Transurethral laser irradiation of urinary bladder tumors. Eur Urol 5: 64–69

Stewart BH, Novick AC (1977) Current perspectives on palliative therapy in cancer of the bladder. Cancer Res 37: 2781–2788

Sullivan RD (1962) Continuous arterial infusion cancer chemotherapy. Surg Clin North Am 42: 365–388 van der Werf-Messing B (1978) Radiation therapy of carcinoma of the bladder. In: Arnoldt F (ed) Verhandlungsbericht der Deutschen Gesellschaft für Urologie, vol 29. Springer, Berlin Heidelberg New York, pp 22–25

Ventafridda V (1981) The management of pain in the cancer patient. Cancer Bull 19(1): 1–3

Vinnicombe J, Abercrombie GF (1978) Total cystectomy—a review. Br J Urol 50: 488–491

Wallace S, Chuang VP, Samuels M, Johnson D (1982) Transcatheter intraarterial infusion of chemotherapy in advanced bladder cancer. Cancer 15: 640–645

Whitmore WF, Batata MA, Ghoneim MA, Grabstald H, Unal A (1977) Radical cystectomy with or without prior irradiation in the treatment of bladder cancer. J Urol 118: 184–187

Subject Index

Previously published volumes in the series

The Pharmacology of the Urinary Tract

Editor: **M. Caine,** Jerusalem

1984. 27 figures. XII, 167 pages
ISBN 3-540-13238-4

This book gives an up-to-date account of the use of pharmacological agents in the management of urinary tract disorders. The emphasis is on the clinical and practical aspects of the subject, but it also includes an account of the underlying mechanisms of the modes of action of the various groups of drugs. This enables the readers not only to approach the treatment of their patients in a fully informed and logical manner, but also, in view of the large amount of research constantly taking place in the field, to assess future scientific developments and new drugs as they appear on the market.

Male Infertility

Editor: **T. B. Hargreave,** Edinburgh

1983. 56 figures. XII, 326 pages
ISBN 3-540-12055-6

"This remarkable monograph distinguishes what is known from what is merely wishful guesswork... we are provided with clear guidelines for the investigations that are appropriate for each type of infertility, and a comprehensive account of their scientific background and sources of error... Anyone concerned in the management of barren couples will find *Male Infertility* excellent, and those engaged in research will find many new questions demanding a solution." *British Medical Journal*

Urodynamics

by **P. H. Abrams, R. C. I. Feneley, M. J. Torrens,** Bristol

1983. 95 figures. XII, 229 pages
ISBN 3-540-11903-5

"It is the only book I have seen which has managed very successfully to combine the detailed practical working knowledge of the subject together with an extensive review of earlier works. For those of us performing urodynamics, or thinking of setting up such a service, this book has admirably crystallized all aspects and knowledge of the subject." *Journal of the Royal Society of Medicine*

Chemotherapy and Urological Malignancy

Editor: **A. S. D. Spiers,** Albany

1982. XVII, 163 pages
ISBN 3-540-11543-9

"This volume is a very useful up-to-date summary of the contribution of chemotherapy to the management of urological cancer... urological tumours range from the exquisitely sensitive Wilms' tumour of the kidney... to those which are almost totally unresponsive, such as renal carcinoma. Such a spectrum of disease makes urological tumours the ideal training ground in the principles of cancer chemotherapy and this book is an excellent introduction to this field."

British Journal of Urology

Urinary Diversion

Editor: **M. H. Ashken,** Norwich

1982. 53 figures. XIII, 143 pages
ISBN 3-540-11273-1

"This book can truly be said to be a landmark in the literature on this subject and brings a much needed review of the advantages and disadvantages to be considered before deciding on diversion. It is essential for surgeons who practice urinary diversion and for the student of urology."

South African Medical Journal

"The editor of this excellent little book has produced a work that must be read by every urologist and general surgeon who practices urology."

British Journal of Surgery

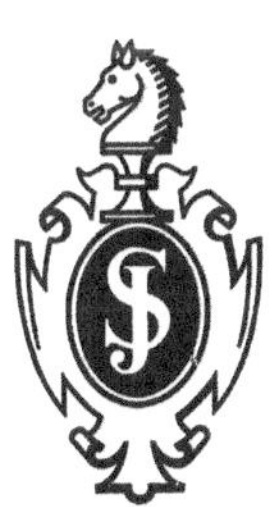

Springer-Verlag Berlin Heidelberg New York Tokyo

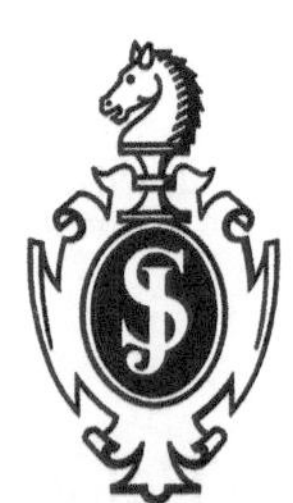